# THE EFFECT OF THE MAN-MADE ENVIRONMENT
## ON
## HEALTH AND BEHAVIOR

LAWRENCE E. HINKLE, JR., M.D.

AND

WILLIAM C. LORING, PH.D.

*Editors*

A Report of the
Inter-University Board of Collaborators

USPHS Contract CPE–R–69–30

Center for Disease Control
Public Health Service
U.S. Department of Health, Education, and Welfare
Atlanta, Georgia 30333

# Collaborating Authors

Robert P. Burden, Ph.D.
Assistant to the Dean for Environmental Affairs, and Director, Environmental Systems Program
Division of Engineering and Applied Physics
Harvard University
Cambridge, MA 02138

John C. Cassel, M.D., M.P.H.
Professor and Chairman,
Department of Epidemiology
The School of Public Health
University of North Carolina
Chapel Hill, NC 27514

Albert Damon, M.D., Ph.D.,* (Physical Anthropology)
Lecturer and Senior Research Associate,
Department of Anthropology
Harvard University

Robert L. Geddes, M. Arch.
Professor of Architecture and Dean,
School of Architecture and Urban Planning
Princeton University
Princeton, NJ 08540

Robert Gutman, Ph.D.
Professor of Sociology
Department of Sociology
Rutgers University
New Brunswick, NJ 08903
    (also Lecturer in Architecture,
    Princeton, University.

*Deceased

Lawrence E. Hinkle, Jr., M.D.
Professor of Medicine, Professor of Medicine in Psychiatry, and Director, Division of Human Ecology
Department of Medicine and Psychiatry
Cornell University Medical College
New York, NY 10021

Stanislav V. Kasl, Ph.D. (Psychology)
Professor of Epidemiology and Psychology
Department of Epidemiology and Public Health
Yale School of Medicine
Yale University
New Haven, CT 06510

Donald A. Kennedy, Ph.D. (Social Anthropology)
Associate Professor, Director of Research
Department of Family and Community Medicine
Hershey Medical Center
Pennsylvania State University
Hershey, PA 17033

William C. Loring, Ph.D. (Urban Sociology), Science Advisor
Environmental Health Services Division, BSS, Center for Disease Control
U.S. Public Health Service, DHEW
Atlanta, GA 30333

Kermit K. Schooler, Ph.D. (Social Psychology)
Dean and Prof. of Social Research
School of Social Work
Syracuse University
Syracuse, NY 13210

DHEW Publication No. (CDC) 77–8318

For sale by the Superintendent of Documents, U.S. Government Printing Office
Washington, D.C. 20402 - Price $3.25
Stock No. 017–023–00110–8

# Preface

The papers published in this book represent an endeavor by the Public Health Service to gain better understanding of the factors in the residential environment which may offer alternative points for intervention to gain reduction of disease and injury. The strategy of controlling disease and injury by environmental changes made under the guidance of the local public health officer has long been accepted practice in community hygiene. The research reviewed and presented by the authors, however, points up that the traditional definition of environment, relating only to the physical surroundings, is too narrow for today in a mobile, impersonal urban community. Their recommendations for further research and for practice of preventive programs may be of interest to epidemiologists; other health professionals; practitioners of design, development, and management of residential environments; and professionals in public recreation and social work.

David J. Sencer, M.D.
Assistant Surgeon General
Director, Center for Disease Control

## Acknowledgements

The Center for Disease Control wishes to express its appreciation of the work done by the authors, and by Professor Lawrence E. Hinkle, Jr., M.D., as principal investigator. For his interest and encouragement the authors thank Mr. Robert E. Novick, (now of the Environmental Health Division, World Health Organization, Geneva), then Director, Bureau of Community Environmental Management, (predecessor to the Center for Disease Control's Environmental Health Services Division), under whose direction the contract for this work was initiated and our chapters drafted. The authors wish to acknowledge their gratitude to Miss Carol Webster for her untiring administrative effort which made their deliberations possible. The helpful contributions of Mr. Richard P. Wakefield, Center for Studies of Metropolitan Problems, National Institute of Mental Health, during all the meetings, and of Richard C. Lee, M.S., now with the Health Resources Administration, are also acknowledged. Mrs. Mildred W. Hershberg also is thanked for her work in proofreading and in preparation of the author index.

# Table of Contents

# List of Figures and Schema

# Introduction

WILLIAM C. LORING

## I. Public Health and the Residential Environment

This book grew out of an endeavor of the Public Health Service (PHS) to identify factors in the physical and social components of the residential environment of urban residents that relate to health and disease or to safety and injury. This residential or living environment is defined as excluding the occupational structures and areas devoted solely to work, but including dwellings, neighborhood, recreation areas, the siting of shopping and other pertinent service facilities (including those for health care, day care, schooling). It is the physical environment in which one lives all, or at least more than half, the average day. An objective of the undertaking was to further the understanding of alternative points for planned change or preventive intervention in aspects of man's environment that should be included in guidelines for planners, architects, developers, social workers and residents. A second objective was to provide criteria for standards and other technical advice for State and local public health agencies to consider in administration of their mission regarding community hygiene. The long range goal of such public health concern is to effect structural and operational changes in human settlements that substantially documented evidence may recommend for disease and injury reduction.

One of the traditional foci of public health administration, to prevent or reduce disease and injury in a human population, has been to change conditions in its physical environment. Historically numerous ideas for such interventions were acted upon before definitive research had determined the nature of the relationship between a particular object and a disease. Someone's incidental observation or some common feeling of a relationship were acted on. If there seemed to be beneficial results, that correction of the physical environment became accepted practice.

One such change might be in some object within the physical environment, like the water source for a town pump. Or it might be in some behavior of the users, like cleanliness around the pump. Again it might affect some nutrition practice relating to the use or handling of the water, such as boiling. Early practice of disease and injury prevention related to interventions in three major components of man's living environment: the physical, the nutrient, and the social.

In other words, what have become known as some of the public health responsibilities of local and State governments related to environmental prevention grew up before the germ theory of disease. In England and North America the practices grew out of the common law tradition for abating public nuisances and out of the evolution of Poor Laws from Elizabethan times on. In Continental Europe the practices grew out of an Eighteenth Century paternalistic concept of pre-industrial communities which in the mid-Nineteenth Century Germanies became known as "medical police."

With the development of chemistry and biology, and the advent of the germ theory, two other major components of environment were added to the first three and rapidly commanded more attention of health professionals and the public: the inorganic, and the biological. Those two areas were the ones in which the new research again and again found direct, linear relationships between environmental phenomena and diseases of the human organism. Research in these areas then determined what sort of disease prevention actions should be taken.

Much progress in infectious disease prevention by environmental means resulted. The very success of the work of the sanitary engineers and sanitarians, changing some facets of environment under the guidance of research findings linking biological and inorganic aspects of physical conditions to health and disease, turned attention for some decades away from further attempts to understand scientifically the roles of the man-made physical and the social components of human environment.

## II. Background Perspective

The present public health concern in the subject of this book goes back to the review of health-effects research in sociologist James Ford's two-volume *Slums and Housing. (1)* Surveying in detail studies of conditions of residential environments in American cities and any direct health consequences, he concluded in 1936 that, except for sanitation and accident hazards, little evidence had been produced directly linking physical conditions of housing or neighborhood to specific disorders or diseases. Ford's study spurred on the work of Dr. C. E. A. Winslow and his Committee on the Hygiene of Housing of the American Public Health Association. That Committee, with help from the Milbank Memorial Fund and the John B. Pierce Foundation, and with Public Health Service representation and participation, developed in 1939 the *Basic Principles of Healthful Housing* and in 1945 an *Appraisal Method for Measuring the Quality of Housing,* followed by a manual for *Appraisal of Neighborhood Environment* in 1950. *(2)* Those publications were primarily intended as tools for urban planning and health department housing code enforcement. The Committee also hoped they would permit research which, with more precise measurements, would test the hypothetical linkages between physical residential environment and health-disease which common sense suggested.

After Dr. Winslow's death the APHA Committee on the Hygiene of Housing experienced difficulty finding private funds to continue its initiatives. Because of continued demand by public health professionals at State and local levels for technical assistance regarding criteria for minimum standards of fitness for human habitation, the Public Health Service with small funds and some discontinuity pursued the identification of residential factors affecting safety and health.

In the ten years immediately preceding the deliberation of the collaborators reported in this volume, the PHS environmental health staff launched several studies to gain more understanding of the role of physical factors in the residential environment in relation to safety and health. The first was a review of the state of the art in their respective professions by an interdisciplinary panel contracted for through the School of Environmental Design at the University of California, Berkeley. Their efforts were summarized by Professor John Dyckman and this editor in presentations to the fiftieth anniversary meeting of the American Institute of Planners. *(3)* Two papers from that group, which were separately published, are particularly pertinent as background to this volume: Janet Abu-Lughod's "The City is Dead—Long Live the City," and Daniel H. Carson and B. L. Driver's "An Environmental Approach to Human Stress and Well-Being: with implications for planning." *(4, 5)*

A second seminar produced papers by various disciplines addressed less to planners and more to the public health preventive professions. Those discussions were summarized in *The Proceedings of the First Invitational Conference on Health Research in Housing and its Environment.* *(6)* Four papers from that group, available in full in photocopy, were particularly useful to the present collaborators. *(7)* In a third effort Ido de Groot, Professor of Epidemiology and Environmental Health Planning, University of Cincinnati, contracted to review the research literature for epidemiological and other bases underlying provisions of the "APHA–PHS Recommended Housing Maintenance and Occupancy Ordinance." *(8)* To the disbelief and shock of the sanitary engineers and sanitarians who had traditionally administered local housing codes, he found little or no epidemiological support for many of the non-sanitation, non-safety provisions. He noted, however, that in most cases the provisions had grounding in either moral or comfort rationales that according to Massachusetts and other court precedents would stand up in court tests.*

From 1965 to 1971 a fourth effort was made to gain some insights by use of research grants. The grant projects concerned with injuries in the residential area from physical hazards presented no new epidemiological insights. As applied studies regarding injury control, however, they typically presented a complex of physical environment and behavioral factors requiring preventive attention, but with the physical factors as "necessary" causes usually meriting priority attention. Two projects based on game-model research sought to develop knowledge of factors in environments outside the dwellings, which might be health-safety criteria for neighborhood standards. These were beginning to be promising at the time the grants program was discontinued. Two other studies were completed successfully dealing with epidemiologic linkage of housing and health. Those were the Burns and the Schooler studies which found there had to be an additive or synergistic mix of physical and social environment factors to account for disease changes noted. (9, 10) Schooler's work is summarized in the first part of Chapter IX.

A fifth effort to find guidance for future research was approximately co-terminous with the final writing of the papers in this book. It consisted of the use of Special Foreign Currency Projects to study the influences of physical elements under different cultural conditions. One such project entailed 23 papers developed for the Polish-American Scientific Symposium on "The Influence of the Micro-environment of Dwellings on the Health of the Residents," held near Warsaw in December 1972. Four American contributions reviewed the impact of the residential environment on physical and mental health, accidental injury, and the problems of noise control. (11) Polish papers reported research on health effects of building materials, particularly on the use of certain plastics, and the dangers of inadvertent use of radioactive material in structural concrete members, and on noise and accoustics control. The symposium again demarcated the limits of direct, unmediated, linear research designs to gain epidemiologic evidence for preventive planning. Another project report authored

---

* The appendix contains a paper Rodney R. Beard, M.D., M.P.H., delivered at the Annual Meeting of the American Public Health Association in November 1972, entitled "Epidemiological Contributions to Environmental Health Policy." It is in part based on discussions at Stanford University in March 1972 of an early draft of one of the chapters in this volume and of photocopies of some of the reports referred to in the above paragraph. The reader will note that Beard's last paragraph before his conclusion implies more can be gained at less cost, with more speed and with more lasting results by pursuing modification of the physical residential environment than seems to be assured by our further reviews and deliberations.

by J. Sadowski and B. Szudrowicz, available in summary through the American Institute of Architects, deals with the acoustic climate in dwellings and its effect on residents' health. *(12)* Another of those projects resulted in a Yugoslav report by Z. Kara-Pesic et al on "Children's Play and Game Areas" in urban sites of different size and density. *(13)* A third project developed an International Conference on Environmental Health in which eight panels dealt with (a) Man's Environments and Health; (b) Natural and Biological Environment: Effect of Pollution on Physical Health; (c) Nutrition as an Environmental Factor; (d) The Built Environment of the Human Settlement; (e) Social Environment and Alienation: Effect on Physical Health, Mental Health, and Social Pathologies; (f) Perceptual Environment and Health; (g) Economic Aspects of Preventive Environmental Interventions to Promote Health and Safety; and (h) Preventive Measures. The 37 papers were presented by authorities from all over the world. *(14)*

Many of the most disabling disease problems scourging mankind in the second half of the twentieth century are not being resolved by the mono-etiologic model, which was so successful in developing preventive strategies to reduce infectious diseases which had plagued earlier populations. Concentration upon simple linkage of a single environmental "cause" to a particular "disease" is often having to yield to multi-etiologic analysis of a web of contributing conditions. This becomes advisable for two reasons. First, for the "new" major diseases, either no "necessary cause," such as bacteria or virus, is involved, or at least none has yet been identified. Secondly, growing knowledge of the identity of the plural contributing conditions leading to their onset suggests there are alternative points for potential intervention strategies. Each of the alternatives may afford some disease reduction in the population, i.e., prevention for some individuals. Thus the identification of those points for intervention and evaluative comparison of their use will offer cost-effective decisions for community hygiene administration.

The present volume, and the selection of the disciplines and practicing professions that contributed to it, resulted from the previous efforts of the PHS to find definitive answers for the questions of local health officers, architects, planners, community developers and residents regarding the subject. The authors are a panel made up partly of experts in the relevant research disciplines, and partly of practitioners of professions needed for planning and effecting environmental changes to reduce the probabilities for disease or injury in populations-at-risk. It had been hoped that it would be possible to undertake an actual research project after the consultation and deliberation here reported. But the funds available for that were cut even before the contract was signed. Relieved of rushing into productive survey and other research our Board of Collaborators, under the able coordination of Dr. Hinkle were able to discuss thoroughly the kind of joint research needed for definitive results. They were also able to review further studies important to them in gauging promising concepts, hypotheses, and methodogy, and finally to propose approaches or even paradigms that could be fruitful in further work.

### III. Authors' Research Design Recommendations

The following chapters reflect the collaborating authors' deliberations, review the applicable value of research reported in their several fields, and present their suggestions of interdisciplinary research designs needed to pursue further the identification or rejection of physical and social factors as environmental hazards to health and safety. Since the subject area and main points of each author's chapter are well reviewed by Dr. Hinkle in Chapters I and X, it is pertinent here only to observe their methodological suggestions for future research.

They arrived at two areas of consensus. First, they agree that their review found that research based on direct, linear cause-and-effect models, usually done within the constraints of one discipline, has not produced definitive identification, positive or negative, of physical factors of man-made environment in human settlements with health-disease outcomes. Gross deficiencies and inadequacies related to minimum standards of basic shelter, basic sanitation, and basic safety have to be excepted from that statement. Often, however, the existence of such gross conditions, violating minimum fitness for human habitation, is as much a result of the human users' behavior as it is of the builders' or providers' design. Secondly, since most environmental stimuli appear to be mediated rather than direct in their influence, the authors agree further investigations may be productive only if one uses multi-disciplinary research designs. Those research programs must be planned for finding how the physical man-made factors may additively or synergistically combine with stimuli from the other major components, especially social environment factors (including cultural and behavioral phenomena) and with nutrient factors, to contribute to the health-disease outcomes. Even in respect to safety-injury outcomes, as Geddes and Gutman suggest, more definitive findings may be attained by such research designs.

In short, they are proposing that researchers test, and that practioners work on the basis of, an hypothesis that—except for some safety-injury physical hazards and some sanitation-pollution phenomena, traditionally attended to by sanitary engineers and sanitarians—physical, man-made environmental factors in the residential environment are part of a web-of-causation only as they may exacerbate or attentuate contributions of the other major components of

xii

man's environment. Perhaps more importantly, these deliberations point to the need to think of the in-put of three types of environmental factors, the nutrient, man-made settlement, and the social, as part of a gestalt of presenting stimuli to which the physiological organism internally responds either normally or in an internal stress-producing manner.

In Chapter IV, Stanislav Kasl points to the need of a program of studies to build cumulatively an understanding of the overall association between health and plural additive, yet mutually mediating, factors in the environment of human settlements. It would be designed to dimensionalize residential environment by factor and cluster analysis, and to use multivariate analysis of data for "causal," path analysis. Unless such identifications of contributing factors, and understandings of their function with others in the environmental process that presents stimuli to the individual, are produced, we will not know what preventive interventions are available and feasible at least cost for the most benefit.

Kasl diagrams a framework for guiding interdisciplinary research designs, so that appropriate questions will be asked, pertinent variables will not be neglected, and types of data analysis with intended kinds of interpretations of results will be suitable. His diagram is provocative, but needs to be put in a full human ecosystem context or perspective. It calls for broader, more interdisciplinary, and more systematic research. He suggests three "compromise" research design strategies:

1. A cross-sectional design comparing individuals, who are comparable in all important respects, living in residential environments which differ in some important aspect (such as low rise vs. high rise), which they always lived in or came to live in without self-selection.

2. A research design made possible by introduction of an architectually designed difference in some feature of a development in which residents are differentially exposed to the physical factor, but are randomly assigned to their dwelling units in the development.

3. A longitudinal design around "natural experiments," particularly those related to some public intervention program which calls for evaluation of the result of the change based on before-after comparisons.

In Chapter V, John Cassel proposes a strategy of "intervention research" carried out by inter-professional teams drawn from agencies charged with improving the urban environment and by research scientists from academic institutions.

Those teams would use the opportunity for working in a residential neighborhood afforded by some need for change in an aspect of its physical environment. Then hypotheses regarding social environment factors would be tested by deliberate alternation of some of them as experimental variables. He offers a four-way classification table of parameters to measure in testing the hypothesis he proposes regarding the linkage of two sets of social factors both to physical residential environments and to susceptibility to a variety of pathologies and disordered behavior.

Albert Damon proposes in Chapter VIII that further research into the relationship of the residential environment to health and behavior is feasible using epidemiologic and anthropologic methods. The populations studied could well be both the primitive and the highly urbanized-industrialized, so as to gain the advantage of contrast in environmental factors—physical and social. He suggests research techniques and strategies suited to modest project budgets. Particularly noted are procedures which ethnographers and applied anthropologists might routinely and inexpensively perform in any study which would permit cross-cultural, comparative analysis of effect of environmental components on health as a by-product of their regular field work. He also tested the utility of applied anthropologic research to analysis of environmental design in a large urban housing project, and was able to report differential effects on health, school studies and delinquency related to excessive traffic noise at one end of the site compared to markedly less noise at the other.

Kermit Schooler in Chapter IX first presents a summary of his research funded by the environmental health services of the PHS (1965–70) on residential environment and health of the aged. Based on data from an area sample of 4,000, he performed path analysis regarding six physical environment factors, seven social relations factors, six morale factors, and three health factors. He discusses interestingly the mediation of the nineteen environmental factors, and some demographic variables, upon each other in their influence as contributing conditions predicting one of the health factors. In the second part of his chapter, Schooler comments on the utilization of social science research in the policy and planning process of administration for the aging. He points out that research findings such as those he reports are useful to the planner in providing insights for some pathways to problem solution, but that much of social research is not sufficiently relevant to the planning and policy process. That process needs to become a goal, or focus, for the work of the social scientist in interdisciplinary undertakings, such as those recommended by the collaborating authors.

Robert Geddes & Robert Gutman in Chapter VI examine problems for the design professions, i.e., architects and planners, in assessing the safety from injury of residents using the built environments which are the products of their professional practice. They conclude that assessment of the built environment from the standpoint of safety is an

applied social science that depends on the development of fundamental knowledge of the interaction of man-made physical environment variables with other environmental variables in influencing behavior and social organization. They set forth a conceptual schema
for furthering that development. They further propose a rudimentary
list of behavioral criteria related to critical elements of human response. Several alternative, interdisciplinary research strategies are
described.

In Chapter VII, Lawrence Hinkle suggests a five point gradient for
measuring the negative effects of observed clusters of environmental
factors upon people. In order of their seriousness of effect, or distance
from an ideal environment, they are the extent to which an environment presents conditions contributing to: (a) shortened life, (b)
disability or impairment, (c) failure to reach full biological potential
for growth and development, (d) constraints upon ability to engage
in necessary or desirable activities, and (e) failure to provide pleasure or satisfaction. He then illustrates the use of the constructs which
define this continuum of environment-health interaction and suggests
methodological procedures pertinent for researching its components.
Such a weighting is needed for quantifying the contributions of the
mix of factors that our ecosystem orientation brings before us as the
conditions to which physiological organisms respond. It would also serve
in setting priorities for administration of change (i.e., environmental
intervention) and for cost-effective evaluation.

In Chapter II Donald Kennedy proposes two interdisciplinary strategies in longitudinal research. One would involve use of a "natural
experimental observatory." The other would call for work in a new
community, using designers' reasoning for site plan and exterior-
interior plans and evaluating the results in terms of safety and health.

In Chapter III Robert Burden suggests an environmental analysis,
evolved from Pareto by the Environmental Systems Program at Harvard University. It is based on identification of a set of "Pareto-
admissable vectors, i.e., technological solutions and surveillance controls." Pareto-admissable means "decisions from which no modification
can be made without making at least one party in the process worse
off." He cites six basic steps in implementation of the analysis: 1)
definition of the decision, 2) identificaton of interested parties, 3) determination of the technological relations between environmental control actions and resultant quality, 4) estimation of new benefit functions, 5) determination of the Pareto-admissable Frontier, and 6) prediction and prescription. This is only good for applied action-oriented
or evaluative studies, not basic research. It requires: (a) the environmental factors related to health be already identified, (b) the processes of their interaction with the physiological organism be understood, and (c) a model of intervention alternatives for decisions be

available, tested and accepted. It could serve as a useful tool, however, both in deciding upon one or a combination of alternative intervention points for administering preventive programs, and in gaining perspective for interpreting cost-effective or cost-benefit evaluations.

## IV. Logical Alternative Points in The Human Ecosystem for Preventive Intervention

As indicated above our reviews and deliberations pointed to a mediative phenomenon among components of man's environment in the process of their interaction with his physiological organism. Any external phenomena which stimulate or produce responses in the individual's physological organism are considered here to derive from one or more major components: the inorganic (including climate), biologic, nutrient, man-made physical (the human settlement and its technology), and social. In that process factors in one component of the environment may have their in-puts for health-disease modified, tempered, constrained, exacerbated or relieved by the concomitant influence of factors in the same or other components. We particularly noted the influence of the social environment (with its relational, cultural, communicative and behavioral factors) in modifying the influence of the built environment stimuli. This mediative phenomenon is suggested as the reason for the inconclusiveness of previous empirical research on the relation to health of the physical man-made environment to produce definitive findings.

We therefore conceive of further work to attain the public health objective, both in research and practice, as requiring a systems setting in which this mediative phenomenon or process can be accounted for. For the epidemiologist, the concept of the human ecosystem, with its two major subsystems—the environmental subsystem and the physiological organism—lends itself for this purpose. The influence of components of man's environment upon each other, in presenting the stimuli to which his physiological organism responds, suggests that they operate as a subsystem. Further, the stimuli produced by the environmental subsystem may be responded to in the physiological subsystem of the individual as synergistic gestalts. These may induce internal responses which can, either at once or over time, overload the tolerance threshold of the organism's adaptive capacity.

Hypothetically, the adaptive capacity of the physiological subsystem functions to hold latent any disease for which an individual has a generalized susceptibility by reason of genetic inheritance or earlier experience. Those homostatic defenses may be penetrated, occasionally by a "necessary and sufficient" inorganic or biologic stresser (as in classic infectious scourges or in accidental poisoning), or more usually

Figure 1. SCHEMA OF HUMAN ECOSYSTEM PROCESSES:

SUBSYSTEM I:
COMPONENTS OF ENVIRONMENT

SUBSYSTEM II:
PHYSIOLOGICAL ORGANISM(S)

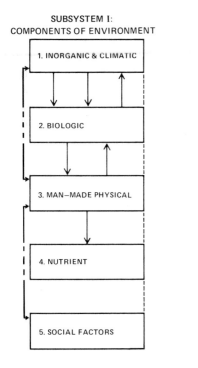

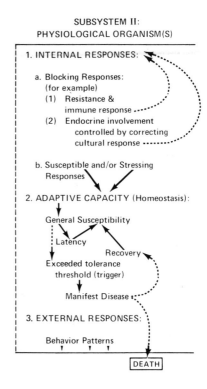

by a web of contributing conditions which contain a plurality of stimuli. The additive or synergistic webs of contributing conditions appear typical of much chronic physical disease and mental illness. The mediated contribution of such stimuli are capable of inducing in the organism one or more endocrinal, hormonal, chemical, or metabolic responses. These responses in turn over time seem to "cause" the particular disease that may onset. The full interaction involves a plurality of stimuli synergistically overtaxing and lowering the homeostatic mechanisms below the organism's tolerance threshold, thus allowing some of the latent disease potential to become manifest. In these "communications" within each subsystem and between the two subsystems, we have alternative points for interventions. Any change that affects one of the synergistically contributing conditions offers the possibility of some reduction in those diseases which the healthy normal adaptive capacity is capable of holding latent.

In the resulting model, then, the environmental factors as a subsystem operate simultaneously or collectively as "stressers" or stimuli. As contributing external conditions, they evoke physiologic responses within the processes of the biological organism. These responses may become, immediately or over time, an overtaxing or undermining internal condition stressful to the person's homeostatic mechanisms and other personal energy-expending adaptive capacities. The human organism produces feedback, both individually and additively as a plurality (read: population), to complete the "communications" in the ecosystem. These processes within the ecosystem are depicted in Figures 1 and 2.

The environmental subsystem is represented on the left in Figure 1. Arrows between the five components suggest some of their dependencies or influence on each other. On the right of Figure 1, the physiological organism as a subsystem is represented, not structurally, but in terms of processes internal to it that schematically relate to environmental stimuli, on the one hand, and to internal health-disease consequences, on the other.

In the middle of Figure 2, between the two subsystems, are long arrows depicting the flow of stimuli presented to the human organism (s). The presenting arrows converge or mingle to suggest two of the possible patterns of mediation of factors in one component by elements in others, which would be characteristic of additive or synergistic action. Each "leg" of a commingled arrow suggests a pair of alternate intervention points to interrupt transmission of stressers, i.e., to change either contributing conditions or "exposure" behaviors.

The "I" group represents stressers from the environmental components most involved in prevention of infectious disease and injury. The "C" group represents those of more concern in non-infectious and chronic diseases. The several addictions are considered as adverse behaviors related to deficiencies in the "C" aspects of environment. The "A" line represents the "health asset" function of time spent daily in a cohesive primary group which, Cassel suggests as a hypothesis, may operate to relieve development of internal stress by stopping responses stimulated by other factors during the day and so reinforcing or recharging adaptive capacity.

The word "stresser" may be helpful as a synonym for "adverse stimulus." But it is doubtful that there is much ecological or epidemiological merit to the word "stress," except when used as in the paragraph above to refer to a specifically describable internal condition that is a precursor to one or more diseases. Stress is variably used by different disciplines and by different writers within the same discipline. It is too easy to use the word "stress" as though it conveyed a complete explanation; but then it becomes a phlogiston-like "entity" deceptively masking the need for more operational investigation and reporting. Instead of employing "stress" as a semantic symbol that communicates fuzzily, it would be a clearer practice, as Hinkle proposes, (15) if we dealt with the specific process the word is presumed to imply, namely: the particular internal condition that has resulted from an internal physiological response to some external stressers and that may become a precursor of some disease. In so dealing, we would have to describe the linkages, or, if some are only hypothetical, we would have to develop research designs that will coordinate evidence from both environment and organism to test the hypotheses.

The physical man-made component is shown in both the I and C groups, although, as discussed in section VI below, it may have more influence in mediating the stimuli of the I group than those of the C group. Anticipating section VI below, it needs to be explained here that our reviews indicate that the man-made residential factors are relatively "passive" rather than "active" contributors to disease when they are defective, but may be considered "active" contributors to health when they function to buffer residents from some I type problems. Except for physical accident hazards, most of the I group's adverse stimuli from the man-made physical component are failures to mediate, i.e., prevent, stressers from the other two components in the group bearing on the physiological organism. In the C group our review noted less certainty about the role of spaces and circulation in mediating, i.e., aiding or hindering, contributions of the other components to disease or health. Indeed in the C group the physical space and circulation conditions appear to be more mediated than mediating, because of the adaptive flexibility of much user behavior.

The mediated, synergistic stimuli of the environmental subsystem may etiologically be analyzed and dealt with separately. But to the physiological organism they present a total ICA gestalt, which also is etiologically pertinent. The individual is able to "reduce" some of that gestalt thanks to "programs" that stem both from personal genetic inheritance or earlier personal environmental experience, and from preventive measures such as immunizations or cultural usages (i.e., habitual behaviors in the use of environmental components learned as norms based on earlier or present generations' group experience). As represented on the right of Figure 2, those physiological and behavioral programs may filter out many stresser-stimuli and cause them to be blocked, ignored, avoided, or adequately neutralized with minimal energy-expenditure on the part of the human organism. It takes some response in the organism to start the internal condition or precursor mechanism, which may be held latent by energy-expending homeostatic mechanisms, but which, if occurring with intensity, frequency or duration, and if not corrected, may lead to dysfunction and disease.

Some culturally prescribed and personally idiosyncratic behaviors in the ecosystem are represented at the bottom of Figure 2 as "feedback" from the physiological organism to the external environment. The relative amount of feedback behavior per individual to the five environmental components is represented by the width of the respective arrows. Those feedback patterns also offer alternative intervention points in the ecosystem processes which may be the focus of public health environmental prevention tactics. In respect to intervention decisions, the feedback of personal use and of cultural usage behaviors related to the nutrient and man-made physical environmental components is often equally as important to change as the stresser stimuli of those components. The feedback of contaminative behavior by one person to the inorganic and biologic "natural" components is relatively slight compared to the amount of his behavioral feedback into the social factors; but the additive contaminative behaviors of a community population is often of enough consequence to warrant change of the behavior in order to correct adverse stressers.

Paranthetically, "social factors" is the name assigned to represent those specific elements of the social environment which in themselves operate "causally" as contributory conditions to health-disease. In that context other aspects of social phenomena, except exposure and feedback behaviors, are present only as background. Before leaving consideration of Figure 2, it should be pointed out that the human ecosystem can be represented in different ways depending on which of its phenomena are pertinent. The disciplines of Geography and Sociology, for example, change the definition of social factors in the environmental subsystem on the left and alter the right subsystem to focus on a population and its sub-groups living in a geographic area rather than on the individual physiological organisms. Here the focus is on health programs, not on, for example, the economics of land use. Many of the secondary (i.e., impersonal) relationships a person has are not included

Figure 2. SCHEMA OF HUMAN ECOSYSTEM PROCESSES: ALTERNATIVE POINTS TO INTERVENE FOR SAFETY & HEALTH

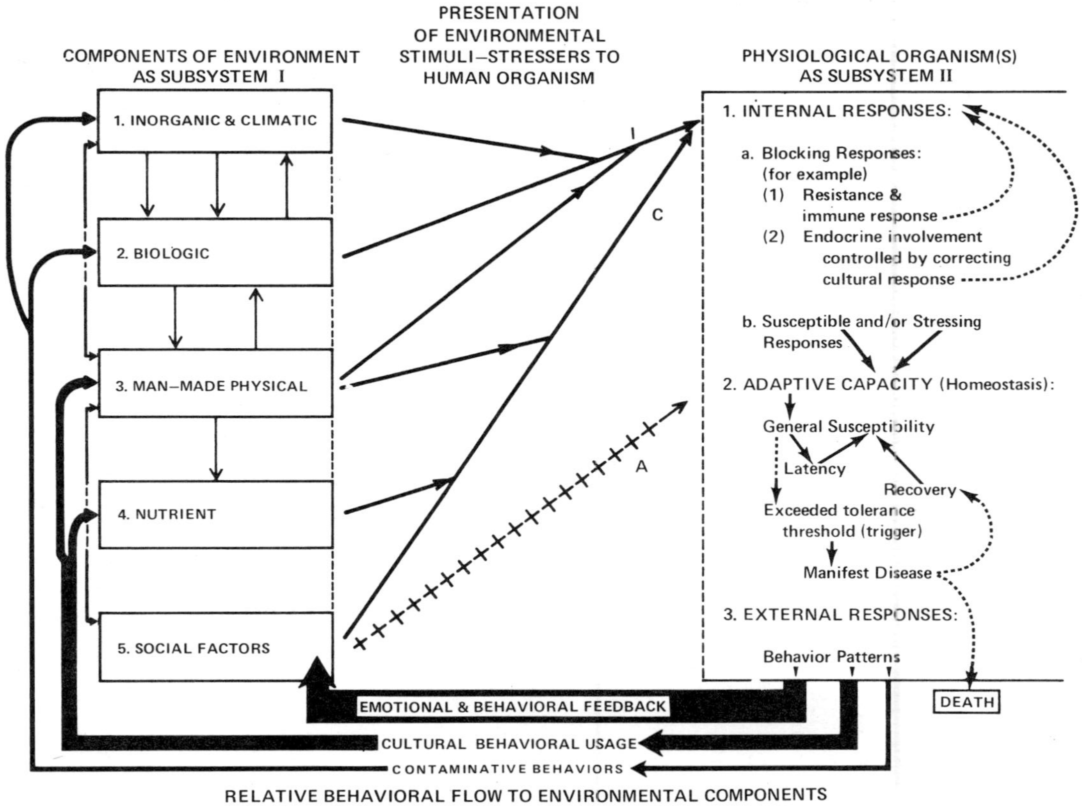

PHYSIOLOGICAL ORGANISM(S) AS SUBSYSTEM II

1. INTERNAL RESPONSES:

a. Blocking Responses:
(for example)
(1) Resistance & immune response
(2) Endocrine involvement controlled by correcting cultural response

b. Susceptible and/or Stressing Responses

2. ADAPTIVE CAPACITY (Homeostasis):

General Susceptibility
Latency
Exceeded tolerance threshold (trigger)
Recovery
Manifest Disease

3. EXTERNAL RESPONSES:

Behavior Patterns

DEATH

PRESENTATION OF ENVIRONMENTAL STIMULI–STRESSERS TO HUMAN ORGANISM

COMPONENTS OF ENVIRONMENT AS SUBSYSTEM I

1. INORGANIC & CLIMATIC
2. BIOLOGIC
3. MAN–MADE PHYSICAL
4. NUTRIENT
5. SOCIAL FACTORS

EMOTIONAL & BEHAVIORAL FEEDBACK

CULTURAL BEHAVIORAL USAGE

CONTAMINATIVE BEHAVIORS

RELATIVE BEHAVIORAL FLOW TO ENVIRONMENTAL COMPONENTS

xxi

here in the social environment factors, since they are not suspect of operating as contributing conditions in the present context.

One role of public health is conceived to be the guidance or performance of interventions at both *stresser* and *feedback* points in the human ecosystem for environmental prevention, as distinct from its medical prevention activities such as immunization. Identification of environmental health-disease factors, understanding their interactions in producing hazard, and estimation of their feasibility as points for preventive intervention are problems that must be pursued in the context of the operation of the whole environmental subsystem of a human settlement.

## V. Social Environment Factors: a Research Design for Definitive Identification

Our collaborators started on a quest to understand the relation of physical factors of residential environment to health and behavior. They found any such relation frequently mediated by or even dependent on the influence of factors from other components of the environmental subsystem. They repeatedly report that the mediation seems to be especially determined by elements among social environment phenomena. What among the phenomena called "social" may be appropriately considered factors or conditions contributing to health-disease? Probably only those which as environmental stimuli can be shown to have some effect on an individual organism's adaptive capacity.

While our collaborators were deliberating and writing their chapters, several other research-review reports were being written that reinforce our work. These reports are noted because with only slight duplication of the literature reviewed they supplement this text. They fill a void in the present volume that may have resulted from two psychiatric and social work researchers having to retire from our collaboration because of pressure of their regular work. From the reviews in our chapters and these other reports, it is obvious that social environment phenomena pertinent to causality in the quality-of-life continuum from well-being and health to disorder, disease and death are only beginning to be analyzed by epidemiologists, applied sociologists and psychologists. Only in the last decade have they begun to identify or sort out to a high level of suspicion specific social factors that support or overtax an individual's adaptive capacity to hold latent those diseases to which the person may be susceptible.

The suspect social factors that our authors or the other reviews find crucial to plan and deal with are not among the aggregated gross data of the present "social indicators." So, the negative side of our question is equally important and perhaps for clarity needs to be answered first. What social phenomena currently available to health planners should *not* be confused as having much bearing on the adaptive capacity of an individual physiological organism?

The social indicators were developed to gauge whether or not there is or should be social change occurring, either "naturally" or by means of some public policy and program. *(16)* The indicators used are not social factors which are causally operative in any analytical system. Rather they are made up of statistical data already available for census and other purposes. As a result they are an eclectic series of data which over time may show some trends more or less indicative of societal symptoms. As is the case with economic indicators, it may be possible from the trends to interpret that some societal change is or is not occurring, but without being able to specify what factors are "causing" the situation.

Several of the standard demographic data are found to be associated with certain populations which typically have more disease than "normal" populations. Areas inhabited by populations with least education and least income report more disease of almost all types. Such statistics do not warrant, however, the assertion that the best and surest preventive intervention is more schooling and more money. Such gross data mask the fact that among the "ignorant" and "poor" are many households that have a "normal" health record. The social factors that are effective (i.e., function) as contributors have to be more specific to distinguish between "healthy" and "sickly" households or between individuals with records of wellness or illness within such disadvantaged parts of a community's population.

The social phenomena studied by medical sociologists, that is, the human relations associated with health (read: illness) care institutions—namely: in-staff relations, staff-client relations, and care agency relations with its service community—are *not* the social environment factors contributing to disease that brings people to those institutions as patients.

Some of the individual or group behaviors, whether culturally expected or idiosyncratic, found by applied anthropologists or practicing health personnel in a population observed to be at-risk of specific diseases or injuries, may be social phenomena requiring change. But there is a distinction between a factor of social environment and a behavior which is a usage related to some other component of environment. In human ecosystem terms a behavior is to be considered etiologically in the context of the environmental component it functionally relates to. Change of adverse exposure and feedback behaviors can be one test of the success of many a preventive program which concerns some aspect of one or more of the other four components of the environmental subsystem. But frequently such behavior change, even when involving change of a pattern of behaviors called a life-style, may *not* entail any change in what are being recognized as social environment factors per se and their health-disease contributions.

So, we come back to the positive side of our question—What are some of the factors of the social component of man's environment that we are now able to point to? Some of them may be relational, and some a meaning or communication mix of social role functions. All of them must be capable of stimulating in the individual physiological organism a demonstrable response which acutely or chronically bears on its adaptive capacity or affects some organic subsystem, and so may be shown to contribute to the web-of-causality of health-disease outcomes.

The following books and articles offer as a group, not separately, the best up-to-date review of research findings about social phenomena that merit our attention. Unfortunately, most of the authors reviewed do not attempt to deal with how the social environmental phenomena may mediate or be mediated by the man-made physical and nutrient stressers in contributing to health-disease outcomes.

Aubrey R. Kagan and Lennart Levi in 1971 considered 183 research reports and commentaries in their useful report entitled "Health and Environment—Psychosocial Stimuli: a review." (17) According to their definitions, "psychosocial stimuli" originate in social relationships, arrangements, and communications. Those stimuli induce "mechanisms" or physiological reactions in the human organism, subject to the individual's reaction propensities or "psychobiological program" which are determined by the person's genetic factors and earlier environmental influences. Those mechanisms "under some conditions of intensity, frequency or duration, and in the presence or absence of certain interacting variables, will lead to psychosomatic disease." The rationale behind much of the research findings and speculations described is that:

> The human organism's pattern of response to a variety of environmental stimuli, including the psychosocial ones, constitutes a phylogenetically old adaptational process preparing the organism for physical activity, usually fight or flight. . . . These activities . . . do not appear to be appropriate in the adaptation of modern man to the endless number of socioeconomic changes, social and psychological conflicts and threats involved in living in a highly industrialized modern, urban society. . . . It is suspected that if this stress pattern of response to psychosocial stimuli and/or this psychophysical discrepancy lasts long enough, it may be pathogenic.

Their review points out that many of the studies, especially those stemming from the work of T. Holmes and R. H. Rahe and their followers, suggest that too great, too swift, and/or too many changes in social relationships can be liabilities overtaxing a person's innate and learned capacities for adaptation. The diseases they find linked to such relational social environment stressers are among the current chronic type, e.g., heart and mental. Where community surveys show relational change in excess of a cultural normal, there is the possibility that elements of a community's population are at more than normal risk of subsequent onset of disease.

Kagan and Levi close their review by concluding:

> In summary, (the) causation of disease by psychosocial stimuli is unproven but at a high level of suspicion. The action of such stimuli on mechanisms and precursors is better, but still rather poorly understood. There is also a high level of suspicion that interacting psychosocial factors and physical factors could prevent some mechanisms, precursors and disease. . . . Nevertheless, there will, no doubt, be occasions when health planners may feel, in the particular circumstances of their community, that action should be taken on the basis of existing level of suspicion.

If the relational changes involve an individual's removal from old ties which afford a form of social support, and if there is failure to establish replacements quickly, three authors (not reviewed by Kagan and Levi) indicate more hazards ensue. John Cassel and his colleagues, (18) S. L. Syme and his co-workers, (19) and Y. S. Matsumoto, (20) report as a health asset function a few hours spent daily in cohesive, primary (i.e., face-to-face) groups, such as family, kin, neighbors, or age-peers. This "asset" seems to serve to relieve tension built up by other stimuli and to recharge adaptive capacity, so that process may function as described in Cassel's Chapter V. Those studies indicate there is need for preventive action when such social support functions are not present in normal amounts among a population.

Barbara S. and Bruce P. Dohrenwend edited a book on *Stressful Life Events: their nature and effects (21)* which includes the later thinking of many of the authors whose studies Kagan and Levi reviewed. Their volume is a reconsideration of research designs that may move us from the high level of suspicion Kagan and Levi describe to more definitive resolution of the health-disease effects of identified social environment factors. With support from the Center for Epidemiologic Studies of the National Institute of Mental Health, they held a conference in June, 1973, out of which grew the papers for the chapters of their 26 authors. Their conclusion is: (1) Life events are, in and of themselves, eminently researchable . . . . (and) (2) (They are) strategic phenomena on which to focus in the study of the role of social factors in health and illness."

Paul M. Insel and Rudolf H. Moos edited a textbook on *Health and the Social Environment* which reviews a wider lot of studies of factors in social environment which may, with further and more definitive research, be identified with health-disease outcomes. (22) The main headings of the book suggest the pertinence of abnormal qualities in a population of an array of social factors, including as incisive social indicators: (1) certain types of relationships and changes therein, (2) certain types of status inconsistency, and (3) certain types of social role fulfillment or nonachievement. The titles to Parts of their book include: psychosomatic disorders and environmental stimuli, social correlates of heart disease, social processes and immunity, social dimensions of obesity, the social environment and mental health, and urban stress and contemporary life. The two editors turn about and become authors Moos and Insel in a companion volume of *Issues in Social Ecology: Human Milieus,* which usefully discusses for planners the "impact that physical and social environments have on human beings." *(23)*

In summary, it appears that a social phenomenon can be health-disease related in one of two ways. First, an individual behavior or a cultural-technological cluster of usage may either be a part of the web of conditions enabling transmission to the physiological organism of stimuli from one of the four non-social components, or be a misuse or an abuse of one of those four components of environment. In either case, intervention to change the behavior or usage may interrupt the communication in either direction sufficiently to achieve some disease reduction. Such behaviors and usages are the typical objects of much health education and other preventive programs. But those exposure and feedback, or life-style, behaviors are not defined as factors of social environment in our present context.

Second, a social phenomenon may be observed to be a contributing condition independent of the other environmental components. If so, then for our purposes it is a social environment factor. Since usually the presently suspect social factors have a relational character, correction in the social environment component may seem at the same time both intimate and complex. Yet those attributes typify much preventive medicine. Unlike many interventions to correct other environmental components, relational corrections in a population at-risk involve no capital investment and can take less time and cost less in operating budget to effect and maintain. Planning, census, or epidemiologic surveys can produce data to indicate whether such relational problems are present among an abnormal number of the individuals in a particular population. When that is the finding, it then becomes possible to administer public (i.e., population-wide) service interventions, rather than the more expensive and time-consuming private (i.e., individually focused) consultation and guidance. The interventions would include encouragement of acquaintance-building and other primary (i.e., face-to-face) relation forming activities among such a population, using the social work techniques of group work and community organization work along with selected recreation and other people-contacting leisure-time pursuits. Incidentally, the community organization work techniques and the resulting groups at the block, neighborhood or village levels often serve four objectives of public health preventive programs: (1) they may broaden and deepen the relational aspects of participants' social environment, (2) they may serve as respected, indigenous sociometric channels for communication and reinforcement of health education messages, (3) they may become means for one's peers to initiate and reinforce changes in behaviors and usages needed to achieve preventive program objectives, and (4) they may develop into vehicles for putting self-help energies of those peers to work at physical environment improvement and maintenance of their area.

The identification and understanding of the functioning of the social environment factors is meaningful for two professional groups. The first are the planners, architects and developers whose professional practice concerns the design, building or management of the man-made physical environment, in both the residential habitat which is the focus of this book and the rest of the human settlement. The identified or suspect social environment factors form an important consideration in developing the reasoning for objectives to guide their work. Any mediating effect of the physical setting they produce should be an aid and not a hinderance to the functioning of the social environment factors relevant to safety or health. As Geddes and Gutman suggest in Chapter VI, those professions need to test their results through evaluation of their product in use, in order to learn by experience how to improve such functionality and consequently the desired safety and health objectives.

The second group are the health planners of environmental prevention programs and the social work group workers. For them more definitive knowledge about the social environment factors that contribute to health-disease will be of interest, if their presence, absence, or deficient functioning offer points for corrective interventions for which feasible procedures can be prescribed and administered. For example, recent in-migrants to a community are easily located by surveys. Because of their mobility, much of their social environment will have been disrupted. To that extent they are a population at-risk of any health-disease problems related to a synergism which includes disrupted or dysfunctional relational factors in their social environment. In neighborhoods in which such a population at-risk are found to be numerous, those residents, with professional social work and recreation advice, can be guided and enabled to self-help themselves to more rapid restoration, replacement, or correction of the primary relational functions of social environment pertinent to health.

When does a social phenomenon merit consideration as a condition or factor contributing by itself to the interface process between the environmental subsystem and the physiological organism? If found by social science and epidemiologic surveys to be a liability or an asset associated with some disease or injury, it can only be considered as highly suspect. To warrant identification it requires demonstration of linkage to an internal psychophysical response which further leads to an internal condition or "mechanism" that may lead to or prevent a disability outcome. This confirmation requires at least clinical, if not experimental, evidence testing the hypotheses suggested by the studies establishing the suspicion.

The liability hypothesis is that under certain conditions the presence of the social factor leads to measurable neural and/or endocrine responses that if continued lead to observed malfunctions which can lead to disability. An hypothesis regarding an asset to health, such as the daily exposure for a few leisure hours to a "cohesive" family, neighborhood or age-peer group cited in the Cassel and Matsumoto studies, requires proof that experience of the asset in some daily amount or frequency maintains normal neural or hormonal mechanisms or reduces to tolerable levels adverse ones set in motion by daily exposure to some of the liability type stimuli from social or other components of the environmental subsystem.

We need research designs that would observe whether the hypothesized internal responses do occur, when a social factor stresser is present in the environmental gestalt stimulating a physiological organism. For example, can responses, such as the turning on or off of endocrinal, hormonal, chemical flows, be verified as occurring in a pattern related to a social environment phenomenon and in a manner that could have health-disease consequences. This will require that the anthropological, sociological and/or psychological observations of the changes in occurrence of social factor stimuli be meshed with clinical observations and tests of occurrence or non-occurrence of physiologic responses.

## VI. Health and Behavior Demands upon the Physical Residential Settlement

There are two conclusions about environmental prevention activities of health and planning departments growing out of our reviews and deliberations. The first is implied. It deals with areas of established epidemiological knowledge regarding physical hazards both to safety from injury and to physical health from insanitation or pollution. Those areas of direct influence of physical man-made environment upon injuries, and of mediated influence of the inorganic and climatic, the biologic, and the physical man-made components of environment in forming the contributing conditions leading to infectious disease, are dealt with in our pages only in passing, because epidemiological evidence and/or professional environmental preventive practice confirm there is no uncertainty about the need for continued efforts in those areas.

The second conclusion is dealt with in each chapter, but perhaps needs to be explicitly emphasized here. In going beyond injury and infectious disease objectives, public health environmental preventive interventions in human settlements will not accomplish much for the expense involved if programs are confined to changes in the physical man-made environment *without* emphasizing both relevant behavioral change and change in any mediating or mediated nutrient and social environment factors.

Only in physical accident hazards and in inorganic or biologic pollution of community air and water supplies does experience indicate we can rely on technological advances to gain such a degree of user acceptance that behavioral usage changes follow with little lag. Those pollution and hazard items that do not permit of automatic change in usage, following technological change, must rely on induced behavior change to break the web-of-causation. As J. Donald Millar, M.D., Director, Bureau of State Services, Center for Disease Control, puts it, to the extent the contributing conditions in a web-of-causation are affected by a particular behavior or by "life-style" patterns of behavior, "interrupting transmission" of chronic as well as infectious disease will increasingly rely on attacking disease reduction through behavior changes. The chronic and mental illnesses that concern us today require prevention strategies that rely heavily on successful health education, social work, community organization work, recreation group work, and other techniques for accomplishing and reinforcing behavior changes in a population at-risk.

Nothing in the research reviewed in the following chapters repeals the logic of most of the 1939 *Basic Principles of Healthful Housing* of the APHA's Committee on the Hygiene of Housing. Disease and injury reduction in any population require housing and neighborhood standards which if observed and enforced will directly prevent man-made physical hazards, whether due to design, construction or maintenance, from putting residents or other users at-risk. Safety demands consideration of physical residential environment conditions which contribute directly to falls, burns, lacerations, poisonings, and to pedestrian or cyclist accidents. Sanitation demands include: (1) control of water supply and sewerage; (2) provision for cleanliness both in food handling, storage and preparation, and in personal and clothing care; and (3) control of vermin vectors, both insect and rodent, and of solid wastes. Shelter demands weather-tightness of roof and freedom from dampness on floors and walls, whether the dwelling is built on stilts or solid foundations. The necessary provision for natural lighting of the interior will vary with latitude and altitude. Depending on the climate, heating and cooling demands for the living areas of the shelter will require attention to ventilation, insulation, safety and effectiveness of equipment, and cultural customs regarding clothing and height of sleeping surface. For some, but not all, of these physical environment requirements, appropriate behavior in their use and maintenance is as important as the physical factors themselves in gaining the environmental prevention objectives.

Nevertheless, it must be pointed out that our deliberations and reviews afford little more definitive grounding of criteria than was available in 1939 for the design and occupancy of dwelling space, divisions of that space, or for circulation between the dwelling and neighborhood common spaces, indoor and outdoor, or regarding access to pertinent service facilities required by the culture of the resident population. In terms of exercise and recreation for development and for health maintenance, we now know from time-distance studies in Finland, Austria and North America that children and adults do not postpone going from their dwelling to outdoor play area or indoor leisure-time facility if the time consumed is under 6 minutes on foot or by vehicle. We understand that the architect-planner of Helsinki intends that some park or recreation facility for common use will by the 1990 Plan be within 5 minutes of every dwelling.

The demands for interior dwelling space or for its separation into common and "private" rooms involve some social environment factors. If a person cannot move easily and effectively from one social role to another, (e.g., from husband or wife role to parent role, from sibling role to child or student roles, or from any of those to an age-peer, friend or neighbor role), because of defect in the design or cultural usage or personal use of the physical dwelling spaces, then our human ecosystem logic suggests that the mediation of the pertinent social environment relational factor by the physical design of dwelling and location of neighborhood common spaces requires corrective change. That change may be indicated by cost-effective considerations to be needed either in the physical space requirements or in the cultural-behavioral practices. Our review indicates that density relates to health, not as physical persons per some square measure, but as overcrowding of social roles, i.e., activities demanding of a person perception and behavior in two or more not easily compatible roles at the same time in the same place. Thus a more cost-effective preventive intervention to conserve social environment functions important to health may be to effect a change as to activities proper for the dwelling. That sort of cultural or behavioral change would shift other activities to alternative spaces provided in the immediate housing environment, i.e., within 1300 to 1500 feet or 5 to 6 minutes from the door of the dwelling. This line of reasoning also suggests that when the economy of a population can not afford more than some minimal amount of space in the dwelling, perhaps suitably sufficient for activities all of the household engage in at the same time, such as sleeping and eating, it becomes essential as an environmental health measure to provide convenient common spaces in the immediate housing environment for the other "home area" activities of household members.

Incidentally, to the extent that perception is influenced by the social role upper-most at the moment in a person's mind, environmental designers planning or evaluating the dwelling and its immediate housing environment for safety, as proposed by Geddes and Gutman in Chapter VI, might well design to minimize the possibility of the over-stimulation and under-stimulation which allow the distraction typical of unintended and often unconscious shifts of social role and so of the context of perception. Such distraction and faulty perception are frequently reported as part of the conditions at the time of an injurious accident. To the extent the physical design cannot guard against such distraction,—e.g., the housewife shifting from cook role to mother role on hearing a child's outcry but completing a now poorly perceived and potentially hazardous cooking activity while thinking about rushing to the child,—the task of prevention of such accidents becomes one for the health educator, the home economist, or the paraprofessional home environment aide.

Anything as precise as a design or occupancy health standard based on some measure of area required per person is too simplistic to withstand changing technology and culture patterns that may occur over the life of the structure. Thus the decision of the APHA's Committee on the Hygiene of Housing to base their *Planning the Home for Occupancy* (1950) on space needed for circulation around furniture conventional to each type of room will continue to be a useful rule of thumb,—but hardly a health-disease criterion for design-occupancy standards. *(24)* The later publications (1957, 1971) of the International Federation for Housing and Planning have had a great influence in Europe on residential standards for both occupancy and building regulations adopted by either national or city governments. But those recommendations, for necessary habitable surface areas for dwelling according to size of family and for accessibility or circulation in the neighborhood environment, are based on users' subjective preferences and some observed behaviors. *(25)* Those data appear to relate "coincidentally" to customary size and number of rooms in European housing existing at the time of the studies. The minimal square meters of space (8 square meters or about 85 square feet) found needed per person in households in which all members are normally healthy happens to coincide with the smallest room conventionally found in French and other Western European working class residential areas. The space per person wanted in a household containing a sickly person or a "difficult" personality happens to be the equivalent of the next largest customary room size (12 square meters or 130 square feet). Like the American considerations of the APHA, these European recommendations of the IFHP will continue to be helpful to designers and code officials. They are suggestive as guides—but hardly proven as health-disease criteria for preventive standards.

Social environment factors per se, (i.e., quite apart from behavioral-cultural aspects of other social phenomena), may upon further research be shown to justify some demands on the space and circulation afforded by the physical residential environment. Of the social environment factors found in our review, or in the reviews noted in section V above, to be stimuli which are presently at a high level of suspicion as conditions contributing to health-disease, those characterized as ascertainable only by subjective responses to interview questions do not lend themselves to change by programs oriented to work with a population at-risk. Those require more personalized corrective effort. But those which allow of objective observation and verification, (i.e., which, though often gathered from a respondent, could be checked in records), are amenable to planning surveys and analyses. Of social environment factors now "suspect," the relational type are the most objective to observe and deal with. An abnormal frequency or amount of relational disintegration or change therein among members of a population beyond what is established to be the normal among a population with an average health record, a fact ascertainable by periodic surveillance typical of both epidemiology and urban and regional planning, is a characteristic which can be noted and mapped to indicate a population at-risk. The relational type includes not only Cassel's primary groups but also the objectively countable breaks or changes in relational ties with kin, neighbors, job acquaintances found among the Dohrenwends' "life events" or among Insel and Moos' three types of data. A frequently met example of such a population at-risk, as Cassel suggests in Chapter V, would be one that dwells in an area demarcated by a large proportion of folk recently in-migrant from some distance. The appropriate preventive program for them may involve use of social work techniques for faster rebuilding of their broken relational ties; or it may be a demand upon their immediate physical man-made environment for a change in either privacy from or accessibility to others.

Our review shows it is not possible presently to offer more definitive detail to the environmental designers and developers who turn to public health sources for guidance regarding space and circulation needed to optimize the physical setting for the health of their clients. They will note in the chapters that follow, however, numerous hints which in the light of their experience they may find helpful.

We hope that our review and suggestions for future research may result in a fuller understanding of physical and social factors in the residential micro-ecosystems of human settlements. We anticipate that development will expand the scope of environmental prevention in public health policy and administration by presenting alternative points and strategies for intervention in the human ecosystems to attain disease-injury reduction objectives.

Is it necessary to await full definitive information before planning and taking preventive measures, at least as exploratory experiments that may do some good and serve as opportunities for applied or evaluation research? The scientists dealing with stimuli of the inorganic and biologic components of environment accomplished much for the reduction of infectious disease in the last 100 years. It was in the two decades before the germ theory era, however, that public health pioneers in Europe, such as Chadwick (1842) and Snow (1855), working on empirical evidence for "a high level of suspicion," planned and got started the administration of the preventive programs of the Sanitary Movement. As described by Mervyn Susser, they relied on rather general and untested hypotheses as to the environmental sources of a considerable number of infectious diseases and were able to interrupt transmission in part of the webs in markedly successful demonstrations. *(26)* Similar inventive enterprise, in the light of current knowledge, hypotheses and reasonable hunches, may now produce, as our authors suggest, demonstrations useful in reducing disease and promoting knowledge of environmental prevention techniques.

## References

1. James Ford, *Slums and Housing* (Cambridge, Mass: Harvard University Press, 2 vol., 1936).
2. Committee on the Hygiene of Housing, (C. E. A. Winslow et al), *Basic Principles of Healthful Housing* (New York: American Public Health Association, Inc., 1st ed. 1939); *An Appraisal Method for Measuring the Quality of Housing*: A yardstick for health officers, housing officials, and planners,
   Part   I: Nature and Uses of the Method (N.Y.: APHA, 1945);
   Part  II: Appraisal of Dwelling Conditions (N.Y.: APHA, 1946); &
   Part III: Appraisal of Neighborhood Environment (N.Y.: APHA, 1950);
   *Principles for Healthful Rural Housing* (N.Y.: APHA, 1957).
3. John Dyckman, et al, "City Planning and the Treasury of Science", in William R. Ewald, Jr., ed., *Environment for Man* (Bloomington, Indiana: Indiana University Press, 1967), Ch. 3, pp. 27–59.
4. Janet Abu-Lughod, "The City is Dead—Long Live the City: Some thoughts on Urbanity." in Sylvia Fava, ed., *Urbanism in World Perspective: A Reader* (New York: T. Y. Crowell Company, 1968), pp. 155–165.
5. Daniel H. Carson and B. L. Driver, "An Environmental Approach to Human Stress and Well-Being: with implications for planning," *Incidental Paper*, Mental Health Research Institute (Ann Arbor, Michigan: University of Michigan, 1968).
6. *Proceedings of the First Invitational Conference on Health Research in Housing and its Environment*, Bureau of Community Environmental Management, PHS (Washington, D.C.: U.S. Government Printing Office, 1970).
7. Raymond Neutra and Ross McFarland, "Accidents and the Residential Environment," 1970;*

John R. Goldsmith and Erland Jonsson, "Effects of Noise on Health in the Residential and Urban Environment," 1970;*

Paul V. Lemkau, "Mental Health and Housing," 1970;* and

Daniel M. Wilner and W. G. Baer, "Sociological Factors in Residential Space," 1970.*

8. Ido de Groot, *Epidemiological Evidence Underlying Provisions of the APHA-PHS Model Code*, 1969.*

*APHA-PHS Recommended Housing Maintenance and Occupancy Ordinance*, Public Health Service Publication No. 1935 (Washington, D.C.: Government Printing Office, 1969) ; the 1975 revision is:

*APHA-CDC Recommended Housing Maintenance and Occupancy Ordinance*, HEW Publication No. (CDC) 75-8299.

See also following related publications of the Environmental Health Services Division, Center for Disease Control, PHS, HEW: *Basic Housing Inspection*, Community Environmental Management Series, Public Health Service Publication No. 2123 (Washington, D.C.: U.S. Government Printing Office, 1970) — a revised edition entitled *Basic Housing Inspection* is HEW Pub. No. (CDC) 76-8315, of the Environmental Health Services Division, BSS, Center of Disease Control, Atlanta, Georgia 30333, in 1976. Also to be issued by the same source in a revised edition in 1977 will be *Community Health Aide: a training resource manual* for paraprofessionals dealing with basic safety and basic sanitation in the dwelling, its premises and immediate neighborhood.

9. Leland F. Burns and Leo Grebler, *The Housing of Nations* (London: Macmillan Company, forthcoming in 1976) ; the reference is to the South Dos Palos, California, and Zacapu, Mexico, case studies in both of which visits to the clinic for acute problems dropped after serendipitous occurrence of relatively inexpensive physical residential environment interventions; one a self-help add-a-room program and the other a rat control and basic sanitation program.

10. Kermit K. Schooler, "Residential Physical Environment and Health of the Aged," final report to PHS on Grant No. EC 00191, Florence Heller Graduate School for Advanced Studies in Social Welfare, Brandeis University, Waltham, Mass., 1970.

11. Michael Brill, "A Survey of Present Research: the Impact of the Residential Environment on Health," 1972;**

Ernest M. Gruenberg, "Housing and Mental Health," 1972;**

Barry Griffith King, "Man, Environmental Hazards and the Control of Accidental Injury," 1972;** and

Theodore J. Schultz, "Noise Control in Dwellings—United States, 1972."**

12. Jerzy Sadowski and Barbara Szudrowicz, *The influence of materials and construction on the acoustic climate in dwellings and its effect on residents' health*: Summary of research report (Washington, D.C.: Office of Research Programs, American Institute of Architects, 1735 New York Avenue NW, 20016, forthcoming) .

---

* (Unpublished; single copies available until supply exhausted from Environmental Health Services Division, BSS, Center for Disease Control, Atlanta, Georgia 30333)

** (Unpublished; single copies available until supply exhausted from Environmental Health Services Division, BSS, Center for Disease Control, Atlanta, Georgia 30333)

13. Zivojin Kara-Pesic, Jasminka Gojkovic, Slobodan Lazic and Bozidar Vlajic, *Children's Living and Play Areas in the Local Community*, (Belgrade, Yugoslavia, January 1975; reprinted by Environmental Health Services Division, BSS, Center for Disease Control, Atlanta, Georgia 30333).

14. *Proceedings: International Conference on Environmental Health* for physicians and allied professionals (Belgrade, Yugoslavia: Union of Medical Societies of Yugoslavia, 1973; printed in English; copies available from Environmental Health Services Division, Center for Disease Control, Atlanta, Georgia 30333). Particularly to be noted in the context of this Introduction are the following papers:

Reuel A. Stallones, "Epidemiological evidence of effect of environment on health," pp. 29–33;

T. Bakacs, "Man and man-made artificial environment; ecological balance: its disruption in cities," pp. 35–56;

Paulo de Almeida Machado, "The ecology of human settlements in the Amazon region," pp. 57–63;

Lawrence E. Hinkle, Jr., "Man's environments and health," pp. 65–73;

Raymond Neutra, "Accident epidemiology and housing policy," pp. 195–215;

Anthony J. Radford and N. R. E. Fendall, "Some effects of social environment on health," pp. 245–268;

Claude Leroy, "Effects of social environment on physical and mental health," pp. 269–283;

Hans Strotzka, "Social environment and alientation, effect on mental and physical health," pp. 285–289;

Irwin Altman, "Social and psychological aspects of man-environment research: relevance for mental health," pp. 309–338; and

Morris Schaefer, "Organization of preventive measures: issues and directions," pp. 377–389.

15. Lawrence E. Hinkle, Jr., "The concept of 'Stress' in the biological and social sciences," *Sciences, Medicine & Man*, vol. I, (Pergamon Press, 1973) pp. 31–48.

16. The following books are typical of the development of social indicators:

Raymond A. Bauer, *Social Indicators* (Cambridge, Mass.: M. I. T. Press, 1966);

Eleanor B. Sheldon and Wilbert E. Moore, *Indicators of Social Change: concepts and measurements* (New York: Russell Sage Foundation, Basic Books. Inc., 1968);

Department of Health, Education & Welfare, *Toward a Social Report* (Washington, D.C.: U.S. Government Printing Office, 1969);

Leslie D. Wilcox, Ralph M. Brooks, George M. Beal and Gerald E. Klonglan, *Social Indicators and Societal Monitoring* (New York: Elsevier Scientific Publishing Co., Inc., 1972);

Daniel B. Tunstall, *Social Indicators, 1973,* Executive Office of the President, Office of Management and Budget (Washington, D.C.: U.S. Government Printing Office, 1973).

17. Aubrey R. Kagan and Lennart Levi, "Health and Environment—Psychosocial Stimuli," report no. 27, Laboratory for Clinical Stress Research (Stockholm, Sweden: Karolinska Institute, 1971); also in *Social Science & Medicine*, vol. 8, pp. 225–241 (Oxford: Pergamon Press, 1974).

Lennart Levi, ed., *Society Stress and Disease: The Psychosocial Environment and Psychosomatic Disease* (London: Oxford University Press, 1971).

Lennart Levi, ed., *Stress and Distress in Response to Psychosocial Stimuli,* (Oxford: Pergamon Press, 1972).

18. John Cassel and H. A. Tyroler, "Epidemiological Studies of Culture Change: Health status and recency of industrialization," *Archives of Environmental Health*, 3:25, 1961; and
    John Cassel, "Physical Illness in Response to Stress," Chapter 7 in Sol Levine and Norman A. Scotch, eds., *Social Stress* (Chicago: Aldine Publishing Co., 1970), pp. 189–209.

19. S. Leonard Syme, et al, "Some Social and Cultural Factors Associated with the Occurrence of Coronary Heart Disease," *Journal of Chronic Disease*, vol. 17, 1964, pp. 277–289.

20. Y. S. Matsumoto, "Social Stress and Coronary Heart Disease in Japan," *Milbank Memorial Fund Quarterly*, XLVIII:1, 1970, pp. 9–37.

21. Barbara S. and Bruce P. Dohrenwend, *Stressful Life Events: their nature and effects* (New York: John Wiley & Sons, 1974).

22. Paul M. Insel and Rudolf H. Moos, *Health and the Social Environment* (Lexington, Mass.: Lexington Books, 1974);
    Gordon E. Moss, *Illness, Immunity, and Social Interaction: the dynamics of biosocial resonation* (New York: John Wiley and Sons, 1973), for a different, interesting but still speculative viewpoint.
    Water McQuade and Ann Aikman, *Stress* (New York: E. P. Dutton & Co., Inc., 1974), for a popularly written introduction to the subject as it relates to many behaviors, but not to social environment factors as discussed here.

23. Rudolf H. Moos and Paul M. Insel, *Issues in Social Ecology: Human Milieus* (Palo Alto, Calif.: National Press Books, 1974).

24. Committee on the Hygiene of Housing, American Public Health Association, *Planning the Home for Occupancy*: standards for healthful housing series (Chicago: Public Administration Service, 1950).

25. International Federation for Housing and Planning, *Cologne Recommendations*, 1957; *Revised Cologne Recommendations*, 1971; *Housing Environment Requirements*, 1973; and *The Immediate Housing Environment*: Vienna Recommendations, 1973 (Luxembourg: General Secretariat of the Standing Committee Rent and Family Income, IFHP).

26. Mervyn Susser, *Causal Thinking in the Health Sciences: Concepts and Strategies of Epidemiology* (New York: Oxford University Press, 1973). This may be an easy orientation to the subject for readers from other professions when preparing for interdisciplinary research teamwork.

# Author Index to Chapter Bibliographies

Bennett, E. M. (1956) 192.
Bennett, R., (1965) 123.
Bensman, J., (1960) 44.
Berenson, J., (1968) 122.
Berger, B., (1960) 121.
Berle, B. B., (1958) 60.
Bernard, J., (1966) 60.
Bernstein, S. H., (1957) 118, 140.
Beshers, J., (1962) 60.
Beyer, G. H., (1963) 124.
Bhandari, N. P., (1960) 119.
Biddle, E. H., (1962) 119.
Bilodean, J. M., (1959) 125.
Blake, R., (1956) 119.
Blalock, H. M., Jr., (1961) 115; (1964) 315: (1968) 115.
Blenker, M., (1967) 122.
Bloom, B. L., (1968) 115.
Bloombaum, M., (1968) 60.
Blum, B., (1949) 140.
Blumenfeld, H., (1969) 112.
Boen, J. R., (1966) 116.
Bogdonoff, M. D., (1962) 142; (1964) 112.
Borgatta, E. F., (1969) 315.
Borhani, N. O., (1965) 141.
Bortner, R. W., (1962) 123.
Boudon, R., (1968) 115.
Bouehler, J. A., (1955) 124.
Boulding, K. E., (1964) 43.
Bracey, H. E., (1964) 120.
Brady, J V , (1959) 142; (1960) 141,
Breckenfeld, G., (1958) 121.
Brennan, T., (1959) 120.
Brett, G. Z., (1957) 114, 140, 261.
Brill, M., (1972) xxxiv.
British Medical Bulletin, (1971) 260.
Britten, R. H., (1934) 139; (1940) 118; (1941) 118, 140; (1942) 118, 140.
Britton, J. H., (1961) 124.
Broadbent, D. E., (1958) 112.
Broady, M., (1969) 60.
Brody, E. B., (1969) 123.
Brooks, G. W., (1966) 122.
Brooks, R. M., (1972) xxxv.
Brotherson, J. H. F., (1957) 120, 140.
Brown, C., (1965) 60.
Brown, J. E., (1940) 118.
Brown, W., (1923) 125.
Brownfield, C. A., (1964) 126.
Bruch, H. A., (1963) 118.
Bryne, D., (1955) 124.
Buck, A. A., (1968) 262.

Buck, C. W., (1955) 116.
Buechley, R. W., (1965) 141.
Bultena, G. L., (1969a) 117; (1969b) 121.
Bureau of the Census, (See U. S. Dept. of Commerce)
Bureau of Community Environmental Management, (See U. S. Dept. of Health, Education & Welfare, Public Health Service)
Burgess, E. W., (1949) 121.
Burns, L. S., (1976) xxxiv.
Burns, N. M., (1963) 112.
Business Week, (1971) 190.

Calhoun, J. B., (1962a) 111, 141; (1962b) 111.
California, University of, (1967) 190.
Camargo, O.. (1945) 121.
Campbell, D. T., (1969) 126.
Campbell, J. S., (1970) 42.
Canter, D., (1969) 124, 190.
Canton, H. R., (1962) 61.
Caplan, N. S., (1968) 60.
Caplovitz, D., (1963) 60.
Caplow, T., (1950) 117; (1952) 190; (1961) 190; (1964) 190.
Carp, F. M., (1966) 120; (1967) 120; (1968a) 120; (1968b) 127; (1969) 117.
Carr, S., (1967) 127.
Carruth, M. L., (1968) 121.
Carson, D. H., (1965) 124; (1968) xxxiii.
Carstairs, G. M., (1965) 202.
Cartwright, D., (1959) 123.
Casler, L., (1968) 126.
Cassel, J. C., (1960) 315; (1961) xxxvi, 116, 142, 315; (1964) 116, 141, 315; (1969) 260; (1970a) xxxvi, 43, 111; (1970b) 142; (1971) 116.
Cavan, R., (1949) 121.
Cestrone, P. F., (1968) 190.
Chagnon, N. A., (1968) 262.
Chalmers, A. K., (1913) 139.
Chamberlain, A. S., (1965) 125.
Chambers, R. M., (1963) 112.
Chance, M. R. A., (1962) 111.
Chapin, F. S., Jr. (1962) 60.
Chapin, F. S., Sr. (1938) 120; (1940) 120, 140; (1951a) 123; (1951b) 123; (1951c) 127; (1961) 141.
Chapple, E. D., (1965) 125.
Chave, S. P. W., (1957) 120, 140; (1964) 120.
Chein, I., (1954) 127.

Nahemow, L., (1965) 123.
Napier, J. A., (1970) 262.
National Academy of Sciences, National Academy of Engineering, (1971) 239.
National Advisory Commission on Civil Disorder, Report of the, (1968) 42.
National Center for Health Statistics, (See U.S.D.H.E.W.: PHS),
National Safety Council, (1968) 193.
Neel, J. V., (1964) 260; (1967) 262; (1968) 262.
Nelson, H., (1945) 140.
Neser, W. B., (1970) 142; (1971) 116.
Neutra, R., (1970) xxxiii; 315; (1973) xxxv.
New York Times, (1970) 41; (1971) 42.
Newman, O., (1972-3) 193.
Nichaman, M. Z., (1969) 261.
Nichols, C., (1962) 142.
Niebanck, P. L., (1965) 117; (1966) 121; (1968) 121.
Norberg-Schulz, C., (1966) 193.
Norman, M. M., (1970) 119.
Norman, R. D., (1952) 125.
Norris, V., (1956) 122.
Novick, L. J., (1967) 122.

Odum, H. T., (1971) 41.
O'Connor, N., (1968) 126.
Opler, M. K., (1962) 115.
Orne, M. T., (1964) 126.
Osborn, F. J., (1969) 44.
Osborne, R. T., (1966) 126.
Osmond, H., (1957) 112; (1966) 193.

Paddock, P., (1967) 41.
Paddock, W., (1967) 41.
Paige, J. M., (1968) 60.
Pan American Health Organization, (1965) 113.
Pardo, A., (1965) 116.
Pareto, V., 58.
Parr, A. E., (1966) 62.
Patrick, R., (1960) 315.
Pemberton, J., (1955) 118.
Perlman, R., (1967) 63.
Perloff, H. S., (1967) 44.
Persky, J. J., (1969) 62.
Peters, R. J., (1933) 139.
Peterson, J. E., (1969) 117.
Pettigrew, M. G., (1951) 140; (1954) 119.
Pettigrew, T. F., (1966) 61.
Pinkerton, T., (1962) 113.
Platzman, R. L., (1958) 239.

Plesaas, D., (1971) 51.
Plummer, N., (1960) 239.
Plutchik, R., (1959) 112.
Polish, E., (1959) 142.
Pollack, M., (1962) 122.
Pollitt, E., (1969) 112.
Polunin, I. V., (1967) 260.
Pond, M. A., (1946) 113; (1957) 13.
Pope, J. B., (1965) 117.
Porter, R., (1965) 261.
Post, F., (1956) 122.
Poster, C. M., (1969) 261.
Power, J. G. P., (1970) 118.
Pozen, M. W., (1968) 121.
Preston, G. H., (1945) 121.
Prior, I. A. M. and Others, (1968) 262.
Prock, V. N., (1965) 123; (1968) 123.
Proshansky, H. M., (1970a) 125; (1970b) 125, 194.
Pugh, T. F., (1967) 114; (1970) 260.

Quastler, H., (1958) 239.

Rabinowitz, F., (1969) 300.
Radburn Management Corp. (n.d.) 194.
Radford, A. J. (1973) xxxv.
Rahe, R. H., (1964) 119; (1967a) 119; (1967b) 119; (1967c) 122; (1968) 119; (1970) 119.
Rainwater, L., (1966a) 63; (1966b) 63; (1966c) 117.
Rand, G. ( 1972-3) 193.
Ratcliffe, H. L., (1958) 111.
Read, C. P., (1958) 141.
Redlich, F. C., (1958) 115.
Redmont, R., (1960) 239.
Regional Plan Association, N. Y., (1962) 194.
Rein, M., (1970) 300.
Reismann, L., (1964) 41.
Reiss, A. J., Jr., (1959) 115.
Rennie, T. A. C., (1962) 115.
Rhead, C. C., (1956) 119.
Rice, A. H., (1953) 125.
Richards, C. B., (1957) 125.
Richter, E., (1971) 315.
Riemer, S., (1943) 127; (1945) 123; (1947) 127; (1951) 124.
Riessman, F., et al., (1964) 63.
Riley, I. D., (1955) 140.
Riley, M. W., (1968) 123.
Rivlin, L. G., (1970a) 125; (1970b) 125, 194.
Robinson, W. S., (1950) 115.

Stamler, J., (1960) 115.
Stang, D. P., (1970) 42.
Stenhouner, J., (1968) 124.
Stein, C. S., (1957) 194.
Stein, L., (1950) 113, 119; (1954) 113, 139.
Stein, M. R., (1960) 43.
Steinman, D., (1970) 115.
Steinzor, B., (1950) 125.
Stephens, P. M., (1967) 141.
Stewart, J. G., (1970) 300.
Stone, G. P., (1954) 117.
Stott, D. H., (1962) 261.
Stouffer, S. A., (ASR, 1940) 84.
Strathclyde, U. of, (1970) 194.
Stratton, L. O., (1964) 125.
Strauss, A., (1968) 194; (1975) 44.
Strotzka, H., (1957) 140; (1973) xxxv.
Struening, E. L., (1969) 260.
Stryker, S., (1964) 190.
Study of Critical Environmental Problems, (1970) 41.
Sturdavant, M., (1970) 125.
Suchman, E. A., (1971) 41.
Surkin, M., (1971) 63.
Susser, M., (1973) xxxvi.
Suttles, G. D., (1968) 63.
Swinyard, E. A., (1961) 141.
Syme, S. L., (1964) xxxvi, 116; (1965a) 116, 141; (1965b) 141; (n.d.) 142.
Szudrowicz, B., (1976) xxxiv.

Taeuber, K. E., (1965) 63.
Taeuber, K. W., (1966) 61.
Tanaka, G. M., (1961) 122.
Tayback, M., (1962) 113, 195.
Taylor, I., (1964) 260.
Taylor, L., (1964) 120.
Tejada, C., (1965) 116.
Theodorson, G. A., (1961) 43.
Thiel, P., (1961) 194; (1969) 63,, 124.
Thiessen, D. D., (1964) 111.
Thiis-Evensen, E., (1958) 112.
Thoma, L., (1961) 121.
Thomas, W. L., Jr., (1956) 41.
Thompson, J. F., (1968) 116.
Thompson, W. R., (1966) 42.
Thursz, D., (1966) 121.
Tillman, W. A., (1949) 142.
Tilly, C., (1960) 117.
Tobin, S. S., (1968) 123.
Townsend, P., (1968) 124.
Train, R. E., (1972) 239.
Trier, T. R., (1968) 122.

Trites, D. K., (1970) 125, 194.
Truelove, S. C., (1947) 140.
Trulson, M. F., and Others, (1964) 261.
Truswell, A. S., (1968) 262.
Tuek, H., (1970) 63.
Tulkin, S. R., (1968) 118.
Tukey, J. W., (1954) 315.
Tunstall, D. B., (1973) xxxv.
Tyroler, H. A., (1961) xxxvi, 116, 142; (1964) 116, 141, 315; (1970) 142; (1971) 116.

Ullrich, R. A., (1968) 126.
U. S. Department of Commerce:
Bureau of the Census, (1970) 260; (1971) 41, 42, 53.
Bureau of Public Roads, (1964) 195.
U. S. Department of Health, Education, and Welfare:
Public Health Service, (1962) 195; (1963) 195; (1964) 195; (1965a) 115; (1965b) 115; (1967a) 115; (1967b) 115; (1968) 239; (1969a) xxxiv; (1969b) xxv; (1970a) xxxiii; (1970b) xxxiv; (1972) 239; (1975) xxxiv; (1976) xxxiv; (1977) xxxiv.
U. S. Department of Housing and Urban Development, (1966) 63; (1971) 195.
U. S. Department of Justice:
Federal Bureau of Investigation, 18.
U. S. Department of Labor:
Bureau of Safety Standards, (1968) 190.
U. S. Environmental Protection Agency, 46.
U. S. National Housing Agency:
Federal Public Housing Authority, (1945) 123.
Urban Land, (1961) 190.

Vail, D. J., (1966) 116.
Van Arsdol, M. D., Jr., (1964) 124.
van Zonneveld, R. J., (1958) 124.
Vásquez, M. A., (1969) 118.
Veitch, R., (1971) 126.
Vidich, A. J., (1960) 44.
Vines, A. P., (1970) 261.
Vissacher, M. B., (1955) 141.
Vistosky, H. M., (1969) 42.
Vlajic, B., (1975) xxxv.

Wacks, M., (1970) 195.
Walkley, R. P., (1955) 119; (1962) 113, 195; (1963) 42; (1968) 121.
Wallace, A. F. C., (1952) 195.

# Chapter I

# The Background and Purpose of This Work

LAWRENCE E. HINKLE, JR.

The effort that lead to the production of this volume began in September, 1969, when the group of authors first assembled in fulfillment of a contract with the Bureau of Community Environmental Management of the U.S. Public Health Service. This contract had been initiated by William C. Loring, Ph.D., who was then Research Director and Science Advisor of that Bureau. The Division of Human Ecology at Cornell University Medical College had been given the responsibility for its administration. The assembled "Board of Collaborators," as it was called, was charged with considering: *(1)* how the man-made part of the physical environment—the cities, the neighborhoods, the buildings, and the other large artifacts of human culture—may influence the health and behavior of people, *(2)* how the effects of this part of the environment may be identified and measured, and *(3)* what strategies of research might be useful for learning more about them.

The members were from the faculties of several eastern universities:

Robert P. Burden, Ph.D., from the Division of Engineering and Applied Physics, Harvard University;

John Cassel, M.D., from the Department of Epidemiology, School of Public Health, University of North Carolina;

Albert Damon, M.D., from the Department of Anthropology, Harvard University;

Robert Geddes, M. Arch, from the School of Architecture, Princeton University;

Robert Gutman, Ph.D., from the Department of Sociology, Rutgers University;

Lawrence E. Hinkle, M.D., from the Division of Human Ecology, Department of Medicine and Psychiatry, Cornell University Medical College;

1

Stanislav V. Kasl, Ph.D., from the Department of Epidemiology and Public Health, Yale University School of Medicine;

Donald A. Kennedy, Ph.D., from the School of Public Health, Harvard University;

Kermit Schooler, Ph.D., from the School of Social Work, Syracuse University.

Dr. Loring, as Project Officer of the contract, participated actively in the discussions of the group and contributed significantly to the concepts that were derived.

During the first two years after the contract was initiated, this group met at intervals of one or two months, at one or another of the universities. The first meetings were given over to prolonged discussions and to intense interchanges of views by men of quite disparate intellectual and scientific backgrounds. A meaningful dialogue and a firm basis for the interchange of information was established with less difficulty than the members had at first anticipated.

It had been hoped by some that the deliberations of the group might ultimately lead to a collaborative effort at research—hence the name "Inter-University Board of Collaborators." It soon became apparent, however, that the field of scientific interest which the group had undertaken to survey was too diffuse and inchoate to allow the members to unite in selecting a concrete and meaningful question to which significant answers might be readily supplied in a relatively short time by the application of the techniques available to them. It was evident that no unifying body of concepts was available to them, nor was there any common body of shared scientific information that they might make use of. It seemed, rather, that each member of the group had approached the general area of their common interest from his own point of view, and that each had asked some questions, or had developed some techniques that might be useful to the others. The common deliberations had stimulated in each of the members an awareness of the potential usefulness of his own information to his colleagues, and a desire to know more about their methods and concepts which might be useful to him.

It was, therefore, agreed that each member should produce for the group a paper bearing on the general area of interest. He was asked to make whatever contribution he thought he could best make to the common charge. Each selected his own topic, and dealt with it as he saw fit. In spite of this, the papers that were produced had a remarkable degree of congruence. Each paper dealt with concepts that the author regarded as important, and these concepts have been regarded important by the group as a whole. Most papers have described methods that the author has developed or used, and many have suggested research strategies that might be appropriately used by other members of the group. The papers, as a whole, represent an unusual series of contributions from a variety of points of view. They have a coherent theme and a remarkable degree of agreement about important concepts, some of which may be quite unfamiliar or surprising to many who have not worked in this field.

In my own role as the more or less informal coordinator of the group's efforts, I have undertaken to arrange the papers in an order which I think develops the main theme of the various contributions. For the interest of the reader, I have summarized these briefly.

In CHAPTER II, "Community Health and the Urban Environment," Donald Kennedy presents a summary of what might be called, in 1973, the conventional view of the problem of health and the modern urban environment.

> "As a central thesis, I would argue that American cities are unhealthy places in which to live, work, play, or visit. All persons using the city environment suffer to some degree from the noise, air pollution, traffic congestion, crowding, and lack of open areas of grass, trees, lakes, and rivers. Depending upon biological endowment and prior medical histories, each person brings to the cities a certain set of vulnerabilities and handicaps. If his residential area has a high crime rate; if his work situation has high levels of toxic chemical exposure; and if his children are denied an adequate education due to racial discrimination, civil disorders, and inadequate tax revenues; then he operates under a burden of stresses and potentially hazardous conditions that are likely to affect his level of health and his longevity."

Kennedy's chapter describes some of the evidence that supports this thesis, discusses some of the questions that are raised, and suggests some strategies for obtaining further information.

In CHAPTER III, "The Forgotten Environment," Robert Burden advances the thesis that "The problems of environmental management for the country as a whole are substantially different from the particular problems of the cities." The health of the environment is not the same as the health of people, and the national effort to improve the environment in general is not immediately relevant to the health or well-being of people in the cities. Burden's central concern is how to manage the environment in the city to improve the quality of life for its residents. He discusses the role of the human community as a determinant of the quality of life in the urban environment, and he presents the thesis that "any program for change in urban environment that will substantially improve the quality of life for the residents must include the residents in its planning and operation." Burden suggests an approach to improving the quality of the urban environment; a method for determining which decisions are likely to be effective under a given set of circumstances; and a way of evaluating the results of actions taken.

In CHAPTER IV, "The Effects of the Residential Environment on Health and Behavior: A Review," Stanislav Kasl has reviewed in detail the English language literature that is pertinent to the question of the effects of the residential environment on human health and behavior. He considers a number of propositions that have been rather uncritically accepted in the past. He discusses the limitations of the "ecological approach" that has been used by urban ecologists. He considers in some detail the reliability of the data that have been employed in various kinds of studies, and the limitations of the methods that have been used. He considers the problem presented by the concomitance of the various kinds of physical environmental conditions that might be relevant to health, and the concomitance of these conditions with significant social and psychological variables, that might also be relevant to health. He describes the inconclusive evidence that has been derived from studies of the effects upon human populations of rehousing, of new housing, and of relocation. He considers the role of satisfactions, attitudes, preferences, and perceptions in determining the response of people to their environments. He considers the role of the physical environment in determining the behavior of people. Throughout his review, he points to the abundant evidence that the social environment is a very important determinant of people's reactions to their physical environment. He concludes with a critique of present methods of investigation, and a suggestion for improved methods.

In CHAPTER V, "The Relation of the Urban Environment to Health: Towards a Conceptual Frame and a Research Strategy," John Cassel states a thesis that is suggested by the Kennedy and Burden contributions and, to a greater extent, by that of Kasl. He points out that, once shelter has progressed beyond the rather primitive level at which housing protects the individual from the hostile elements and does not directly contribute intrinsic hazards of its own, there is great difficulty in demonstrating any close correlation between the physical quality of the housing and the health of the inhabitants. Considering the processes that may relate housing to health, he puts forward the thesis that in all cases the social environment—the social characteristics of the individuals who live in the housing and the relationship between them—is the essential link in the chain. He goes beyond this and draws upon evidence from the observation of both humans and animals to support, first, a conclusion that it is the relation of the individual to other members of his own social group, and to other individuals of his own species, that is the primary determinant of the health of members of communities; and, second, its corollary that the physical characteristics of the housing or neighborhood in which he lives are important only as they affect the relationships within the social group. Cassel then

4

develops a second corollary thesis that the nature and strength of available primary group supports are of fundamental importance in determining the health of individuals living in the urban environment. He suggests a strategy of research for obtaining more information on these points.

Robert Gutman and Robert Geddes in CHAPTER VI, and Lawrence Hinkle in Chapter VII, turn their attention to problems of measurement, in a complementary manner. In Chapter VI, "Environmental Assessment: Research and Practice," Gutman and Geddes have approached the question of how one identifies and measures those features of the man-made environment that may have important effects upon people who live in and use this environment. After reviewing the present state-of-the-art of environmental assessment as it applies to the "urban" or "man-made" environment, and after considering what is required for the classification of the attributes of an environment, they present in detail their proposition that "there are eight properties of the physical environment which, in our judgment, have some significance for the behavior of people." These are: spatial organization, circulation and movement systems, communications systems, ambient properties, visual properties, amenities, symbolic properties, and architectonic properties. They also consider the dimensions of a behavioral classifications system that might fit into this system of evaluating the environmental properties, and they give examples of research design and strategy which are quite detailed.

Lawrence Hinkle in CHAPTER VII, "Measurement of the Effects of the Environment Upon the Health and Behavior of People," has approached the problem of measurement from the opposite direction. He has asked the question, How does one identify the effects of the environment upon the individuals who live in it, and how does one measure these effects? He begins with a theoretical consideration of the nature of man-environment interrelations from a biological point of view and the mechanisms by which the interactions of men with their environment may affect their health. In the course of this, he discusses in some detail the evidence bearing on the physiological processes by which the interactions between men and their social environment affect their health. Hinkle proposes that the effects upon health and behavior that are created by the environment be classified as lethal effects, disabling effects, effects upon growth and development, constraints upon behavior, and effects upon pleasure and satisfaction. He suggests means by which these may be identified, counted, and measured, using as his methods those that have been developed by epidemiologists, sociologists, and psychologists. In illustrating the usefulness of these methods, he describes their application to urban and rural populations in various societies, and suggests that the conventional view that modern urban societies are unhealthy for humans is quite contrary to some of the available evidence.

Albert Damon, in CHAPTER VIII, "The Residential Environment, Health, and Behavior: Simple Research Opportunities, Strategies, and Some Findings in the Solomon Islands and Boston, Massachusetts," has drawn both upon the methods of the epidemiologists and upon methods of environmental assessment like those of Gutman and Geddes. He considers many of the problems and propositions pointed out by the other authors, and he has used these to suggest how one can find many opportunities within American society to use available data and special populations to answer questions about the relations between health and the urban environment. He also presents evidence that comparable studies in other societies can yield data of great value in the interpretation of observations made during studies in our own society, and he provides evidence on this from studies that he and his associates have carried out. He also considers many of the practical pitfalls involved in research of this nature.

In CHAPTER IX, "Residential Environment and Health of the Elderly: Use of Research Results for Policy and Planning," Kermit Schooler has used a national sample study of the effects of the residential environment upon the health of elderly people and multi-variate factor and path analyses as a framework for considering how such studies may be carried out, and especially the problem of how to analyze the data from the many intercorrelated variables that are usually considered. He goes on from this to provide some concrete suggestions for the use of information of this sort in the policy and planning areas.

In arranging these papers for publication, this editor had the authors' permission to separate the body of some papers into two parts when this has seemed to be desirable from the point of view of the reader. Under these circumstances, the first part of the paper is made up of the author's primary contribution in terms of concepts or methods, and the second part includes his more detailed suggestions for (or examples of) the application of the methods or concepts in certain concrete situations.

# Chapter II

# Community Health and the Urban Environment

DONALD A. KENNEDY

## Orientation

After nearly a century of cumulative growth in scientific knowledge concerning the physical environment and the diseases of man, we find ourselves in a deteriorating environment and lack the precise scientific evidence we need for the justification of corrective policies and the implementation of significant social reform. Our cities and metropolitan areas are in serious trouble, and their difficulties directly affect the health of the people who use them.

For at least 100 years, man has been aware of major connections between his environment and his health status and from time to time social reforms have been made on the basis of intuitive knowledge in advance of precise findings based upon scientific study. This was certainly the case in the late 1800's when the "sanitary movement" in England resulted in the Public Health Act of 1875, and in Germany when public hygiene measures were encouraged during the same era. Rene Dubos illustrates this point in his description of the changes in the city of Munich at that time:

> In Germany the most picturesque and influential of the pioneers in sanitation was the chemist Max von Pettenkofer, who regarded hygiene more as an all-embracing philosophy of life than as a laboratory science. In Munich he persuaded the city fathers to bring clear water in abundance from the mountains to clean streets and houses, to carry away refuse and garbage, to dilute the sewage downstream in the Isar, and even to plant trees and flowers, which he regarded as essential to the mental well-being of the population because they satisfy esthetic longings. Following these measures, the typhoid mortality in Munich fell from 72 per million in 1880 to 14 in 1898. The city soon became one of the healthiest in Europe, thanks to the efforts of this imaginative and enterprising hygienist who was not a physician and did not believe in the germ

7

theory of disease. Max von Pettenkofer's lectures, "The Health of a City," conveyed to the general public the view that collective cleanliness was the surest approach to health. (1)

The situation today is not fully analogous with the situation at the end of the last century. There has been a shift in the disease profile away from infectious diseases to chronic diseases as causes of death and handicap. Environmental pollution is much more massive now. Man has considerably increased his ability to add pollutants to the land, water, and air that surround his habitations. And the scale of man's impact has increased to the point where the survival of many species of living organism are clearly threatened. (2) With a sudden increase in the human population, these effects are now magnified.

Man's dependence upon the burning of fossil fuels to heat dwelling places, to manufacture "essential" goods, and to transport people and supplies has now begun to change the chemical and physical composition of the earth's atmosphere and to visibly affect the airshed over metropolitan communities. (3) The dumping of muncipal sewage and industrial waste into rivers has combined with the runoff of agricultural fertilizers to produce major changes in large lakes and river systems. With the influx of large volumes of nutrients, the plant life in lakes multiplies rapidly, changing the previous ecological relationships between plant life and fish by reordering the oxygen cycle and the food chain that support the dominant species of fish. Soon the lake will no longer yield fish or provide clear water for swimming or drinking. These transformations have been observed in small bodies of water for years. Now they are seen in bodies of water the size of Lake Erie with a surface area of 10,000 square miles.

Man's development of nuclear energy and petrochemicals has produced a new realm of threats in the contamination of the environment. The wide dispersion of DDT and of mercury are only two of the better know recent examples of how hazards to environmental health have multiplied. Although the poisonous effects of mercury have been known for centuries, it was not until 1968 that the micro-organisms living in the oxygen-free mud of lake bottoms were known to be capable of converting inorganic mercury into the highly toxic form of methylmercury. (4) Once in an organic form, the mercury spread rapidly through the food chain in the aquatic environment. And thus methylmercury found its way into man through his consumption of poisoned fish.

In addition to these changes in the environment, there is mounting pressure on both resources and environment stemming from the population avalanche. (5) According to most authorities, our planet is now seriously overpopulated and the presence of this large and expanding population seriously hinders the search for solutions to most significant social problems. Despite dramatic improvements in agriculture productivity we are nearing the limit of food production capability using traditional methods. Intemperate efforts to increase food production will cause serious deterioration of land and water resources. *(6)* There are no technological solutions for this set of problems associated with population-food-environment; adaptive solutions are locked in by a set of values and attitudes, widely shared by people in nearly all parts of the world.

The problems of health and environment noted above, differ sharply in their impact, their priority, and their visibility for people on different continents. Nearly all cities with large amounts of fuel consumption experience increasing dangers from air pollution. Population growth varies considerably by continent and region. Levels of poverty and malnutrition vary widely among families. The effects of noise generated by jet aircraft is related to location in relation to airports. Persons in each behavior setting are aware of a specific set of health hazards and a special set of priorities for social action. But in most parts of the world, there are now signs of the threshold effects described above. The web of connections is more clearly visible now in every corner of the world. The interconnections are now more easily perceived because of television communication, foreign travel, world trade, mobility of military personnel, and the increasing severity of ecological disturbances.

Within a worldwide context, this paper focuses upon the particular problems of environmental health associated with cities in the United States. The approach taken attempts to blend the physical, biological and social dimensions of the problem into a single frame of reference. Each of the health and environmental issues raised in this paper can be seen as operating at several different scales. The worldwide scale is used in the initial presentation of the problem. Then the problems are traced through the societal to the metropolitan scale. Although the scale changes, the central themes remain with minor variations in patterning.

As a central thesis, I would argue that American cities are unhealthy places in which to live, work, play, or visit. All persons using the city environment suffer to some degree from the noise, air pollution, traffic congestion, crowding and lack of open areas of grass, trees, lakes and rivers. Depending upon biological endowment and prior medical history, each person brings to the city a certain set of vulnerabilities and handicaps. If his residential area has a high crime rate; his work situation high levels of toxic chemical exposure; and his children are denied an adequate education due to racial discrimination, civil disorders and inadequate tax revenues: then he operates under a burden of stresses and potentially hazardous conditions that are likely to affect his level of health and his longevity.

My purpose is to explore various interconnected dimensions of health and environment in the context of the contemporary American city. The hope is to find new approaches for both research and social action.

The perspective taken is that of general systems and human ecology. *(7)* The fields drawn upon include sociology, economics, city and regional planning, biology, public health, ecology, demography, psychology, anthropology, zoology, and several of the environmental sciences. The orientation is one of synthesis from several bodies of knowledge. In developing this approach, I have taken quite seriously the recommendation of John Kenneth Galbraith:

> The boundaries of a subject matter are conventional and artificial; none should use them as an excuse for excluding the important. Nor can one be indifferent to practical consequences of an effort such as this—whatever the tendency to celebrate such indifference as a manifestation of scientific detachment. *(8)*

The purpose of this exercise is to suggest a composite strategy that blends scientific research with social reform and cultural development. As Suchman has commented:

> The emphasis today is clearly upon the application of knowledge to the amelioration of social problems. The same scientific methodology that (has) been so successful in discovering knowledge (is) now to be brought to bear upon the utilization of that knowledge. Social change could be planned and implemented by scientific research upon the causes of society's ills and by the development of intervention programs to meet these causes. Man, it seems, has now entered a period of widespread planned social change or innovation. *(9)*

### The Urban Community: Ecological, economic, and demographic perspectives

In terms of physical environment, the city differs from the rural town in the near total dominance of man-made structures. The city is a man-constructed environment with little evidence of plant life. The rural town is a small group of man-made structures dominated by a rural landscape of woods and fields with earth and rocks clearly evident. The suburban community represents a blend of both city and town. It has a more equal balance of plant life and man-constructed structures. *(10)*

From an ecological perspective, each of these community types—urban, suburban, and rural—represent a different mix of environmental factors. The city poses the most difficult challenge to the natural circulation of water, air, oxygen, and energy. There is less modification of these circulatory and exchange processes in the rural towns, suburbs, or wilderness areas. The concentration of human beings with their attendant consumption of food and energy, without the presence of plant life, generates by-products and waste products that seriously challenge the circulatory and regenerative processes of the biosphere and geosphere. *(11)*

From an economic perspective, the city represents one part of a large geographic division of labor and economic activities within the society

10

as a whole. *(12)* City dwellers must be supplied with volumes of water, food, textiles, and construction materials. Their sewage and solid wastes must be removed. Large amounts of fuel must be supplied to heat their plentiful dwellings, cook their food, and provide vehicular transportation. All of these materials, goods, and services must be obtained from a variety of economic activities that take place at considerable distances from the city. In exchange the residents of the city must produce goods and services that are wanted by persons in other communities and locations. Workers in the city produce: manufactured goods; art museums, radio and television communication; higher education; government services; professional sporting events; large conventions; highly specialized trade; financial services; advertising services; and terminals for the trans-shipment of goods and people. *(13, 14)* Cities are tied into most of the economic relationships that operate in the larger society.

Under current conditions of economic well-being in a post-industrial society, the economy is developing with an emphasis upon tertiary services. Efficiencies achieved in producing a surplus of food to meet the requirements of a population of 200 million, and in meeting their mining and manufacturing needs with a smaller fraction of manpower, yields expansion of activity in the service sector. *(15)* These changes in the economy can be seen in the employment statistics for major sectors of activity in the United States during the past twenty years.

### Employment by Major Sector of Activity
(Number of workers in millions)

|      | Agric. | Mines | Const. | Manuf. | Trans. | Trade | Finan. and insur. | Misc. serv. | Govt. | Total civilian workforce |
|------|--------|-------|--------|--------|--------|-------|-------------------|-------------|-------|--------------------------|
| 1950 | 7.2    | .9    | 2.3    | 15.2   | 4.0    | 9.4   | 1.9               | 5.4         | 6.0   | 62.2                     |
| 1960 | 5.5    | .7    | 2.9    | 16.8   | 4.0    | 11.4  | 2.7               | 7.4         | 8.4   | 69.6                     |
| 1970 | 3.5    | .6    | 3.3    | 19.4   | 4.5    | 15.0  | 3.7               | 11.6        | 12.6  | 82.7                     |

Agriculture and mining are using less manpower. Construction and transportation show little change. Manufacturing has increased slightly. But trade, financial services, and government show large increases in manpower employed. The tertiary services clearly show the greatest growth. This pattern gives continuing support for the development of activities normally associated with cities and metropolitan areas.

From a demographic perspective, the picture is more complicated. In 1970 there were 203 million Americans. Of that total, 43 million lived outside of community places designated by the census. The remaining 160 million lived in 21,000 communities. The census classified 7,000 of these as urban places and 14,000 as rural communities. The distribution and changes between 1950 and 1970 are as follows: *(16)*

11

## Settlement Pattern

### (Communities)

| Places | 1950 | 1960 | 1970 | Differences |
|---|---|---|---|---|
| Urban | | | | |
| 1 million + ............. | 5 | 5 | 6 | 1 |
| 100,000-1,000,000 .... | 101 | 127 | 150 | 49 |
| 10,000-100,000 ......... | 1,156 | 1,767 | 2,143 | 987 |
| 1,000-10,000 ............. | 3,479 | 4,142 | 4,762 | 1,283 |
| Total .................. | 4,741 | 6,041 | 7,061 | 2,320 |
| Rural | | | | |
| 1,000-5,000 ............. | 4,158 | 4,151 | 4,193 | 35 |
| Under 1,000 .............. | 9,649 | 9,598 | 9,514 | −135 |
| Total ...................... | 13,807 | 13,749 | 13,707 | −100 |
| Grand total ..................... | 18,548 | 19,790 | 20,768 | +2,220 |

## Settlement Pattern

### (Populations)

| Population (in millions) | 1950 | 1960 | 1970 | Differences |
|---|---|---|---|---|
| Urban | | | | |
| 1 million + ............. | 17.4 | 17.5 | 18.7 | 1.3 |
| 100,000-1,000,000 .... | 26.9 | 33.6 | 37.7 | 10.8 |
| 10,000-100,000 ......... | 29.6 | 46.4 | 56.0 | 26.4 |
| 1,000-10,000 ............. | 22.5 | 28.0 | 36.9 | 14.4 |
| Total .................. | 96.4 | 125.5 | 149.3 | 52.9 |
| Rural | | | | |
| 1,000-5,000 ............. | 6.5 | 6.5 | 6.7 | .2 |
| Under 1,000 .............. | 4.0 | 6.5 | 3.9 | −.1 |
| Other ........................ | 43.7 | 43.7 | 43.4 | −.3 |
| Total ...................... | 54.2 | 54.1 | 54.0 | −.2 |
| Grand total ..................... | 150.6 | 179.6 | 203.3 | 52.7 |

These figures show an increase of nearly 53 million persons in total population for 1950–1970. The population of 54 million living in rural communities and rural areas remained remarkably stable during twenty years. Most of the growth took place in the medium size communities of 10,000 to 100,000 population. Within that size range the greatest growth occurred in the smaller size communities as shown in the following chart:

## Number of Places

| Size of community | 1950 | 1960 | 1970 | Differences 1950-1970 |
|---|---|---|---|---|
| 50,000-100,000 .................... | 126 | 201 | 240 | 114 |
| 25,000-50,000 ..................... | 252 | 432 | 519 | 267 |
| 10,000-25,000 ..................... | 778 | 1,134 | 1,384 | 606 |
| 5,000-10,000 ...................... | 1,176 | 1,394 | 1,840 | 664 |

**Population**
(in millions)

| Size of community | 1950 | 1960 | 1970 | Differences 1950-1970 |
|---|---|---|---|---|
| 50,000-100,000 | 8.9 | 13.8 | 16.7 | 7.8 |
| 25,000-50,000 | 8.8 | 15.0 | 17.8 | 9.0 |
| 10,000-25,000 | 11.9 | 17.6 | 21.4 | 9.5 |
| 5,000-10,000 | 8.1 | 9.8 | 12.9 | 4.8 |

It is interesting to note that the numbers of "urban places" increased as well as the aggregate population in communities of a given size.

An analysis of population changes in the ten largest cities of the country provides further evidence of this trend towards deconcentration. Five of the cities have lost population in the range of 120,000 to 340,000 persons; three cities have remained fairly stable in size for twenty years; and only two have grown. The two that have increased in size, Houston and Los Angeles, have also grown in land area. Houston increased its land area by adding 113 square miles between 1960 and 1970. Los Angeles added 9 square miles during the same time period.

**Population**
(in millions)

| Rank (in 1950) | Name | 1950 | 1960 | 1970 | Differences |
|---|---|---|---|---|---|
| 1 | New York | 7.89 | 7.78 | 7.90 | + 10,000 |
| 2 | Chicago | 3.62 | 3.55 | 3.37 | −250,000 |
| 3 | Los Angeles | 1.97 | 2.48 | 2.81 | +840,000 |
| 4 | Philadelphia | 2.07 | 2.00 | 1.95 | −120,000 |
| 5 | Detroit | 1.85 | 1.67 | 1.51 | −340,000 |
| 6 | Baltimore | .95 | .94 | .91 | − 40,000 |
| 7 | Houston | .60 | .94 | 1.23 | +630,000 |
| 8 | Cleveland | .91 | .88 | .75 | −160,000 |
| 9 | Washington | .80 | .76 | .76 | − 40,000 |
| 10 | St. Louis | .86 | .75 | .62 | −240,000 |

Source: 17.

In summary, the aggregate population is growing at the rate of approximately 2 million per year and this increase is being absorbed primarily in suburban communities in the size range of 10,000 to 50,000. The rural population is remaining remarkably stable in terms of absolute numbers. The largest cities are tending to lose population. The growth of suburban communities near and between major cities has become the dominant pattern in the re-distribution of the residential population. Both highway construction and extensions in the system

13

of commercial air service have followed this population growth so that some of the best transportation services are now available in suburban and exurban residential areas.

## Distribution of Minority Groups

Large cities have historically served as entry points for immigrants entering the country. The processes of acculturation and adjustment between the majority and minority groups have been concentrated in the larger cities. (18) This was particularly true for the decades immediately following the era of heavy immigration (1840–1910). (19)

During the past thirty years a variation on this process has been taking place with the Negro population within our country. There has been a major increase in the size of this population and an important geographical re-distribution as shown in the following table:

### Regional Distribution of Black Population (1940-1970)
(Population in millions)

|  | 1940 | Per-cent | 1950 | Per-cent | 1960 | Per-cent | 1970 | Per-cent |
|---|---|---|---|---|---|---|---|---|
| United States .... | 12.9 | 100 | 15.0 | 100 | 18.9 | 100 | 22.7 | 100 |
| Northeast ......... | 1.4 | 11 | 2.0 | 13 | 3.0 | 16 | 4.3 | 19 |
| North Central .... | 1.4 | 11 | 2.2 | 15 | 3.4 | 18 | 4.6 | 20 |
| West ................ | .2 | 1 | .6 | 4 | 1.1 | 6 | 1.7 | 8 |
| South ............... | 9.9 | 77 | 10.2 | 68 | 11.3 | 60 | 12.1 | 53 |

Source: 20.

The percentage of each region's population that is black has changed in the following way:

### Black Percentage of Regional Populations

|  | 1940 | 1950 | 1960 | 1970 |
|---|---|---|---|---|
| United States ....................... | 10 | 10 | 11 | 11 |
| (Percent of |  |  |  |  |
| all classes) |  |  |  |  |
| Northeast ....................... | 4 | 5 | 7 | 9 |
| North Central ................. | 4 | 5 | 7 | 8 |
| West ............................. | 1 | 3 | 4 | 5 |
| South ............................ | 24 | 22 | 21 | 19 |

Source: 21.

There has also been an important shift in the rural and urban location of residence. Over half of this minority group now lives in the central cities of the nation:

## Location of Residence of Black Population

| Residence | 1950 Pop. | Percent | 1960 Pop. | Percent | 1968 Pop. | Percent |
|---|---|---|---|---|---|---|
| Metropolitan areas | 8.3 | 56 | 12.2 | 65 | 15.1 | 68 |
| Central cities | 6.4 | 43 | 9.7 | 52 | 11.9 | 54 |
| Urban fringe | 1.9 | 13 | 2.5 | 13 | 3.2 | 14 |
| Smaller cities, towns | 6.6 | 44 | 6.6 | 35 | 6.9 | 32 |
| | 14.9 | 100 | 18.8 | 100 | 22.0 | 100 |

Source: 22.

By far the most impressive feature of black migration has been the concentration of population in the central cities. To quote the Kerner Commission Report:

> Almost all Negro population growth is occuring within metropolitan areas, primarily within central cities. From 1950 to 1966, the U.S. Negro population rose 6.5 million. Over 98 percent of that increase took place in metropolitan areas— 86 percent within central cities, 12 percent in the urban fringe. *(23)*

As described earlier the white population is leaving the central cities with a resulting segregation of blacks in the central city and whites in the surrounding suburbs. Again quoting the Kerner Commission:

> The 12 largest central cities (New York, Chicago, Los Angeles, Philadelphia, Detroit, Baltimore, Houston, Cleveland, Washington, St. Louis, Milwaukee, and San Francisco) now contain two-thirds of the Negro population outside the South, and one-third of the black population in the United States . . . In 1968, seven of these cities are over 30% Negro, and one (Washington, D.C.) is two-thirds Negro. *(24)*

The degree of residential segregation within all of these cities is very strong. The segregation pattern is similar in the suburbs as well and is stronger than that found with other minority groups, including Puerto Ricans, Orientals, and Mexican-Americans.

Unlike earlier patterns of immigrant assimilation and dispersion out from the central cities through the adjacent suburbs, the black population is not moving in the same way. Racial discrimination produces a combination of residential exclusion from white suburban neighborhoods and a rapid white withdrawal from neighborhoods when blacks begin to move in. Under these conditions dispersion and integration seldom occur.

Since unemployment and poverty rates are much higher for nonwhite families, the concentration of blacks in the central cities provides a strong demand for various governmental and community services. The demand for housing, education, welfare support, employment, manpower training, and health services place heavy burdens on municipal, private, and voluntary service agencies.

All of the serious problems associated with the black minority group are becoming concentrated in the central cities just at the time when the cities are bombarded with a whole set of threatening events.

## Cities in Crisis

Most of the large cities in this country are in serious trouble. They suffer from: air pollution; traffic congestion; high noise levels; poor public schools; high crime rates; sharp segregation of residents by race, income, and marital status; and a large proportion of residents receiving welfare support. (25) In addition these cities suffer from strikes by municipal employees, including school teachers and policemen; civil disturbances; bombings in public buildings; and inadequate tax revenues to meet rising costs.

Many of the physical facilities in the cities have deteriorated to the point where they must be replaced. This applies to the underground facilities such as water and sewer mains, electric and telephone lines, as well as visible constructions such as sidewalks, public transportation systems, housing, public schools, municipal hospitals, and recreation facilities.

In the private sector, there is a sharp discontinuity between commercial property and residential property. House construction lags far behind new construction for business and industrial purposes. (26) The lack of adequate housing for poor families then generates an increase in the construction of public housing by municipal governments. (27) This housing then reinforces the concentration of culturally handicapped persons in specific residential neighborhoods, thus cutting them off from neighborly contact with healthy and well-adjusted families. The scale of this housing effort, with its segregation and impersonal management, violates essential requirements for the healthy functioning of human communities.

In a certain sense public housing projects resemble mission-oriented organizations like schools, hospitals, and prisons, and yet they have no educational, therapeutic, or correctional mandate within the community. They are merely clusters of "adequate" housing in the center of the city. And yet a family does not enter a housing project the way it enters a house or an apartment in the suburbs. Persons are admitted and discharged from housing projects according to income level, race, and family composition. Since there are no employed staff and few non-handicapped neighbors around to assist the residents of the project, it must be assumed that residents of public housing projects can change their way of life on their own. "Helping services" come exclusively in the form of government housing and subsistence welfare checks to pay for food, clothing, and transportation.

The amount of criminal behavior within the city represents another component of the urban crisis. The differences in crime rate between rural, suburban, and urban communities are striking. Ramsay Clark has commented on the differences in this way:

> Crime is not spread evenly over the nation. The chance of being a victim of violent crime is much greater for the city dweller. Robbery is the most urbanized of all violent crimes. Robberies per capita in cities of more than 250,000 people occur ten times more frequently than in surrounding suburban jurisdictions and thirty-five times more frequently than in outlying rural areas. The mur-

der rate in big cities is four and a half times higher than in the suburbs and two and a half times above the rural rate. The big city rates for aggravated assault, rape, burglary, larceny, and theft exceed both suburban and rural rates by two to four times. The rate of auto theft is fourteen times greater in urban than in rural areas . . . Crime is heavily concentrated in small geographic areas of the inner city and pockets of rural poverty. Here, where fewer than one-fourth of the people live, more than three-fourths of all arrests occur. *(28)*

In the last few years the crime rates have been increasing rapidly. This has been especially true for crimes such as burglary, auto theft, robbery, and larceny where the percent increase in rate per 100,000 rose between 83% and 125% during the years 1960 through 1968. In the same time period the murder rate increased 36% and there were 67% more aggravated assaults. *(29)*

In spite of the widespread skepticism concerning the validity of the Uniform Crime Reports of the FBI, a national survey of victims of crime indicated that these figures under-report criminal acts. A survey of 10,000 households in 1966 revealed the following crime rates:

Forcible rapes were more than three and one-half times the official rates, and burglaries three times. The high crime districts in Washington, D.C., Chicago, and Boston, revealed from three to ten times more offenses than were reported in police statistics. The survey figures suggest that in high crime districts, between 10,000 and 24,000 offenses per 100,000 persons are committed against individual residents in one year. This figure is roughly four times as great as police figures would suggest. *(30)*

These results further reinforce the warnings expressed by a variety of commissions, government agencies, professional groups, and legislative committees at both state and federal levels of government.

The daily experience of people living in areas with high crime rates is difficult to capture in a set of statistics. But the mounting threat to security of person and property must be emphasized as one of the major indicators of a deteriorating urban environment in contemporary American society.

In terms of both political process and administrative procedure, the management of the city has become very difficult. *(31)* The government system of controls and decision-making is too centralized in certain respects and too diffuse in other respects to produce effective and timely actions. *(32)* The relationships with both state and federal governments are out of balance. Most cities have inadequate control over their tax income to meet rapidly increasing expenditures for essential community services. The public services of the city are used by residents, workers, visitors, and travelers, but not all of these groups produce a fair share of tax revenues to pay for the services they use. *(33)* Cities are expected

18

to cope with social problems that surrounding suburbs can comfortably exclude from consideration. The provision of low-cost housing is an obvious example, as is the strong pattern of *de facto* racial segregation in housing and public education. (*34*) The need for fundamental rearrangement in the organization of local governments within metropolitan areas is now quite apparent and well-documented. The need for decentralized control and strong community participation at the neighborhood level is also very evident.

The problems of management have become so severe that a proposal has been made to have the President convene an "Urban Constitutional Convention." This unusual proposal was made by Lloyd N. Cutler as part of a staff report to the National Commission on the Causes and Prevention of Violence. (*35*) Cutler argued that the management and control of urban problems has reached a level of truly national concern. Convening a "constitutional convention" would focus much needed attention and resources on the problem. He believes that the recent British experience in changing the government of metropolitan areas could be of assistance in coping with the changing urban environment in this country.

Whether a "constitutional convention" is called or not, the difficult conditions in the cities have become of increased concern to the federal government. Funds for urban renewal and improvement in model city neighborhoods have been provided. Congress is currently considering major changes in welfare assistance for poor families, expansion of health insurance coverage, and revenue-sharing with both cities and states. The reports from Presidential Commissions have been quite valuable in defining central issues and identifying alternatives in remedial approach. The reports from the Commission on Urban Problems (Douglas Commission), the Commission on Civil Disorders (Kerner Commission) and the Commission on the Causes and Prevention of Violence (Eisenhower Commission) contain important observations and candid assessments of our contemporary urban situation. These reports serve a unique function in bringing together information from many different fields of knowledge and from highly specialized disciplines and professions. The formulation of legislation and executive action requires just such a composite picture of urban phenomena.

## Goals for an Urban Society

The enumeration and documentation of problems associated with urban environments is insufficient for our purpose. It is necessary to develop a perspective and a problem-solving strategy. Lyle Fitch has

19

provided a set of goals that may serve to focus our attention in terms of objectives. (*36*) A summary of his goals follows:

1. To create an urban society with values, environment, and services that respond fully to the needs and wants of families and individuals . . . a society drawn to the human scale . . . a pluralistic society that honors cultural differences . . . that provides freedom to move-up occupational and social ladders.

2. A national commitment to the work of developing the urban frontier, as pervasive and compelling as the national commitment to developing the western frontier in the nineteenth century . . . based on a heightened sense of common interest among all urban dwellers, with increased communication and mutual understanding across class lines, and a general concern for the well-being of each community.

3. The eradication of poverty and the increase in productivity through providing job opportunities for all who wish to work . . . and raising the levels of social insurance and public assistance to promote stable family life of high quality.

4. Extending new meaning to the traditional American ideal of equality of opportunity by making available to all citizens lifelong educational opportunities, adequate housing, health and medical services adequate to allow each person to achieve his full potential and sense of well-being, and a variety of recreational and cultural outlets.

5. Extend the meaning of individual freedom to include:

(a) freedom from personal aggression in public and private places;

(b) freedom from the physical and psychological damage caused by environmental aggression, including obtrusive noise, polluted air, and overcrowding;

(c) freedom from the threat of uncompensated losses by public action for the benefit of others, whether in the name of public welfare or progress;

(d) freedom from discrimination under the law—assurance of opportunity for defense against prosecution and protection against loss of rights owing to poverty or other personal circumstances.

6. Application of modern technology to the improvement of amenity, efficiency, and beauty of the urban environment and the development of new concepts and techniques for guiding metropolitan growth.

7. Maintenance of central cities as vital, healthy centers of knowledge and culture, of management, and commerce, and of residence for city-lovers.

8. Metropolitan development planning for efficiency and aesthetic appeal, and for conservation of urban natural resources and regional ecology.

The goals are clearly stated. Many of them sound like the cultural goals originally enunciated in our most treasured national directives, others have a more modern sound and emphasis. A strong concern for health and environment is found throughout the series.

## The Daily Round of Life

Up to this point, the presentation has been made at a high level of abstraction and in a societal or metropolitan frame of reference. It is now necessary to examine the question from the viewpoint of the family unit. There are 51 million families in this country and only 2.5 million of them live on farms. Each family is a decision-making unit. The choices of residential location, of employment, of school, and the allocation of personal income for goods and services—all of these decisions are made by families, not by business firms or governments.

The choice of residential location is one of the significant decisions made by each family. Let us examine the factors that enter into the question of residential location. The size and needs of the family vary according to its stage in the life cycle. Newly married couples without children; parents with school age children; parents with grown children; couples living in retirement: all have different requirements.

The amount and type of economic support plays a major part in this decision. Families can support themselves by: (1) raising their own food; (2) selling the time of adult members for wages; (3) making products for sale; and (4) investing their money and property to yield income. Farmers usually live close to their fields; wage earners live close to their work locations; and investors live where the climate matches their preference.

The amount of income per year is a significant determinant. People with little income often have to live where they can walk to work or use public transportation. People on welfare subsistence may have to live in a public housing project. Wealthier families can have several homes and good transportation to move between places of work, residence, and recreation. The availability of housing of the right size and price level will also affect the decision on residential location. Since there has been a general shortage of housing for decades in this country, this factor has often been the most significant one in shaping the location decision.

Since all children between the ages of 7 and 16 years must attend school and eligibility for public school attendance is usually based upon geographic area of residence, many families select their residential neighborhood so as to optimize the quality of educational services available to their children.

Transportation services and traffic congestion may also enter into the decision. To some degree, climate and the availability of mountains, lakes, or the ocean may also play a part.

But the most fundamental questions concerning location revolve around income level, work, and school. For adults, the time spent in their place of work is considerable; for children the time spent in school is also a large fraction of their waking hours. The home should be reasonably convenient to both work and school or too much time will be spent in commuting. We can estimate that most people spend between 30 and 100 minutes per day commuting to work or school for 180 to 235 days per year.

The choices made by families concerning residential location are not independent of choices being made by business firms concerning preferences in location. An industrial organization wants to find a large piece of land zoned for business, near a good labor supply, and in a community that provides good transportation and utilities at a low tax rate. With the gradual development of a rich network of all weather roads and good airports, trucks, cars, and airplanes can now transport people and goods in nearly any direction at low cost and with great convenience. The earlier dependence upon waterways and railroads has diminished. This means that both business firms and families are leaving the large central cities and decentralizing throughout suburban areas. As suburban residential populations and densities increase, the retail stores and business firms soon follow, and then major industrial organizations begin to construct larger facilities at major intersections of the interstate road network.

The process of suburban growth continues. It works fairly well for most families. It does not work well for poor families or black families. When a family is both poor and non-white there is serious trouble because there is little opportunity for participation in the general pattern of mobility, development, and improvement. In 1969, 16.7 million whites had incomes below poverty level. (37) They represented 9.5 percent of the total white population. In the same year, 7.6 million non-whites were defined as poor and that represented 31 percent of all non-whites in the country. Perceptions and attitudes differ sharply when proportions differ to this degree. Nearly a third of all black people are very poor and only 10% of whites experience the same level of poverty.

In the daily round of life with its biological rhythms, people spend a large fraction of their time in or near their homes. Most people probably spend more than half of their total life time of waking hours in or near their place of residence. Due in part to this time investment, the household dwelling and the immediate neighborhood area acquire significant meaning for most families. Territorial security and control become linked with a group identity and this is reinforced by interaction with friends in the locality. This is quite evident in the studies of working class families conducted in England and the United States over the past 20 years. (38, 39, 40)

The health status of family members is in some significant measure related to this home environment. And in the case of a sudden illness or injury, home becomes the first site of medical care. Instead of going out to work or school the person "stays home sick." Therefore our residential neighborhood ought to be sanitary, the air we breathe ought to be clean, and we should not feel threatened by criminal assault or harrassment on or near our property. Encounters between pedestrians and vehicular traffic should be arranged to give a high probability of safety for both parties. And in terms of what we know about the importance of exercise in the prevention of chronic heart disease the pathway facilities ought to encourage walking between home and most other locations of daily use.

But there are logical, physical, and political incompatibilities that hinder the development of an open and flexible matrix for simultaneously achieving these multiple goals. John Gardner has commented "there are no easy victories" in the reform of ancient social institutions, and Edward Banfield feels strongly that government cannot solve the central problems of urban environment—the very attempt to correct a specific difficulty will mobilize a coalition of other interest groups and these in turn will produce results that both neutralize the original reform movement and make several other conditions worse. (41, 42) The problems are much larger than the resources and managerial expertise presently allocated to cope with them. Until that central reality is widely appreciated and a re-allocation in priorities is made, it is safe to predict that there will be only "rhetorical solutions" and little change in the stubborn underlying realities of the urban situation.

It is in this sense that the chronic imbalance in spending between the private and public sectors of the economy must be re-adjusted and the large expenditure for warfare and national defense must be sharply reduced. (43) Violence is no longer an effective technique for conflict resolution in either the international or domestic scene. From a moral perspective it has been unacceptable for a long time; now it is unacceptable for economic and political reasons. (44) The United States cannot fight a war in Indochina and effectively cope with serious problems in American cities at the same time. (45) Mankind has arrived at a new set of boundary conditions. As Kenneth Boulding has assessed the situation, we have to replace warfare as the means for settling international disputes, bring our population increase to zero, and convert our economy to a closed-cycle use of natural resources. (46) And we have to accomplish all of these fundamental reforms, simultaneously, within a span of 25 years. The interconnections between domestic difficulties in urban areas and these "large-scale" problems are becoming increasingly visible.

## A Sense of Family and Community

All of the description and analysis to this point refers to populations, artifacts, and environments as abstract forces without specific reference to psychological, social, and cultural processes. It is time to add these dimensions to the frame of reference.

The starting point is the realization that a person's health and well-being depend in a significant way upon his perceptions, attitudes, and expectations about the world in which he operates. His health also depends upon his pattern of participation in the activities and needs of various groups, organizations, communities, and societies that compose the sociosphere. The evidence assembled over the past thirty years makes these points unmistakably clear. Illness is both a social and biological affair. And it is socially relevant in terms of both cause and effect. Social events such as warfare or industrialization can cause biological disruptions; the loss of a parent or worker due to illness can seriously interfere with the performance of a family or a work group. As suggested by the work of Alexander Leighton and associates, (47, 48, 49) two features of the social environment stand out as significant for our purposes: the family and the community.

The family is important both as a central point of interaction in the kinship network and as the primary group that begets, rears, protects, and maintains the individual in various ways throughout his lifetime. (50) Families are important both as small groups and as nodes in in a kinship network. Each person participates in two family groups during his lifetime, and these two household groups meet a continuing set of essential needs for each family member at every age level. At the same time each family member participates in a set of interlinked activities outside the home. This "open-system" of collective and coordinated activities produces a tremendous range of results that we refer to as "the economy," "society," and "mankind." The intricate and exquisite patterning of many social organizations makes it possible for each person in a family, as a consuming unit, to use an expanding realm of goods and services. The cumulative advantages in remaining a participant in the post-industrial economy far outweigh the alternative condition of returning to a pattern of self-sufficiency on the land with hunting and farming as the only means for producing food, shelter, clothing, and transportation.

Family groups are located within communities and linked in meaningful ways with work organizations, schools, stores, churches, and government agencies. In spite of the multiplicity of relationships and activities operating simultaneously in a post-industrial society, it is possible to sort out those activities that absorb a great amount of time for most individuals. Translated into space and time coordinates, we can estimate that people spend most of their time in the following places:

24

|     |                       | Percent |
| --- | --------------------- | ------- |
| 1.  | at home               | 50      |
| 2.  | at work or school     | 25      |
| 3.  | travelling            | 10      |
| 4.  | playing or socializing| 10      |
| 5.  | other activities      | 5       |
|     |                       | 100     |

In terms of concepts, the next major unit of analysis beyond the family is the "community." Communities are geographically organized, self-integrating social units, anchored to clusters of family residences. Alexander Leighton has given a description in the following terms:

> If one flies over the Northeast (United States) and looks down, he can see human patterning very plainly. Here are towns, villages, and hamlets interconnected with rail and road . . . Here, over and over again from one node in the network to another can be seen the reduplication of homes, stores, factories, schools, and church spires. These physical arrangements reflect the patterning of group living on the part of the people who inhabit the land below.
>
> The community is not only a unit; it is a living unit. By this, I mean to emphasize that it is a system consisting in energy exchange, of dynamic equilibrium . . . energy sources are extracted from the sea and the land, partly used or stored within the unit and partly exported in exchange for energy sources and potentials for energy sources derived from other areas . . . Wherever there is work, wherever there is action, biological energy is transit through the system.
>
> Embedded in this patterning are activities having to do with promoting a satisfactory psychological state of existence among the persons who make up the community . . . Ordinarily it provides resources whereby the needs and desires of most of the individuals can be met to some degree. . . .
>
> Part of the functioning of a community unit, in short, is concerned with providing opportunity for the psychological functioning of the individual persons of which it is composed.
>
> More than this, the community system plays a part in shaping instincts through experience into basic urges and, ultimately, sentiments. Hence the community unit functions both to meet personality needs and to shape and even create them. This occurs as part of the process of replacement in the continuous loss and gain of individual death and birth. (*51*)

Leighton and his associates then classify communities on the basis of their influence on the health of their residents. Communities that are socially integrated enhance health and those that are disintegrated create a noxious or negative effect. The indices of *community disintegration* are: (1) high frequency of broken homes; (2) few and weak associations; (3) few and weak leaders; (4) few patterns of recreation; (5) high frequency of hostility; (6) high frequency of crime and delinquency; (7) weak and fragmented network of communication.

There are additional features that may indicate social disintegration. They are: (1) a recent history of disaster; (2) extensive poverty; (3) cultural confusion; (4) widespread secularization; (5) extensive migration; (6) rapid and widespread social change. This last set of indicators are associated with situations that can create disintegration if they operate over long enough periods of time and/or with sufficient severity.

It is important to note that most of the indicators of community disintegration would yield very high readings for the residential neighborhoods of central cities, as described in the first section of this paper.

There is debate among experts on the relative importance of the concept of community in understanding essential features of the sociocultural environment as experienced by contemporary man. But let us stay with the concept of community and listen to what Maurice Stein, a sociologist, has to say about the subject. His book, *The Eclipse of Community*, presents a very intensive analysis and interpretation of the major community studies done by anthropologists and sociologists in the United States during a period of thirty years. (52) His use of the word "eclipse" in the title indicates his concern about the neglect that this process has received in recent decades. His central conclusion is as follows:

> By now the fundamentals of (my) position ought to be clear. It rests upon the assumption that human communities exist to provide their members with full opportunities for personal development through social experimentation. This experimentation presupposes sufficient openness in personal identity so that an expanding range of possibilities is appreciated, sufficient closure in personal identity so that an integral personal style gradually evolves, and sufficient dramatic perspective so that alien styles espoused by others can be appreciated without weakening one's own commitments. . . .

These conclusions about the central function of high performance communities echo the findings of Edward Sapir published in 1924. (53) Despite slight differences in terminology his conclusions are similar:

> The genuine culture is not of necessity either high or low; it is merely harmonious, balanced, self-satisfactory. It is the expression of a richly varied and yet somehow unified and consistent attitude toward life, an attitude which sees the significance of any one element of civilization in its relation to all others. It is, ideally speaking, a culture in which nothing is spiritually meaningless, in which no important part of the general functioning brings with it a sense of frustration, of misdirected or unsympathetic effort. It is not a spiritual hybrid of contradictory patches, of water-tight compartments of consciousness that avoid participation in a harmonious synthesis. . . .

It is not enough that the ends of activities be socially satisfactory, that each member of the community feel in some dim way that he is doing his bit toward the attainment of a social benefit. This is all very well so far as it goes, but a genuine culture refuses to consider the individual as a mere cog, as an entity whose sole *raison d'etre* lies in his subservience to a collective purpose that he is not conscious of or that has only a remote relevancy to his interests and strivings. The major activities of the individual must directly satisfy his own creative and emotional impulses, must always be something more than means to an end. The great cultural fallacy of industrialism, as developed up to the present time, is that in harnessing machines to our uses, it has not known how to avoid the harnessing of the majority of mankind to its machines.

In our post-industrial society a great majority of our people are indeed harnessed to "social machines" that Galbraith calls techno-structures.(54) The large organizations of business and government have come to dominate the social landscape. Their effective control by the dominant values of our culture is the central issue of the day. Etzioni has defined the situation as follows: (55)

> A central characteristic of the modern period has been continued increase in the efficacy of the technology of production which poses a growing challenge to the primacy of the values these means are supposed to serve. The post-modern period, the onset of which may be set at 1945, will witness either a greater threat to the status of these values by surging technologies or a re-assertion of their normative priority. Which alternative prevails will determine whether society is to be the servant or the master of the instruments it creates. The active society, one that is master of itself, is an option the post-modern period opens.
>
> In the social realm, a two-step development may be recognized. The first societal revolution came with the development of the corporation, or modern organization in general, which provided the sociological machine, the more effective way of "getting things done." The second societal revolution involves the control by second-order organizations of first-order organizations which do the work—in other words, the introduction of a comprehensive overlay of societal guidance. . . .
>
> Societal guidance differs from the overlayer which automation imposes on machines in that it has itself two layers: control and responsiveness. One layer controls the member units, specifying their commitment to the values of society. The other layer's function is to insure the responsiveness of the control to the members of society. Weakness of the first layer causes drifting, with the society moving wherever the vectors of corporate ambition (or somnolence) push it; the weakness of the second layer implies either internal rigidities in the mechanism or subjugation of most members by some who monopolize access to societal control centers.

A similar re-arrangement in our thinking and our priorities is recommended by Galbraith:

The preoccupation of economists now continues to be with the volume of output of goods and services both for itself and as the remedy for unemployment. Once again underlying change has made the preoccupation partially obsolete; as a result, the recommendations of economists are again either irrelevant or damaging . . . if education is deficient, regional development is unequal, slums persist, health care is inadequate, cultural opportunities unequal, entertainment meretricious or racial inequality is glaring . . . all of the conditions for a shift from the preoccupation with unemployment and growth do exist. The primary prescription must henceforth be for the improvement of what may broadly be called the quality of life. This should now be the foremost goal. *(56)*

In addition to the need to assign highest priority to improving the quality of life, there is need to correct the imbalance between the resources allocation in the public and private sectors of the economy. Galbraith puts the issue in the following terms:

We identify economic performance with the production of goods and services. Such production is, in the main, the task of the private sector of the economy. As a result, privately produced goods and services, even of the most frivolous sort, enjoy a moral sanction not accorded to any public service except defense. Desire for private goods is subject to active cultivation . . . And the equation of psychic with physical need excludes any notion of satiety. It is a mark of an enfeebled imagination to suggest that two automobiles to a family is sufficient. Public services, by contrast, are the subject of no similar promotion; that there are severe limits to what should be expended for such services is, of course, assumed.

The consequence of this difference in attitude is a sharp discrimination in favor of one and against another class of needs. Meanwhile a series of changes in the society increases the pressure for public services. A growing population, and particularly a growing urban population, increases the friction of person upon person and the outlay that is necessary for social harmony. And it is reasonable to suppose that a growing proportion of the requirements of an increasingly civilized community—schools, colleges, libraries, museums, hospitals, recreational facilities—are by their nature in the public domain. *(57)*

If we put this economic perspective with psychological and social requirements we arrive at a position which requires a basic re-definition of the relationship between the individual person and society. Etzioni has attempted such a re-definition in the following words:

Man is *not* unless he is social; what he is depends on his social being, and what he makes of his social being is irrevocably bound to what he makes of himself. He has the ability to master his internal being, and the main way to self-mastery leads to his joining with others like himself in social acts. Potentially, every man is free to choose; social laws, unlike those of nature, can be flaunted and, above all, re-written. In fact, however, social laws penetrate individual existence so deeply that most escapes are limited in scope and often lead from compliance with one set of laws to even fuller compliance with another.

The confines of social life are frequently composed of other people in the same predicament; hence, in principle, the transformation of social life can be propelled by give-and-take among the subjects themselves. While individual action is possible, it cannot be understood except against the background of the social action of which it is a part, on which it builds, or against which it reacts. (58)

This interpretation leads Etzioni to an interesting conclusion concerning the development of a general strategy for social reform and modernization:

In his pains to master his fate, man is reaching a new phase in which his ability to obtain freedom, as well as his ability to subjugate others, is greatly extended. Both of these build in his increasing capacity to transform social bonds rather than accommodate to, or merely protest, the social patterns he encounters.

The post-modern period will be marked, in addition to a continued increase in the potency of instruments available and an exponential growth of knowledge by man's potential ability to control both. An active society, one which realizes this potential, would differ most from modern societies in this key way: it would be a society in charge of itself rather than unstructured or restructured to suit the logic of instruments and the interplay of forces they generate. Hence, this study seeks to develop a theory of societal self-control. (59)

## Participation, Competence, and Control

In the preceding commentary about community health and the urban environment, few specifications have been given in terms of the landscape, daily rhythms of living, and the patterning of interaction and social relationship. It is necessary to make such translations at this point.

We start with the significance of the home and residential neighborhood to all persons. This is where people spend most of their lifetime. It is where all children acquire their first five years of socialization. As they grow older they move out of the house to explore the neighborhood, to make friends, and to interact with other children who live nearby. Once they are of school age, they attend elementary schools in the neighborhood. At the same time the homemaker, usually the children's mother, spends most of her time at home or shopping for goods and services in the community. Only the head of the household, the wage earner, travels outside the vicinity of the home on a regular basis and for long periods of time. In off-duty hours, various members of the family attend church services, go to the library, use the recreational facilities or visit friends in their homes.

All of the activities mentioned require a primary forum of communication, namely direct interaction in a face-to-face situation, supplemented by telephone conversation, and some correspondence. Through this direct interaction, ideas, attitudes, needs, values, and expectations are formed, transmitted, and re-defined. Because of the frequency, timing, and duration of these interactions, a large spectrum of the biological-psychological-social needs of the participants are satisfied, modified, or restrained in these behavior settings.

It is within these direct interactional networks of people engaged in socially meaningful activity in and near their homes, that the images and controlling ideas about distant events in the world are developed, mediated, and revised. (60)

Recent studies in social psychology have provided convincing evidence on the importance of feelings of competence and effectiveness in the healthy performance of these daily activities. Smith has commented on this process in the following words:

> In a first approximation to a formulation of the competent self, then, we would look for distinctive features in the person's attitudes toward self and world. The self is perceived as casually important, as effective in the world—which is to a major extent a world of other people—as likely to be able to bring about desired effects, and as accepting responsibility when effects do not correspond to desire. In near equivalent, the person has self-respect. . . .
> Coordinate with the feeling of efficacy is an attitude of hope— the world is the sort of place in which, given appropriate efforts, I can expect good outcomes. Hope provides the ground against which planning, forebearance, and effort are rational. . . .
> With these positive attitudes toward self and world goes a characteristic behavioral orientation that throws the person into kinds of interaction that close the benign circle. . . .
> The person is attracted to moderate challenges that have an intermediate probability of success. By setting his previous performance, he reaps the maximum cumulative gain in sensed efficacy from his successes. This is, in effect, an active, coping orientation high in initiative, not a passive or defensive one characterized by very low goals. . . . (61)

Participation and personal effectiveness are essential features in the experience of daily living if people are to avoid feelings of distress and frustration.

Most family members are interested in decisions that affect the landscape, the air shed, and the availability of goods and services in the vicinity of their homes or along frequently used pathways. Changes in roads, sidewalks, utility lines, buildings, and fences are immediately noticed. The same is true for changes in levels of environmental pollution whether it be trash lying on the ground, foul smells in the air, visible pollutants in the air, loud noises, or dirty water in streams and lakes. Changes in the activity patterns associated with the schools, police, and fire protection, churches, and shopping centers are also readily noticed. Since many changes in the physical environment have a direct impact upon the tax bill paid by family units, there is a reinforcement of interest in environmental changes produced by business firms and government agencies.

Most persons are aware and concerned about their environment but they lack a sense of participation and effective influence in the decision-making process. This condition holds for many people living in cities and towns. Citizens generally feel that important changes in the environment are beyond the control of the people who inhabit or frequently use a given geographic area. In distant and unknown locations, landlords, industrial executives, and government officials make decisions that directly affect both the physical and social environment of residential communities. This experience is likely to generate apathy, alienation, protest, or violence.

For most citizens a strong, comfortable, and continuing participation in community decision-making is missing. Families seldom have an opportunity to experience the role of legislator at the neighborhood or community level. Neither the educational system or the typical community provide realistic opportunities for citizens to acquire political skills and to learn how to mobilize responsible political action to cope with significant social and environmental issues at the local level. When active political participation is missing at this level, where there is the richest network of face-to-face communication, a sense of frustration and impotency often develops in reference to decisions being made at more remote locations in the society. (62) Under these conditions the family often perceives a change in residential address as the only decision remaining within its realm of control. This decision, resulting in residential mobility, then ruptures the network of personal interactions with familiar landscape and familiar persons. If this migration process goes beyond a certain threshold for a given family or a given community there are usually disturbing repercussions to the healthy functioning of families and communities as open-linked social systems.

## Health in the Urban Environment

There are four distinctive population groups of interest in a study of health in the urban environment; residents, workers, students, and visitors. Each group experiences a different amount and kind of exposure to health hazards generated by the urban environment. And each group has a different bio-social characteristic that affects its disease profile and restricted activity pattern. For the purposes of this chapter, we will focus our attention upon the residential population in the large city environment. This population category contains family units that experience the full impact of the urban environment for the entire 24-hour daily round of life. This is also the population group with a large number of health problems and a shortage of health care services.

Health problems in the residential urban population can be classified into three groups: *first,* those disease conditions where the prevention and treatment is known but the clients are not receiving needed services; *second,* where the health hazards are partially understood but this tentative knowledge is not effectively utilized in policy formulation and effective social action; and *three,* where the etiology or treatment of the health hazards is so mysterious that a strategic program of research is needed before any effective socio-political or administrative action can be initiated.

These distinctions are worth making because many important professional and public discussions of the topic have given ample evidence that confusion frequently occurs on this conceptual point. The major cities of this nation have a concentration of medical personnel and facilities. They also have a large number of low-income families with serious health care needs. But in most of their cases, the disease conditions are well-known and the appropriate techniques of medical intervention are known; there is no mystery about either etiology or effective medical intervention. The key issue is political and economic, not biomedical. As the country moves to change the eligibility rules with reference to health care services for all segments of the population, these health problems well begin to diminish. Since there has been a large migration of black families with a backlog of health problems into the large cities, there is a new demand for improvement in the delivery of primary and environment health services to benefit this residential population.

In the second category where we have partial knowledge, the central requirement is to simultaneously conduct appropriate research projects, initiate well-designed demonstration projects, and carefully evaluate alternative intervention programs. Heart disease, lung cancer, automobile accidents, alcoholism, obesity, and drug addiction, and many psychiatric disorders fall into this category.

In the third category where we have no knowledge or effective treatment, the priority issue is allocation of resources for supporting basic and applied research projects. Most of the forms of cancer should be considered in this class.

Once the populations, environments, and general types of health problems have been specified, it is necessary to define the scope of events referred to by the term "health." We assume that the following set of events represent an inclusive set of categories within the general rubric: (1) unnecessary death; (2) preventible injuries; (3) correctible handicaps; (4) unnecessary restrictions in normal activity due to illness, crime, or discrimination; and (5) dangerous or unpleasant levels of stress as registered in perturbations of psychological or social events.

The category of "unnecessary deaths" would include: accidental death; suicide, homicide; deaths due to negligence on the part of physician, patient, or guardian; deaths due to violence in police or military action; and deaths resulting from severe, acute or chronic illness where the effective therapeutic or preventive intervention was known but not applied within an appropriate period of time. This excludes natural death due to old age; deaths due to uncorrectible congential defects, and voluntary euthanasia. Preventible injuries and poisionings are self-explanatory. Correctible handicaps run the spectrum from congenital biological handicaps through remedial deficiencies of the special senses, the addictions of obesity, alcoholism and drug abuse, to learning disabilities and cultural handicaps. Unnecessary restriction in activity would cover preventible illnesses such as poliomyelitis, or lack of prompt medical treatment, unnecessary hospitalization or bedrest, and discriminatory behavior associated with race, sex, religion, or native language.

The category of "dangerous or unpleasant stress" refers to a diverse set of events that are presumed to be unhealthy and are experienced as noxious, unpleasant, or disturbing to most people. Disturbances in normal patterns of sleep, eating, or elimination; sensations of pain within the body; increased frequency of emotional outbursts; extended periods of anxiety, frustration, or fatigue; and high levels of interpersonal conflict: all are indicators of the presence of undesirable levels of stress.

This means that events that have nuisance value are to be included within this definition of health. The noise of jet aircraft passing overhead can be loud enough to interrupt a classroom discussion. The sound does not impair the hearing of the students in the classroom, but it does intrude upon and interrupt their discussions. Threats that are invisible and undetectable by the natural senses of man also pose a significant threat. This applies to radioactivity; chemical contaminants of food, air, water; certain types of air pollution; and high levels of electromagnetic radiation.

There is a sharp contrast between the "disease-specific" orientation of modern medicine with its extensive differentiation into clinical specialties and multiplication of autonomous servicing activites; and the "holistic-ecological" orientation of public health. Galdston has defined this as the problem of creating the "third revolution" in medicine:

> Here we confront the third revolution in medicine. It is a revolution which few anticipate or conceptualize . . . Medicine pro-

poses to deal with the now emergent morbidities prevalent among the people in the ways it so successfully dealt with the infectious diseases. It attempts to use a specific disease approach, in contrast to an ecological approach. But is it not one task, involving one technique to control typhoid and yet another task involving yet another technique to control, say, obesity or cigarette smoking?

The major crowd diseases have been effectively controlled. What we face now as the great challenge are the disorders of bad hygiene, of insalubrious environments, of a malign physical and moral ecology. These are not to be dealt with as were the infectious, epidemic diseases. They are disorders engendered by malign environments and man's corrupt relations to his immediate world and his individual existence. These disorders are not to be remedied by sterilization, vaccines, immune serums, nor by medicinal specifics. They are, in the broadest sense of the term, *ecological disorders,* arising from a disordered ecology, both physical and moral. (63)

These two perspectives do not combine easily, as the use of the term "revolution" implies. The autonomy of professional schools for "medicine" and "public health" in the universities gives institutional evidence on this point. But now we are faced with the combination of difficulties associated with the delivery of services to a larger and more demanding public and a significant shift in the disease profile of the population. This situation forces us to carefully examine our frames of reference and our allocations of effort.

Perhaps there are composite strategies of intervention that could produce significant improvements "across the board" in terms of improved health status for specific residential populations. Such intervention strategies would be directed to primary prevention of several organic and mental disorders by means of synchronized changes in social relationships and important features of the physical environment (especially the man-made environment).

Modifications in the design of buildings and the layout of community facilities could be coupled with changes in organizational service programs to provide new kinds of relationships between healthy and handicapped families. Instead of concentrating low-income families in public housing projects in the central city, one could provide relocation services to distribute low-income families throughout suburban communities and support these families with a composite package of employment-training-medical-housing services. Neighborhoods with high social integration could easily absorb a small number of handicapped families and provide a natural set of development opportunities. As Smith has observed:

> Underlying my search . . . is a view of causation in personal and social development as inherently circular or spiral, rather than linear in terms of neatly isolable causes and effects. As the very concept of interaction implies, developmental progress or deficit is typically a matter of benign circles or of vicious ones, not of persistent effects of clear-cut single causes. . . .

. . . Launched on the right trajectory, the person is likely to accumulate successes that strengthen the effectiveness of his orientation toward the world while at the same time, he acquires the knowledge and skills that make his further success more probable. His environmental involvements generally lead to gratification and to increased competence and favorable development. Off to a bad start, on the other hand, he soon encounters failures that make his hesitant to try. What to others are challenges appear to him as threats; he becomes preoccupied with defense of his small claims on life at the expense of energies to invest in constructive coping. And he falls increasingly behind his fellows in acquiring the knowledge and skills that are needed for success on those occasions when he does try. (64)

Or to take an example from current clinical research, how do we intervene in the epidemic of coronary artery disease? We can launch a composite research and treatment program that simultaneously copes with the multiple factors of smoking, high blood pressure, cholesterol level, and physical exercise. Such a composite strategy involves important modifications of behavior in the areas of smoking, eating, and exercise. To change these fundamental habits of daily living will require combining educational and medical techniques and creating new opportunities for exercise.

Composite strategies of this kind are not unreasonable given the recent findings from the general field of medical ecology. Changes in social relationships and environment are found to be associated with a wide range of organic and emotional disturbances. A major study in this area was conducted by Hinkle and his associates and reported in 1961. A summary of the findings and an assessment is provided by John Cassel:

In study groups of men all working for the same company and all holding similar positions as managers, they found marked differences in the disease prevalence in those groups who had completed college as opposed to those who had not completed college prior to coming to the industry.

Those who had completed college, were, with few exceptions, fourth-generation Americans, sons of managers, proprietors, and white-collar workers, and had grown-up in families with middle to high incomes and in good neighborhoods.

In contrast, the group who had not completed college were hired as skilled craftsmen and later advanced to managerial status. They were sons and grandsons of immigrants, their fathers were skilled or unskilled laborers with an average of grammar school education or less, and they had grown-up in families of low-income in modest to sub-standard neighborhoods.

This latter group shared a significantly greater number of illnesses of all sorts than did the former group. It is important to note that they were more susceptible to major, as well as minor illnesses, to physical illnesses, as well as emotional illness, to illnesses affecting every organ of the body, and to long-term as well as to short-term illness.

In addition, therefore, to supporting the notion of the importance of "preparedness" for a situation, this study of Hinkle's raises a further possibility. The clustering of so wide a variety of disease syndromes in the unprepared group would suggest that to the extent exposure to unfamiliar situations is important as a determination of disease or as a factor leading to increased susceptibility to disease, it need not be expected that it will necessarily be related specifically to any particular disease classified according to current nomenclature.

In other words, the possibility must be entertained that social factors may increase the risk of ill-health by increasing general susceptibility to disease. The manifestation or form of the disease may well be due to an entirely different set of factors (including genetic make-up and the physical and biological pathogens with which the susceptible groups come into contact). (65)

Discoveries of this kind highlight the importance of explorations that proceed in an interdisciplinary fashion. The traditional compartments of knowledge and occupational specialization have pushed us to new frontiers. These frontiers require the creation of quite new forms of research and action strategy. It is now apparent that these biological, behavioral, and environmental events are often coupled in ways that can yield a critical outcome in terms of health status for individual persons and for families. Standards for judging healthy and unhealthy performance are beginning to emerge in the fields concerned with personality development, family dynamics, work organization, community settlements, and habitable environments. The integration of these areas of fragmented knowledge and empirical testing of hypotheses in composite programs of research and social action is a central task in the decade ahead.

## Strategies for Action and Research

Our frame of reference leads to a proposal to combine the quest for new knowledge with social action programs aimed at improving the health status of families living in urban environments. We offer two strategies that seem to offer strong possibilities for success within the cultural heritage and situational dynamics of American society.

The first proposal is to establish a series of "Community Health Observatories" in contrasting residential environments. Pair communities would be selected to give maximum comparative contrast and to yield data on strong stressful events in the environment. The time commitment would have to be for a minimum of ten years.

There are several types of scientific field stations that can provide experience for the establishment of these community observatories. Many of the field sciences such as astronomy, meteorology, archeology, geology, botony, zoology, and primatology have had to establish long-range support for specific observation sites to collect data. In the realm of applied research there are the field stations, and demonstration farms supported by land-grant colleges and the U.S. Department of Agriculture. Data recording activities associated with the construction of dams and the development of river systems show some of the same features of continual monitoring of environmental events. The worldwide activities of the weather bureau and the monitoring of production in an oil refinery represent additional parallels. Long-term social science research activities in specific communities also represent essential components in our proposal for the establishment of composite "Community Health Observatories." The work of Vogt in Chiapis, Mexico; of Leighton in Nova Scotia; of Kluckhohn in New Mexico; of Holmsberg in Vicos, Peru: all of these long-term programs of investigation involved the establishment of field stations and maintenance of strong rapport with the indigenous communities.

The types of data to be collected would include: essential features of the physical environment known to be noxious or detrimental to the health of man (gases, particles, noise, chemicals, smells, pollen, air pressure); the numbers and proximities (crowding) of human beings; the proportions of natives and strangers; tensions and conflicts between groups and families; levels of health and crime; mobility of families and individuals in various statuses; modifications in land use (activities associated with buildings and constructed areas); information on the daily round of life; perceptions of threat and sets of images, value orientations, sentiments, attitudes, that may influence the adaptation of the human body to its environment. The indicators of "social integration" developed by Leighton and his associates should be used, plus selected items from the inventory of "social indicators" developed by Eleanor Sheldon, Wilbert Moore, Raymond Bauer, and others. (*66, 67, 68, 69*)

Some features would have to be monitored regularly or continuously while others would be needed much less frequently on a total community basis. Other data collection efforts would be triggered by events such as a new family moving into the area, a criminal action, a riot, a strike, or a fire.

The field stations would require specific sites for automatic recording instruments—especially of the physical environment, noise, air pollutants, wind, and time sampling of the human vocalization levels, sounds of sirens, and roar of passing aircraft.

For the behavioral data collection it would be necessary to have living quarters for students and research staff. Just as anthropological field stations have at least one "scientist-family" resident in the community at all times, a similar arrangement would be required here. This family household would have accommodations for guests. The family would be expected to participate in community activities. There

37

would be a strong tie with local schools and local newspapers so that optimal relationships with the public were maintained. An exchange program of students or families might be established between the paired observatory communities to produce evidence from "initial impressions" by visitors and to encourage a diffusion of successful innovations.

There should be a research advisory group at the national level that would select the sites; specify the minimum requirements of funding, equipment, and data collection; and invite the participation of various single and multi-disciplinary research groups from several universities to utilize the observatories for their own studies. Cooperative research would be essential. To maintain the integrity and continuity of the basic research program it would be necessary to have long-term investments by specific universities as part of their responsibility for training graduate students and promoting relevant research programs.

It would be advisable to search for opportunities to add the observatories to other federal or regional programs. A good example is that of Operation Breakthrough of the Department of Housing and Urban Development. In HUD, one program office has had management responsibility for land assembly in eleven different American cities and the setting of specifications on the types of residential buildings to be constructed on those sites using mass production techniques. It would seem relatively easy to add one or two paired "Community Health Observatories" to the Breakthrough Program. The metropolitan plan of Detroit to pair suburbs with urban neighborhoods might provide a similar opportunity.

These programs of data collection would be tied to management and development efforts within the communities. Projects that would change the physical environment or the objectives of ongoing human service programs would become connected with the action-research-evaluation activities, so that new scientific findings would be immediately implemented through education and legislation at the community level. There are models for this community development approach in the work of John L. Kennedy and Allan Holmberg, (70, 71)

The second strategy concerns the development of a set of new communities. With the strong increase in population there is a large amount of residential housing being constructed. Most of this is being added in suburban or urban fringe communities. Only a small fraction of it is being added in the form of new communities. Although the "new towns" movement started in England at the turn of the century and many of the essential requirements were written down in 1898 by Ebenezer Howard, there has been relatively little interest in "new communities" in the United States until recently. (72) Probably the two best-known "new communities" are Reston, Virginia, and Columbia,

Maryland. Now there are signs of growing interest in this field and various kinds of "new communities" are being proposed. (73, 74, 75)

A great number of writers and advisors on urban life have been suggesting a mobilization of effort behind this approach. So far the federal government has not assigned a high priority to this area within the programs of the Department of Housing and Urban Development. New support for this field may come from the recently released Report of the Commission on Population Growth and the American Future which recommends the establishment of a new Department of Community Development. Questions concerning the distribution of populations are considered in major sections of this Report. The problems of population size are linked in important ways with patterns of migration and settlement. (76)

The essential features of the new community are: (1) a pre-set maximum size and residential density; (2) putting work, school, home, shopping, and recreational areas close together; (3) eliminating the conflict between pedestrian and vehicular traffic; (4) maintaining social diversity among the residential population; (5) encouraging strong community participation by residents; (6) providing for a smooth transition between the phases of planning, construction, and municipal operation of the community; and (7) providing a greenbelt surrounding the community.

The key in this approach to community development is the use of a single organization in developing a comprehensive community on open land. Instead of developing something within the matrix of an established community with its historical landmarks, investments in man-constructed facilities and buildings, and the vested interests of various landowners, it is possible to start fresh.

For our purposes it is only necessary to know that new communities are being developed and that our interests could be served by strong participation. Concern with creating and maintaining a healthy community is widespread. The new housing developments are making efforts to respect essential ecological processes, to develop new means of waste re-cycling and/or disposal, to be concerned about the elimination of racial discrimination, and to meet the needs of poverty families. What I am suggesting is a stronger partnership in the sense of testing specific hypotheses about the links between health and community process. New communities will be developed with different policies and styles of operation. These differences in policy and program can be compared. The developers and managers of these communities are eager to acquire information about health that will increase their chances of attracting families, businesses, and visitors.

It ought to be possible to approximate an experimental research strategy through strong collaboration with the management and development groups that launch such communities. To answer key questions in the real world, natural history studies comparing populations and environments will never suffice, nor will controlled laboratory experiments. We need larger blocks of socio-cultural activity in natural field laboratories. This is possible as Holmberg and his associates have shown in their work in Vicos, Peru. (77) Our ability to maneuver large blocks of socio-cultural events is crucial. And the public climate has now shifted so that reform revitalization, and modernization are high priority features in the contemporary scene. If there is a cooperative strategy, with strong participation by "resident clients" in the control of information gathering and application, then this approach is acceptable. Control by an elite group of scientists and developers would not be acceptable. This represents a new type of self-directed change with open collaboration among three interest groups: community developer/ managers, community resident-clients, and health researchers.

We are arriving at a stage of need and knowledge where man can assume an impressive degree of self-control over the larger sociocultural events of deep concern to him.(78) The community as a piece of land and interconnected human activity represents the basic unit of study. Human beings grow to full personhood only through lengthy and multiple involvements with determining their own affairs. It could be that properly developed communities would effectively reduce disease and crime rates across the board. Environmental pollution, interpersonal conflict leading to violence, racial discrimination, population control, criminal behavior, mental illness, and a number of the major chronic diseases—all are known to be affected by certain features of community life. A new community, designed with inputs from all relevant areas of knowledge, might be quite capable of solving in one stroke a whole set of disturbing social problems.

It must be realized however that many of the essential controls available in large corporations are not available in most communities. Communities are open social systems in an important sense. If you have the money to buy property you can enter, unless you are the target of discrimination. You can live in a community without participating in any political activities other than paying your taxes on time. You do not have to attend church. You do have to send your children to school when they are between 7 and 16 years of age. You do not have to purchase goods and services at stores in town. With the mobility of the auto and plentiful highways you can spend most of your time away from home, out of town as well. This leaves a small set of "native residents" pretty much in charge of the local government. (79) They, in combination with the business firms in the community, will control the use of land and decide most of the major changes in the environment.

But these typical conditions of community life are not inherent or necessary. Communities, like organizations, vary in their levels of integration, performance, and *esprit de corps*. A specific community can acquire

40

a strong sense of purpose like "improvement in the quality of life." Improvement in health, self-actualization, and life-long learning can become focal points of priority and consensus. *(80)* A more comprehensive pattern of health services might be developed as part of such plans for a series of "new communities" and thus expand the alternatives presently available. Health scientists ought to be alert to the potentialities for participation in the new communities movement.

## References

1. Rene Dubos, MAN ADAPTING, New Haven, Connecticut: Yale University Press, 1965, pp. 352–353.
2. William L. Thomas, Jr., MAN'S ROLE IN CHANGING THE FACE OF THE EARTH, Chicago: University of Chicago Press, 1956.
3. Report of the Study of Critical Environmental Problems: MAN'S IMPACT ON THE GLOBAL ENVIRONMENT, Cambridge, Massachusetts: The MIT Press, 1970.
4. Peter and Katherine Montague: "Mercury: how much are we eating?" Saturday Review: February 6, 1971, pp. 50–54.
5. Paul and Anne Ehrlich: POPULATION, RESOURCES, ENVIRONMENT, San Francisco: W. H. Freemand and Co., 1970, pp. 321–324.
6. William and Paul Paddock: FAMINE—1975, Boston: Little, Brown and Company, 1967.
7. Alan Sheldon, Frank Baker, and Curtis P. McLaughlin, SYSTEMS AND MEDICAL CARE, Cambridge, Massachusetts, Massachusetts Institute of Technology, 1970.
   See also—Frederick Sargent's article, "The Human Habitat" in Architecture, Environment, Health, Volume 25, October 1972, pp. 229–233.
8. John K. Galbraith, THE NEW INDUSTRIAL STATE, New York: Signet Paperback, 1968, p. 19.
9. Edward A. Suchman. "Action for What? A Critique of Evaluative Research," in THE ORGANIZATION, MANAGEMENT, AND TACTICS OF SOCIAL RESEARCH, edited by Richard O'Toole, Cambridge, Massachusetts: Sehenkman Publishing, 1971, p. 98.
10. William H. Whyte, THE LAST LANDSCAPE, Garden City, New York: Doubleday and Company, 1968.
11. Howard T. Odum, ENVIRONMENT, POWER, AND SOCIETY, New York: Wiley-Interscience, 1971.
12. Scott Greer: "Urbanization and Social Character," in THE QUALITY OF URBAN LIFE, Edited by Henry Schmandt and Warner Bloomberg, Beverly Hills, California: Sage Publications, 1969, pp. 95–127.
13. Jane Jacobs, THE ECONOMY OF CITIES, New York: Random House, 1969.
14. Leonard Reismann, THE URBAN PROCESS, New York: The Free Press, 1964.
15. Bureau of the Census, U.S. Department of Commerce: THE STATISTICAL ABSTRACT OF THE U.S., 1971. Government Printing Office, Washington, D.C. Table 327, p. 201, and Table 341, p. 217.
16. *Ibid*. Table 16, p. 17.
17. Loc. cit. Also, New York Times, September 2, 1970, p. 27.
18. Oscar Handlin: BOSTON'S IMMIGRANTS, A STUDY IN ACCULTURATION, New York: Atheneum Paperback, 1968. (Originally published by Harvard University Press, 1941.)

41

19. Bureau of the Census, op. cit., Table 130, p. 89.
20. New York Times, March 4, 1971, p. 20, and Bureau of the Census, op. cit., Table 18, p. 20.
21. Bureau of the Census, op. cit., Table 19, p. 20.
22. New York Times, March 4, 1971, p. 20.
23. REPORT OF THE NATIONAL ADVISORY COMMISSION ON CIVIL DISORDERS, New York: Bantam Books, 1968, p. 243.
24. Ibid.
25. Leo Levy and Harold M. Vistosky: "The Quality of Urban Life: An Analysis from the Perspective of Mental Health," in THE QUALITY OF URBAN LIFE, edited by Henry Schmandt and Warner Bloomberg, Beverly Hills, California: Sage Publications, 1969, pp. 255–267.
26. Alvin L. Schorr: "National Community and Housing Policy," in URBAN PLANNING AND SOCIAL POLICY, edited by Bernard J. Frieden and Robert Morris, New York: Basic Books, 1968, pp. 107–118.
27. Preston David, "The Human Dimension in Public Housing," in URBAN PLANNING AND SOCIAL POLICY, edited by Bernard J. Frieden and Robert Morris, New York: Basic Books, 1968, pp. 96–106.
28. Ramsey Clark, CRIME IN AMERICA, New York: Simon and Schuster, 1970, pp. 49–50.
29. Bureau of the Census, op. cit., p. 137.
30. Edwin M. Schur, OUR CRIMINAL SOCIETY, New Jersey: Englewood Cliffs, Prentice Hall, 1969, p. 26.
31. Sam Bass Warner, Jr., editor, PLANNING FOR A NATION OF CITIES, Cambridge, Massachusetts: The MIT Press, 1966.
32. Edward C. Banfield and James Q. Wilson, CITY POLITICS, Cambridge, Massachusetts: Harvard University Press, 1966.
33. Wilbur R. Thompson, "Toward a Framework for Urban Public Management," in PLANNING FOR A NATION OF CITIES, edited by Sam Bass Warner, Jr., op. cit., pp. 229–245.
34. Eunice and George Grier, "Equality and Beyond: Housing Segregation in the Great Society," in URBAN PLANNING AND SOCIAL POLICY, edited by Bernard J. Frieden and Robert Morris, New York: Basic Books, 1968, pp. 124–147.
35. James S. Campbell, Joseph R. Sahid, and David P. Stang, LAW AND ORDER RECONSIDERED, Report of the Task Force on Law and Law Enforcement to the National Commission on the Causes and Prevention of Violence, New York: Bantam Paperback, 1970, pp. 137–148.
36. Lyle C. Fitch, "Eight Goals for an Urbanizing America," pp. 1141–64 in DAEDALUS issue on "The Conscience of the City," Fall, 1968.
37. Report of the National Advisory Commission on Civil Disorders, op. cit., p. 258.
38. Marc Fried, "Grieving for a Lost Home," in THE URBAN CONDITION, edited by Leonard Duhl, New York: Basic Books, 1963, pp. 155–171.
39. Daniel Wilner and Rosabelle Walkley, "Effects of Housing on Health and Performance," in THE URBAN CONDITION, edited by Leonard Duhl, op. cit., pp. 215–228.
40. Oscar Lewis, "The Culture of Poverty," in ON UNDERSTANDING POVERTY, edited by Daniel P. Moynihan, New York: Basic Books, 1968, pp. 187–200.
41. John W. Gardner, NO EASY VICTORIES, New York: Harper and Row, Paperback, 1968.
42. Edward C. Banfield, "Why Government Cannot Solve the Urban Problem," in DAEDALUS issue on "The Conscience of the City," Fall, 1968, pp. 1231–41.
43. James A. Donovan, MILITARISM, U.S.A., New York: Charles Scribner's Sons, 1970.

44. Ernst B. Haas, BEYOND THE NATION-STATE: Functionalism and International Organization, Stanford, California: Stanford University Press, 1964.
45. John K. Galbraith, "Foreign Policy: The Plain Lessons of Bad Decade," in ECONOMICS, PEACE, AND LAUGHTER, edited by John K. Galbraith, Boston: Houghton, Mifflin, 1971, pp. 165–183.
46. Kenneth E. Boulding, MEANING OF 20th CENTURY, New York: Harper and Row, 1964.
47. Alexander H. Leighton, MY NAME IS LEGION, New York: Basic Books, 1959.
48. Charles C. Hughes et al., PEOPLE OF COVE AND WOODLOT, New York: Basic Books, 1960.
49. Dorothea C. Leighton et al, THE CHARACTER OF DANGER, New York: Basic Books, 1963.
50. Gerald R. Leslie, THE FAMILY IN SOCIAL CONTEXT, New York: Oxford University Press, 1967.
51. Alexander H. Leighton, op. cit., pp. 195–197.
52. Maurice R. Stein, THE ECLIPSE OF COMMUNITY, Princeton, New Jersey: Princeton University Press, 1960.
53. Edward Sapir, "Culture, Genuine and Spurious," in SELECTED WRITINGS OF EDWARD SAPIR, edited by David G. Mandelbaum, Berkeley, California: University of California Press, 1958, pp. 308–331.
54. John K. Galbraith, THE NEW INDUSTRIAL STATE, New York: Signet Paperback, 1968, pp. 77–82.
55. Amitai Etzioni, THE ACTIVE SOCIETY, New York: The Free Press, 1968.
56. John K. Galbraith, "Economics and the Quality of Life," in ECONOMICS, PEACE, AND LAUGHTER, edited by John K. Galbraith, Boston: Houghton, Mifflin, 1971, pp. 3-25.
57. Ibid., p. 19.
58. Amitai Etzioni, op. cit., p. 2–3.
59. Amitai Etzioni, op. cit., p. 4–6.
60. George A. Theodorson, STUDIES IN HUMAN ECOLOGY, New York: Harper and Row, 1961.
61. M. Brewster Smith, "Competence and Socialization," in SOCIAL PSYCHOLOGY AND HUMAN VALUES, edited by M. Brewster Smith, Chicago: Aldine Publishing Co., 1969, p. 219.
62. Anton C. Zijderveld, THE ABSTRACT SOCIETY, New York: Doubleday, 1970.
63. Iago Galdston, "The Third Revolution: Prelude & Polemic," in ETHICAL ISSUES IN MEDICINE, edited by E. Fuller Torrey, Boston: Little Brown and Company, 1968, pp. 8–9.
64. M. Brewster Smith, loc. cit.
65. John Cassel, "Physical Illness in Response to Stress," in SOCIAL STRESS, edited by Sol Levine and Norman A. Scotch, Chicago: Aldine Publishing Company, 1970, pp. 189–209.
66. Charles C. Hughes et al, PEOPLE OF COVE AND WOODLOT, New York: Basic Books, 1960.
67. Raymond A. Bauer, SOCIAL INDICATORS, Cambridge, Mass.: MIT Press, 1966.
68. Eleanor Sheldon and Wilbert Moore, INDICATORS OF SOCIAL CHANGE, New York: Russell Sage, 1968.
69. Eleanor Sheldon and Wilbert Moore, THE HUMAN MEANING OF SOCIAL CHANGE, New York: Russell Sage, 1972.
70. John L. Kennedy, "A Transition-Model Laboratory for Research on Cultural Change," in HUMAN ORGANIZATION RESEARCH, edited by R. N. Adams and J. J. Preiss, Homewood, Illinois: Dorsey Press, 1960, pp. 316–323.
71. Allan R. Holmberg, "The Research and Development Approach to Change: Participant Intervention in the Field," Ibid., pp. 76–89.

72. Frederic J. Osborn, GREEN-BELT CITIES, New York: Schocken Book, 1969.
73. Harvey S. Perloff, "Modernizing Urban Development," pp. 789–800 in *DAEDALUS* issue on "Toward the Year 2000," Summer, 1967.
74. Kevin Lynch, "The Possible City," in ENVIRONMENT AND POLICY: The Next Fifty Years, edited by William R. Ewald, Jr., Bloomington, Indiana: Indiana University Press, 1968, pp. 137–157.
75. Percival and Paul Goodman, COMMUNITAS: Means of Livelihood and Ways of Life, New York: Random House, Vintage Paperback, 1960.
76. Report of the Commission on Population Growth and the American Future, New York: Signet Paperback, 1972.
77. Allan R. Holmberg, "Changing Community Attitudes and Values in Peru: A Case Study in Guided Change," in SOCIAL CHANGE IN LATIN AMERICA TODAY: Its Implications for U.S. Policy, edited by Richard N. Adams et al, New York: Harper and Brothers, 1960, pp. 63–107.
78. Ward H. Goodenough, COOPERATION IN CHANGE: An Anthropological Approach to Community Development, New York: Russell Sage, 1963.
79. Arthur J. Vidich and Joseph Bensman, SMALL TOWN IN MASS SOCIETY, Garden City, New York: Doubleday Anchor, Paperback, 1960.
80. Jan Howard and Anselm Strauss, eds., HUMANIZING HEALTH CARE, New York: John Wiley & Sons, 1975.

# Chapter III

# The Forgotten Environment

ROBERT P. BURDEN

Major national attention is presently focused on the environment. Documentation of the need to improve environmental quality can be found everywhere. Countless indications of the widespread concern of individuals, as well as records of recent legislative hearings, attest to the need to address the problem of environmental quality control. But assuming success in all of the existing programs, as well as programs currently proposed, only a minimal improvement will be achieved in the environments where a substantial percentage of Americans spend their lives—the deteriorating sections of urban areas.

The problems of environmental management for the country as a whole are substantially different from the particular problems of the cities. A direct analogy is not possible. An examination of the two kinds of environmental problems, however, yields some useful observations on an approach to the concern of this paper: improvement in the quality of life in urban environments.

It has been stated in the Congress and Federal agencies that environmental pollution can be controlled with the application of existing knowledge. The only two needs cited are money and political action. There is some truth in this view for water pollution, air pollution, and noise pollution with the validity decreasing in that order. While extensive additional research will be required, the application of current technology can solve major pollution problems.

In water pollution, there are several pollutants that must be dealt with, but the source of pollution is concentrated at a limited number of points. For example, the liquid wastes of a city are collected and ultimately discharged at one or a few points into the receiving waters. Tens of thousands of individual sources are thus reduced to what in effect is one source. The collection process makes it possible to treat these wastes at a limited number of points.

The whole thrust of the water pollution program is, however, aimed at the protection of the water rather than the population. The national objective is to raise the quality of the water. There will be attendant benefits from increased recreation, reduced water treatment costs for industries and municipalities, and improved aesthetics. Certainly the quality of the environment will be improved. But the health of the people in the cities or in the river basin will not be affected materially one way or the other.

Air pollution is a bit different but shows some of the major characteristics of water pollution. Almost all air pollution can be traced to the waste products of energy use as, for example, in transportation and electric power generation. Automotive air pollution in a city is generated by tens of thousands of point sources which discharge directly into the air and cannot be collected. New vehicles, however, can be fitted with control devices at a very few points so that in time only local inspection will be required to maintain performance in compliance with the standards. Power stations and certain large industries discharge their wastes to the air at a limited number of point sources and are thus relatively easy to control, granted adequate technology. The resulting improvements in air quality will affect urban residents directly, in fact primarily. In this case, health benefits can be demonstrated in addition to aesthetic and economic benefits.

Thus, under the stimulus of public concern, a system is evolving to combat the gross effects of pollution. Control of pollution has been recognized as the responsibility of government. The unprecedented industrial growth since World War II has increased the stress on the environment. At the same time, there has been a corresponding increase in the resources that can be allocated to the environmental protection sector. As a result, Federal agencies have evolved rapidly over the last decade. The direction of the change, leading through several intermediate steps to the creation of the Environmental Protection Agency in 1971, has been to establish an agency with clear-cut responsibility to undertake the job. Standards have had to be set and mechanisms for enforcement established.

The decision to take action at the Federal level establishes a focal point for attention, research, funding, liaison with the states, and a mechanism to provide analyses upon which policy actions can be taken and rational political decisions made. Analytical and descriptive methods must be extended to make them applicable to decisions in which a global objective does not exist and in which a cost-benefit ratio based on the national income objective has limited usefulness. The processes of the body politic, like the facts about treatment cost functions of industrial polluters and physical systems, must effectively be taken into account in contending with questions of environmental quality. These steps are beginning to be taken for water pollution, air pollution, and in a very preliminary fashion for the solid waste and noise problems. As we shall see later in this paper, these types of approaches are going

46

to become increasingly important for analysis of urban environmental quality.

Once the requisite Federal action is taken an increased State role generally follows. This is already happening in connection with the more general environmental problems. A number of states have completed or begun the reorganization of their environmental protection activities. The new consolidated State environmental activities will have a stronger role in monitoring and enforcing standards. The main characteristic of the new State institutions is that there is a much more conscious effort to have an organization which matches the Federal organization. To this match, adequate legal authority is being added to ensure that action is possible.

Similar organizational patterns are beginning to emerge in some cities. While it is too soon to measure the result, it is clear that new patterns of public action for environmental protection will emerge. What is not clear is whether the reorganization at the city level will result in effective agencies for the management of micro-environmental problems (environmental problems at the neighborhood and building levels) within the urban areas. At the present time, effective mechanisms do not exist for constructive approaches to community organization and programs of local agencies for urban environmental improvement. This is primarily a managerial problem rather than an economic problem.

While the Federal task is enormous, the setting of standards, policies, research directions, and various forms of funding assistance is relatively amendable to large-scale analysis. At the State level the tasks get more difficult as the problems become more specific. The immediate questions about how much pollution, and where it should be controlled, get down to stretches of a given river, particular industrial plants with real addresses, and municipalities by name. Within a city, the resultant shifts in organization for environmental management may be directed at matching the State and Federal programs at the expense of solving more difficult, longer range environmental problems relating to quality of life for the residents.

In some basic fashion, the program response thus does not reflect the real needs of the people. The environmental degradation of the neighborhood is occurring right where the residents live; yet in most cities at the present time, the management and resources for amelioration are physically and administratively remote from the neighborhoods. Consequently, remedial steps are separated from any active participation and intervention by community people who should be working much more closely with local government. A further difficulty is the lack of effective, research and development studies that provide methodologies for new approaches to these problems. As these studies are relatively capital intensive, they continue to be channeled to the remote agencies

—a practice which tends to continue the separation of the resident's problems from the official problem solvers.

An example of program remoteness is typified by solid waste problems in the City of Boston. The inner city neighborhoods are dirty. The major contributor to this environmental fouling is litter that escapes the solid waste collection service. Many of the community leaders believe the attitude of the residents regarding social change is partially dependent on their perception of the quality of their local environment. The Public Works Department, which is responsible for solid waste collection and disposal, runs an efficient curbside collection service. The Department views their major solid waste problem as ultimate disposal, which is indeed a pressing problem. The solution of this problem, however, will have no impact on the environmental quality of the inner city neighborhoods. Thus, even if the City is successful in finding an efficient ultimate disposal system, the residents will have no evidence of any perceptible change. Unfortunately, this difficulty is not limited to solid waste problems. It cuts across many of the environmental areas related to quality of life in American cities.

This example of one environmental problem of one city serves as a useful reminder of the general problem of waste disposal and treatment within an urban area. While it is well recognized in the technology of treatment of particular wastes, and by environmental management specialists in general, there is one factor underlying most methods that has great import for city environments. This factor is the assimilative services provided by the environment itself. Self-purification of rivers, dispersion of stack discharges over large distances, dissipation of noise energy, all form part of environmental control in macro-environments.

In the micro-environments of cities, and inner cities in particular, there is not enough assimilative capacity to provide effective natural treatment. People, their wastes, the waste of supporting services, and industrial wastes are inextricably interlocked. Waste products that are not collected and exported or managed directly at the source affect the quality of life for the residents adversely. If the concept of minimal pollution has any meaning, it is in the cities. Once a waste escapes into the commons of a city, it remains part of the city until it is degraded or removed.

## The City Environment

The central concern of this paper is how to manage the environment of the city to improve the quality of life for the residents. More specifically, within the city, the main concern is with the neighborhood environments in which the less affluent people live. This includes the poor people, ethnic groups who may not all be poor, and those eco-

48

nomic groups who by choice or necessity remain in the city but cannot afford the high rent districts. In the major cities an increasing number of black people in particular areas are affected.

For these people and their areas of the city, the benefits of the new programs in environmental protection discussed in the first section are not apparent. There are two major reasons for this. First, the new programs are primarily directed at protecting nature rather than people. Second, the causes of degradation of the environment of inner and older city areas are not understood. The explanations usually advanced are a mixture of symptoms and causes. But even separating these factors does not provide a rational explanation. Poverty, changing tax bases, flight to the suburbs, crime, traffic congestion, bad schools, bad housing, racial conflicts—all these are some of the reasons cited for urban problems. In many urban areas some or many of these conditions exist at any one time. And where they do, they are very real problems. They do not, however, provide a rationale for structuring a research instrument to get at the underlying causes of the decay of the urban environment.

In the urban setting we are dealing with an environmental system which is much more complex than a rural environmental system. Furthermore, we are dealing with an environment in which people are the most important part. Most national, state, and local environmental programs exclude consideration of people or the immediate impact of the environment on its residents.

In any neighborhood the physical environment is part of the individual's identity. In inner city neighborhoods this is of greater importance than in other city neighborhoods or the suburbs. The reason for the increased importance is simply the decreased environmental choice that is available to the children and adult residents of the inner cities. They do not get away from the city to a second home for the weekend. They may not get away for vacations. In fact, they may not get away at all unless or until they move. In the latter case, they are likely to move to a similar neighborhood where a similar lack of choices exist.

Thus the noise, the litter, the lack of accessible urban recreational space, the crowding, the impact of vacant and decaying buildings all remain part of the physical environment. Consequently, they continuously affect the urban dweller. Insofar as these factors or their combination are deleterious, damage to the identity and health of the dweller results.

## Environmental Health Effects of Urban Neighborhoods

In health work, there is a strong tradition based on controlled clinical trials for the evaluation of new disease control methods. By the very nature of these trials, there is a prior requirement to understand the causative agent for the illness or dysfunction so that therapeutic means can be developed. Chemotherapy, vaccines, diet, surgical procedures all fit this pattern.

The provision of safe water for municipalities preceded a complete understanding of waterborne diseases, but conventional evaluation methods have long since formalized our understanding of control measures in a traditional form. By and large, however, progress in medical care and public health has occurred along single lines.

Where progress has been less spectacular—in understanding heart disease, mental health, or cancer, for example—the underlying causes are either not clear or perhaps multiple. Nevertheless, extensive research on these problems is underway in Federal laboratories, universities, private industries, and health agencies. By contrast, in spite of the magnitude of the problem, there is a very great deficiency in the allocation of research and study funds to the problems of urban microenvironments and their relation to health.

There are several reasons which bear on the lack of research in this area. A principal difficulty is that of measuring how the quality of human life is affected by the environment. Hinkle discusses this problem elsewhere in this monograph.[1] One reason for this lack, as he stresses, is that the question is not well enough understood to permit the standardization of methods so that causality can be established and change measured. In fact, this area is one of the main research efforts needed.

A second major difficulty is the large number of competing local and Federal agencies dealing with various parts of the health and environmental problems in the cities. The increased number of agencies in recent years is in some measure a recognition of the need, but not the nature of the problem. Densely populated urban areas are very complex systems. If we have learned one fact in the analysis of complex systems, it is that you cannot understand a system by studying bits and pieces as isolated segments.

A third difficulty has been pointed out separately in this monograph by Cassel [2] and Kasl.[3] Their independent reviews of the literature do not support conclusions that there are simple and direct relationships between the urban environment and health. This does not say that health in the inner city areas is as good as in other city areas or in the suburbs. In fact it is not. What these reviews do demonstrate is that it is

---

[1] See Chapter VII, *Measurements of the Effects of the Environment upon the Health and Behavior of People*, by Lawrence E. Hinkle, Sr.

[2] See Chapter V, *The Relation of the Urban Environment to Health: Toward a Conceptual Frame and a Research Strategy*, by John Cassel.

[3] See Chapter IV, *Effects of Residential Environment on Health and Behavior: A Review*, by Stanislav V. Kasl.

almost impossible to draw causal inferences from the analysis of existing data on the effects of physical aspects of the micro-environment on human health and behavior.

These difficulties pose major problems to separating 'out the environmental factors which may produce deleterious effects. But the lack of knowledge may not pose insuperable difficulties in affecting beneficial change in the health and behavior of inner city residents. A new approach may enable progress to be made if a very pragmatic procedure is adopted.

At the present time, the proliferation and duplication of health-related undertakings in the cities of this country interfere with such a new approach. A brief summary of some of the activities currently underway is illustrative of this point. Table 1 shows the difficulty of effective study of health-related programs because of the fractionation of activity and coordination at the city level.

TABLE 1—Competing Local and Federal Coordinating Agencies *

| Local coordinating agency | Federal coordinating agency |
| --- | --- |
| Community action agencies | OEO |
| Model neighborhood areas | HUD |
| Model neighborhood health programs | HEW & HUD |
| Comprehensive neighborhood health centers | HEW & OEO |
| Economic development districts | Commerce |
| Overall economic development program | Commerce |
| Cooperative area manpower planning system | Labor |
| Concentrated employment program | CEP |
| Comprehensive health planning agencies | HEW |
|  | OEO |
| Neighborhood service centers | HUD |
|  | Labor |
|  | HEW |

* *Toward Rationalization and Integration of Urban Health Bureaucracies,* J. L. Falkson, Demetrius Plessas, RHSMHA Reports, Vol. 86, No. 6, June 1971.

There is a continuing effort to provide top level coordination in Washington and at the regional level. At the local level, where services and activities take place, coordination all too often gives way to competition. Inputs, data, services, and needs all become badly complicated through such diversification. When one adds parallel municipal activities, and experimental community health services sponsored by yet another set of institutions, the search for definitive relationships becomes hopelessly complex.

The most important fact about inner city environmental quality that can be stated is that the aggregate effect of the environmental factors involved in inner city housing and its immediate neighborhoods is detrimental to health. One may then suggest that priority should be directed toward ways to effect change now without waiting for the results of research studies which might eventually identify and rank deleterious factors.

## Characteristics of Inner City Areas

The demographic, economic, and social conditions of urban America over the next twenty years will be characterized by a period of quickening technological and social change. The social dynamics that now operate in the urban areas of this country have important consequences for health maintenance and health improvement activities.

Low income groups are heavily concentrated in cities. The black communities in cities are segregated. The size of these communities in central cities is increasing and will continue to do so. The communication networks and political activities of these communities will have an increasing importance in environmental change in cities. The social and political activities organizing these neighborhoods will provide increased leverage for environmental change for its residents within the larger system. This will occur even in the absence of demonstrated causality between environmental and health factors. The developing political activity of inner city residents will have substantial effects on health programs, just as it will on housing and education.

The homogeneous character of the less advantaged, as seen by the outside, will be broken as individual, group, ethnic, and neighborhood identities shift from their seemingly helpless static condition in regard to entering the system. The shift will produce a vital, ego-asserting state regarding environmental needs and the means of providing for these needs.

At present roughly 69 percent of all families in the United States live in metropolitan areas, including about 31 percent who live in central cities and about 38 percent who live outside central cities; approximately 31 percent live in non-metropolitan areas. The overall distribution has not changed markedly since 1960, but the concentration of blacks in central cities has increased. The trend toward an increase in the size of small cities and suburbs and a decrease in rural areas does not alter the major distributional aspects. The major shift is in the distribution patterns of the black and white populations, as shown in Tables 2 and 3. The black and white populations have strikingly different distribution patterns.

## TABLE 2 *—Distribution of the Black Population

|  | 1960 | | 1970 | |
|---|---|---|---|---|
|  | Millions | Percent | Millions | Percent |
| Metropolitan residence | 12.8 | 68 | 16.8 | 74 |
| Inside central cities | 9.9 | 52 | 13.2 | 58 |
| Outside central cities | 2.9 | 15 | 3.7 | 16 |
| Non-metropolitan residence | 6.1 | 32 | 5.9 | 26 |

* 1970 Census of Population and Housing, U.S. Dept. of Commerce, Oct. 1971.

## TABLE 3 *—Distribution of the White Population

|  | 1960 | | 1970 | |
|---|---|---|---|---|
|  | Millions | Percent | Millions | Percent |
| Metropolitan residence | 106.3 | 67 | 121.2 | 68 |
| Inside central cities | 50.1 | 32 | 49.5 | 28 |
| Outside central cities | 56.3 | 35 | 71.8 | 41 |
| Non-metropolitan residence | 52.4 | 33 | 56.0 | 32 |

* 1970 Census of Population and Housing, U.S. Dept. of Commerce, Oct. 1971.

In 1970, 58 percent of the black population was living in central cities in contrast to 28 percent of the white population. This is an increase of 6 percent of the black population and a decrease of 4 percent of the white population. The black population in the central cities represents almost 21 percent of the total population of the central cities. These trends are expected to continue for the next decade or two; thus, the concentration of blacks in central cities will continue to increase.

The distribution of total low-income families by place of residence is proportional to the distribution of total United States families. Nearly one-third of the low-income families in the United States live in central cities. There are significant differences between the distributions of the non-white and the white low-income population by residence, with a heavy concentration (47%) of low-income non-white families in central cities.

As population growth continues, there is little or no unused land within city limits for new construction; land prices and construction costs will remain high. The resulting cost of renewal and redevelopment produces an income-correlated out-migration from central cities to less densely populated urban areas. These migrants are principally from lower-middle to upper-middle income classes; they are also white. Between 1960 and 1966, 1.2 million whites left the twenty largest central cities while 3.2 million blacks moved in.

Residential mobility is related to income among white families. At any income level white families can move to any area of the cities, suburbs, or towns they choose. The only constraint is ability to pay. So as white family income rises, moves to the suburbs or less densely populated urban areas are a question of personal choice for whites.

Black families, however, have and will continue to have to improve their economic status faster than their residential mobility. Blacks in cities will continue to live in black areas. As their percentage of the total city population rises, the pattern of residence will be expanding black areas growing outward from one or more centers. Where distance between centers is not great these areas will tend to become contiguous.

In planning for environmental work in the central cities, it is also important to understand the perceptions of the residents and the patterns of life. The degradation of the visible neighborhood environment is likely to cause misconceptions on the part of outside workers about the patterns of life inside the low-income areas of the central cities. The apparent decay or lack of concern may be misleading about the actual attitudes of inner city residents.

In northern cities, by 1970, the median income of black families was over $6,000 a year. More than three-quarters of the residents are motivated toward economic and social improvement. Migration forces, community organizations, voter registrations, and voluntary recognition of the power gained through self-selected residence and economic independence are important characteristics of inner city areas that will influence the life style of these communities over the next two decades.

Low-income inner city residents are block dwellers. Their interest in the physical features, facilities, and membership in a social network of an area, center around the block where they live, the stores they patronize, and the few institutions that have particular use for them. People tend to be concerned with a limited number of people in the area, but they are generally connected to groups in the larger neighborhoods by interacting social networks.

Low-income groups identify neighborhoods in a physical rather than social sense. Territory is the base of a poor society. People live where they do because of such reasons as convenience to work and local stores, low rents, proximity to public transportation, and social homogeneity. Where economic considerations allow, preferences for types of housing or areas is expressed; such alternatives, however, are not common. Long-term residence brings security from knowing the territory.

There is great variety or variability in the amount of esprit de corps and sense of community in low-income neighborhoods. The degree of this spirit is probably the key to improving micro-environmental conditions. The sense of community varies even within a single city from area to area. The major factors affecting this variation are the size of the area, its location, its physical and environmental characteristics, length of residence, incidence of home ownership, rentals, ethnicity, kinship ties, and freedom, or lack of freedom, of movement. When an area is physically separated from the surrounding area, when rents are low and fixed, when residence is stable, and there are internal voluntary associations, then the sense of local community approaches that of a village community. Even in those areas where some of these factors are lacking, a sense of territoriality develops which sets off the area from the rest of the city.

Low-income groups frequently view the world in terms of "we" and "they." "They" is the world of most public and private institutions, employers, professionals, middle-class city government workers, and, with few exceptions, middle-class society. "We" includes those people in local neighborhoods and, to a lesser degree, other poor people. Most agencies, including health and environmental agencies, are viewed as external to the local society. The staff are viewed as non-members of the neighborhood whose behavior is not influenced by the peer groups in the community. As a result, services may be used if they are considered necessary or desirable, and ignored or fought if they seek to change the group or community. For example, welfare is accepted and fought simultaneously in many communities where mothers try to optimize the service for their need but also try to eliminate as many aspects of the delivery of the service as possible, such as welfare workers in their homes.

There is a tendency among low-income residents toward evasion of government operations and institutions. This stems in a large part from historical experience. The result is often justified but leads to ill-understood reactions toward new institutions and services designed to help the residents. Furthermore, as part of their successful survival, low-income groups have established many kinds of informal institutions to deal with problems and conditions that they have not been helped with in the past. They are thus more independent of outside institutions than economic conditions alone would suggest.

The educational system in low-income neighborhoods is often at odds with the environment in which the children live. In most low-income neighborhoods, family and street-corner society teach children implicitly to be sensitive to people rather than ideas. In general, words are not used as concepts but rather to impress people and get things. The local environment teaches pragmatic, intuitive problem-solving rather than logic and reason. These factors and other circumstances of day-to-day living often make the educational system seem irrelevant to the children and the community at large. If external efforts, made to improve local environmental quality factors, are introduced in an educational mode, they are likely to fail.

Much low-income family behavior has a strongly pragmatic cast, essentially non-class and non-culture in its derivations. The diversity of low-income family behavior patterns across ethnic groups suggests that behavior patterns develop around problems which are frequently economically based, rather than built around ethnic or other subgroup distinctions. In general, the problems and the needs of low-income groups are more similar than unique or distinct among subgroups.

Economic factors are the major influence on life style among all low-income groups. Low wages, chronic unemployment and underemployment lead to low income. Lack of prosperity, ownership, absence of savings, absence of food reserves, and a chronic shortage of cash are the usual conditions of life. These conditions place severe restriction on all low-income groups in their efforts to operate within the larger system.

In summary, the changing demography and mobility patterns in the major metropolitan areas have, and will continue to have, a major impact on the quality of life in the inner cities. The migration to the suburbs, the industrial relocation, and the resultant shifts in commerce all tend to reduce the tax base of the central cities. With the shift in population, new patterns of housing emerge, age groups shift, and demands for health and welfare services increase drastically. Municipal service costs rise at the same time that the tax base is decreasing.

In addition, the new population does not have the knowledge of available services, and accessibility of these services is decreased. Further complicating the problem is the fact that the existing services were set up to handle a different and older set of problems. Municipal bureaucracy is slow to change, so that response to the new needs lags. In general, the new Federal programs have at best set up parallel programs and at worst competitive programs.

The Model Cities Program was addressed to a recognition of many of these problems. It has a broad base. Yet it does not seem to be affecting change where it matters—in the inner city. There are many reasons for its failure. In one sense it almost duplicates municipal planning and services for specific areas of the cities. The funding requirements resulting from the planning activities are enormous and unlikely to be realized, at least in the short run. In many places the leverage of the program was applied to urban renewal type activities. New sidewalks, sewers, and parking lots were constructed. All of these improved parts of the urban environment, but the impact on the residents is marginal. If this program is replaced with some form of revenue sharing, it will be difficult for the community to maintain even its limited voice in the allocation of the funds against the rising need for general municipal funds.

## A Program for Change

Any program for change in urban environments that will substantially improve the quality of life for the residents must include the residents in the planning and operation of the services. Similar words can be found in most of the Federal programs introduced in the last 5 to 10 years. What cannot be found are working examples, on any significant scale, where this approach has been implemented and has succeeded.* A new way must be found to organize the communities and the services so that effective planning and operation will occur. In effect, a new form of community organization with a new form of management must be found. To organize the task around improving environmental quality will be difficult, in contrast to public education for example, as so many more agencies and services are involved.

The primary concern of such a new community organization should be their own urban micro-environment, but the focus should not be concerned solely with the management of residual pollutants. As the example shows, the interdependencies of inner city problems require an approach which crosses the boundaries of various specific problems. In effect, the groups should constitute themselves as environmental quality organizations or perhaps even as quality-of-life groups. They could then work with the categorical agencies to define their problems and set priorities for the programs. Such community groups must work with the municipal environmental services, the housing agencies, the schools, the Model Cities Programs, the training programs, and all other agencies that affect the community's self-perception and its political actions.

The necessity for starting in advance of having a clear-cut understanding of the multiple causal relationships must be clearly understood. The reasons for this have been set forth earlier in this chapter. The objectives should be real problem solving for real people. At the same time, however, parallel research efforts should be undertaken on both the management systems and the health systems. There are two reasons for this. First, the process should evolve continually based on assessments of the efficacy of multiple activities. Second, as a better understanding of interdependencies and causalty evolves through research efforts, changes should be made in the setting of priorities and

* A useful example of the interdependencies of inner city problems, and the difficulties of effective community organization to deal with them, is the current difficulty in Boston of getting residents to evening meetings concerned with community problems. Many program activities have been established with community groups. These programs include welfare, education, housing, medical care delivery services, and others. Participation, originally strong, is now difficult to get. Since the resident members have to work during the day, the meetings must be held at night. However, many of the participants do not now dare venture from their houses to the meetings after dark—even if the distance to be traveled is only 2 or 3 blocks. The reason is simple: they are afraid of being assaulted and robbed. Police and community statistics show that the assailants are primarily drug addicts—and young. What is called a law-and-order problem is thus at some level a health problem. The net effect is a breakdown of community organizations painstakingly achieved. To complicate the problem even further, when a community group does manage to get together the only topic they want to discuss is drugs, regardless of the original purpose for the meeting.

the design of action programs. The research should be in the form of intervention and include community members with the representatives from the outside research institutions. The research institutions would then become part of the cooperative effort, as involved and committed as the residents. A successful approach will require a synthesis of technical, economic, environmental, social, health, and political factors. Successful intervention will also require simultaneous substantial investments of energies and dollars in the community organizing and intervention research. A design is suggested here for both action and research to give an operational framework.

The suggested approach would be derived from Paretian [1] environmental analysis, a method of analysis which has evolved through efforts of the Environmental Systems Program at Harvard University.[2] The method identifies decisions—technological solutions and social controls—for environmental problems that are Pareto-admissible, that is, decisions from which no modification can be made without making at least one party in the political process worse off. The analysis would focus on the problems of a local organization concerned with environmental quality—use of different zones of the environment, treatment or remedial requirements, setting of local quality standards, etc. The analysis predicts how the agency will operate in given circumstances and how its action will change when those circumstances change. It also assists the agency in making decisions that respond to the wishes of its constituency. In addition, it provides a structural framework in which the research workers and the community workers can organize their joint efforts.

The analysis identifies a set of Pareto-admissible decision vectors, any of which is a likely candidate for being the one actually selected. This set is much smaller than the set of all feasible decision vectors and shows the agency the range of choice of decisions that are economically and technically efficient, as well as practical from the political viewpoint. The end product is a set of technological solutions, with associated policies for environmental management. These solutions can be useful at the local level. They indicate to local authorities what data are pertinent and how the various elements interact.

This analysis requires no evaluations other than those of the people affected by the decision of the agency. Moreover, unlike benefit-cost

[1] Important concepts upon which this analysis depends were developed by Vilfredo Pareto (1848–1923), an Italian engineer, mathematician, economist, and sociologist.

[2] The seminal papers are Robert Dorfman, "General Equilibrium with Public Goods" in *Public Economics*, J. Margolis and H. Guitton, eds. New York: St. Martin's, 1969; Robert Dorfman and Henry Jacoby, "A Model of Public Decisions Illustrated by a Water Pollution Policy Problem" in *The Analysis and Evaluation of Public Expenditures: The PPB System, Vol. I*, A Compendium of Papers Submitted to the Subcommittee on Economy in Government of the Joint Economic Committee, 91st Congress, 1st Session, Washington, D.C.: U.S. Government Printing Office, 1969.

analysis it is explicitly noncommital with respect to the importance of different participants in projects for environmental control. It requires data upon which the people and the agency concerned base their evaluations and decisions, but unlike benefit-cost analysis it does not assume that anyone has a formula for overall social evaluation. The analysis does not yield a single final recommendation, but it does describe how the participants in a political process relating to environmental issues will interact to produce a decision, and which decisions can be expected to evoke the support and cooperation they need to be effective.

There are six basic steps in implementation of the analysis.

1. *Definition of the Decision.* The first step is to delineate the decision or set of decisions to be made by the community quality-of-life groups. Dimensions and boundaries of the decision space, within which a particular choice must be sought, are established. These include:

Physical system boundaries;

Environmental quality indices;

Policy instruments and control measures;

Constraints and factors beyond the control of the community group.

2. *Identification of Interested Parties.* The interests and concerns of affected parties are introduced into the analysis explicitly.

3. *Determination of the Technological Relations between Environmental Control Actions and Resultant Quality.* The scientific and technological knowledge of environmental processes are introduced into the analysis at this stage.

4. *Estimation of Net Benefit Functions.* A net benefit function is derived for each interested party. The relevant benefit and cost measures used are those perceived by the participants themselves. Transfer payments are considered explicitly.

5. *Determination of the Pareto-Admissible Frontier.* From the estimates of net benefit and the technological relations, it is possible to identify a range of Pareto-admissible outcomes that is likely to result from the decision processes within the community agency.

6. *Prediction and Prescription.* The solution to the prior five steps gives a range of environmental control measures that is Pareto-admissible. In these steps, the random probing vectors of step 5 can be weighted to reflect more nearly the relative political influence of the participants to further narrow the range of likely outcomes for the decision being considered.

This approach has a unique potential. It can have great utility to the decision agency itself (or to one or more of the interested parties) as a means of mapping out, in a consistent manner, the opportunities at its disposal and the implications of different alternatives. In framing the problem and in the preliminary screening of possible solutions, the analysts are led to consider a larger number of physical alternatives and a larger variety of technological solutions than in conventional analysis. At the same time many human factors largely ignored in conventional analysis can be considered.

By adopting this framework for both the community groups and the intervention research group, a high order of complementarity would be possible. The community group could handle all the steps with word models and numerical calculation. The parallel and participating research agency or group could develop the full mathematical richness of the analysis in a completely compatible form. Thus, the action and the research could contribute each to the other.

## References

Abrahams, Frederick F., "Sociology of Poverty." Course Outline and Annotated Bibliography, Department of Sociology, Brandeis, 1968.

Allport, Gordon W., The Nature of Prejudice, Cambridge, Mass., Addison Wesley, 1954.

Barresi, Charles, and John H. Lindquist, "The Urban Community Attitudes toward Neighborhood and Urban Renewal," Urban Affairs Quarterly, Vol. 5, no. 3, 278–290, March 1970.

Becker, H. S., "Education of the Lower Class Child." In: Gouldner, A. S., et al, Modern Sociology: An Introduction to the Study of Human Interaction, Harcourt, Brace, and World, 1963.

Bellush, Jewel, and M. Hausknecht, Urban Renewal: People, Politics, and Planning, New York, Anchor, 1967.

Berle, Beatrice B., 80 Puerto Rican Families in New York City: Health and Disease Studied in Context, New York, Columbia University Press, 1958.

Bernard, Jessie, Marriage and Family Among Negroes, Englewood Cliffs, N.J., Prentice-Hall, 1966.

Beshers, James, Urban Social Structure, New York, Free Press, 1962.

Bloombaum, Milton, "The Conditions Underlying Race Riots as Portrayed by Multi-dimensional Scologram Analysis: A Reanalysis of Liberson and Silverman's data," ASR:30:no. 1, 76–91, Feb. 1968.

Blumenfeld, Hans, "Criteria for Judging the Quality of the Urban Environment." In: The Quality of Urban Life, edited by Schmandt, H., and Bloomberg, W. Urban Affairs Annual Reviews, Vol. 3, 137–164, Sage Publications Inc., California, 1969.

Broady, Maurice, "The Social Context of Urban Planning," Urban Affairs Quarterly, Vol. 4, no. 3, 355–378, March 1969.

Brown, Claude, Manchild in the Promised Land, New York, Macmillan 1965.

Caplan, Nathan S., and J. M. Paige, "A Study of Ghetto Rioters," Scientific American, Vol. 219, no. 2, 15–21, 1968.

Caplovitz, David, The Poor Pay More, Free Press of Glencoe, 1963.

Chapin, F. S., and S. Weiss, "Livability of the City." In: Urban Growth Dynamics, F. S. Chapin (Ed.), New York, Wiley, 1962.

Clark, K. B. Dark Ghetto: Dilemmas of Social Power, New York, Harper, 1965.

Coleman, James S., et al. "Equality of Educational Opportunity," U.S. National Center for Education Statistics, U.S. Government Printing Office, Washington, D.C., 1966.

Conant, James B. Slums and Suburbs, New York, McGraw-Hill, 1961.

Davies, S. Clarence III, *Neighborhood Groups and Urban Renewal,* New York, Columbia University Press, 1966.

Downs, R. M., The Cognitive Structure of an Urban Shopping Center." In: *Environment and Behavior,* Vol. 2, 13–39, 1970, Beverly Hills, Calif., Sage Publications Inc.

Drake, St. Clair, and H. R. Canton, *Black Metropolis: A Study of Negro Life and Northern Cities,* New York, Harpers: New Series, 1945 and 1962.

Duhl, Leonard. *The Urban Condition,* New York, Basic Books, 1963.

Eddy, Elizabeth M., "Urban Education and the Child of the Slum," Project, Hunter College, 1965.

Fellman, Gordon, and Roger Rosenblatt, "The Social Costs of an Urban Highway: Cambridge and the Inner Belt Road." Unpublished paper, 1969.

Foley, Donald L., "The Use of Local Facilities in a Metropolis." In: Cities and Society, edited by P. K. Hiatt and A. J. Reiss, Free Press, Illinois, 1951, pp. 607–616.

Freeman, Howard E., J. Michael Ross, David Armor, and Thomas F. Pettigrew, "Color Gradation and Attitudes Among Middle-Income Negroes." ASR 31 no. 3, 365–374, June, 1966.

Fried, Marc, "Grieving for a Lost Home." In: *The Urban Condition,* edited by Leonard J. Duhl, pp. 151–171, 1963.

Fried, Marc, Progress Report and Study of Demographic and Social Determinants of Functional Achievement on a Negro Population, OEO, Div. Res. and Plans, April 22, 1968.

Fried, Marc, and Peggy Gleicher, "Some Sources of Residential Satisfaction in an Urban Slum," *JAIP,* Vol. XXVII, no. 4, Nov. 1971.

Galle, O. R., and K. W. Taeuber, "Metropolitan Migration and Interviewing Opportunities," ASR 31, no. 1, 5–13, Feb. 1966.

Gans, Herbert, "Planning and Social Life: Friendship and Neighbor Relations in Suburban Connecticut," JAIP, Vol. XXVII, no. 2, May 1961.

Gans, Herbert, "Subcultures and Class." In: Ferman, L. A., et al. "Poverty in America," Ann Arbor, University of Michigan Press, 1965.

Gans, Herbert, *The Urban Villagers Group and Class in the Life of Italian Americans,* Free Press, Glencoe, 1962.

Glazer, Nathan, and D. P. Moynihan, Beyond the melting pot: The Negroes, Puerto Ricans, Jews, Italians, and Irish of New York City. Cambridge, Mass., MIT Press and Harvard University Press, 1963.

Gordon, Margaret S., "Poverty in America," Proceedings and National Conference, 1965, San Francisco, Chandler.

Gottmann, Jean, "Environment and Ways of Life in the Modern Metropolis." In: *The Quality of Urban Life,* edited by Schmandt, H., and W. Bloomberg. *Urban Affairs Annual Reviews,* Vol. 3, 61–94, 1969, California, Sage Publications Inc.

Gross, Bertram M. "The City of Man: A Social Systems Reckoning." In: *Environment for Man: The Next Fifty Years,* edited by William R. Iwald, Sr. Bloomington, Indiana University Press, 1967, pp. 136–157.

Handlin, Oscar, "The Newcomers: Negroes and Puerto Ricans in a Changing Metropolis," Garden City, Doubleday, 1962.

Hannah, John A. et al., "Racial Isolation in the Public Schools," U.S. Commission on Civil Rights, U.S. Government Printing Office, 1967.

Hartman, Chester, "The Limitations of Public Housing," *JAIP,* Vol. XXIV, no. 4, November 1963.

Harvard Business School, "Roxbury Development Corporation and New England Community Development Corporation." Mimeographed.

HAEYOU (Harlem Youth Opportunities Unlimited, Inc.), "Youth in the Ghetto: A Study of the Consequences of Powerlessness and a Blueprint for Change," New York, Harlem Youth Opportunities Unlimited, Inc., 1964.

61

Heller, Celia S., "Mexican American Youth. Other Youth at the Crossroads." New York, Random House, 1966.

Hunter, David R., *The Slums: Challenge and Response*, Free Press, Glencoe, 1964.

Irelan, Lola, (Ed.) Low Income Life Styles, U.S. Department of Health, Education, and Welfare, U.S. Government Printing Office, Washington, D.C., 1966.

Jacobs, Paul, *Prelude to Riot—A View of Urban America from the Bottom*. Random House, 1966.

Kain, John F., and Joseph J. Persky, "Alternatives to the Gilded Ghetto," *The Public Interest*, 14:7487, Winter 1969, N.Y. National Affairs, Inc.

Keller, Suzanne, *The Urban Neighborhood: A Sociological Perspective*, New York, Random House, 1968.

Kriesbug, Louis, "Neighborhood Setting and the Isolation of Public Housing Tenants," *J. of the American Institute of Planners*, Vol. XXXIV, No. 1, 1968, Washington, D.C.

Lamanna, Richard, "Value Concensus Among Urban Residents," *JAIP*, Vol. XXX, no. 4, November 1964.

Langner, T. S., and S. T. Michael, *Life Stress and Mental Health*, Glencoe, Free Press, 1963.

Leacock, Eleanor, "The Culture of Poverty: A Critique," New York, Simon and Schuster, 1971.

Leacock, Eleanor, "Distortions of Working—Class Reality in American Social Science," *Science and Society*, 31:1–21, 1967, New York, Science and Society, Inc.

Lee, Terence, "Urban Neighborhood as a SocioSpatial Schema," *Human Relations*, 21:241–268, London, Plenum Press, April 1968.

Lefcowitz, Myron J. "Poverty and Negro-White Family Structures," Unpublished manuscript, 1965.

Lenman, Paul, "Individual Values, Peer Values and Subculture Delinquency," IFSA, 33:219–235, April 1962.

Lewis, Hylan, "Culture, Class, and Family Life Among Low Income Urban Negroes." In: Employment Race and Poverty, A. M. Ross, (Ed.), New York, Harcourt, Brace, and World, 1967.

Lieberson, Stanley, and Arnold R. Silverman, "Precipitants and Underlying Conditions of Race Riots," *ASR*, 30:6, 887–898, Dec., 1965.

Liebow, Elliot, *Tally's Corner: A Study of Negro Streetcorner Men*, Little, Brown, Boston, 1967.

Long, Norton E. *The Policy*. In: "The Local Community as an Ecology of Games," Chapter 10, Chicago, Rand McNally, pp. 139–155, 1962.

Mann, Peter H. "The Concept of Neighborliness," *American Journal of Sociology*, Vol. 90, no. 2, 163–168, Sept. 1954.

Marquis, Stewart, "Ecosystems, Societies, and Cities," *American Behavioral Scientist*, 11:6, 11–15, July-Aug. 1968.

Michelson, William, "An Empirical Analysis of Urban Environmental Preferences," *JAIP*, Vol. XXVII: No. 6, Nov. 1966. 3M

Miller, S. M. "Poverty and Self Indulgence: A Critique of the Non-Deferred Gratification Pattern." In: "Poverty in America," L. A. Freeman et al., Ann Arbor Michigan Press, 1965.

Moguy, John, *Family and Neighborhood*, London, Oxford Press, 1956.

Moynihan, Daniel P. "Education of the Urban Poor," Cambridge, Mass., Harvard Graduate School of Education Association Bulletin XXI, No. 2, 1967.

Moynihan, Daniel P., The Negro Family: The Case for National Action, Washington, D.C., U.S. Department of Labor, 1965.

Parr, A. E. "Psychological Aspects of Urbanology," *Journal of Social Issues*, Vol. 22, no. 4, 39–45, 1966.

Perlman, Robert, and David Jones, Neighborhood Service Centers, Washington, D.C., U.S. Dept. of Health, Education and Welfare, U.S. Printing Office, 1967.

Rainwater, Lee, "Crucible of Identity: The Negro Lower-Class Family." In: Daedalus, Vol. 95: Richmond, Va., American Academy of Arts and Sciences, 1966.

Rainwater, Lee, "The Problem of Lower-Class Culture," Pruitt-Igoe Occasional Paper, St. Louis, Mo., Washington University, 1966.

Rainwater, Lee, "Poverty and Deprivation in the Crisis of the American City," Pruitt-Igoe Occasional Paper 9, Washington University, St. Louis, Mo., 1966.

Riessman, Frank, et al., *Mental Health of the Poor: New Treatment Approaches for Low-Income People,* Glencoe, Free Press, 1964.

Rodman, Hyman, "Middle Class Misconceptions about Lower-Class Families." In: Blue Collar World, by A. B. Shostak and W. Gomberg, Englewood Cliffs, N.J., Prentice Hall, 1964.

Schorr, A. W. *Poor Kids, A Report on Children in Poverty,* New York, Basic Books, 1966.

Schorr, A. "Slums and Social Insecurity: An appraisal of the effectiveness of housing policies in helping to eliminate poverty in the U.S." U.S. Department of Health, Education and Welfare, Social Security Administration, 1963 and 1965.

Schwartz, M., and G. Henderson, "The Culture of Unemployment: Some Notes on Negro Children." In: "Blue Collar World," by A. B. Shostak and W. Gomberg, Englewood Cliffs, N.J., Prentice Hall, 1964.

Seeman, Melvin, et al. "Community and Control in a Metropolitan Setting." In: *Race, Change, and Urban Society,* edited by Orleans, P., and W. Ellis. *Urban Affairs Annual Review,* Vol. 50, Sage Publications, Inc., California, 1971, pp. 423–450.

Sommer, Robert, "Man's Proximate Environment." *J. Social Issues,* Vol. 22, no. 4, 59–70, 1966.

Surkin, Marvin, "The Myth of Community Control: Rhetorical and Political Aspects of the Ocean Hill-Brownsville Controversy," In: *Race, Change, and Urban Society,* edited by Orleans, P., and W. R. Ellis, Vol. 5, *Urban Affairs Annual Reviews,* California, Sage Publications Inc., 1971, pp. 405–422.

Suttles, Gerald D., *The Social Order of the Slum,* Chicago, University of Chicago Press, 1968.

Taeuber, Karle E., and F. Alma, *Negroes in Cities: Residential Segregation and Neighborhood Change,* Chicago, Aldine, 1965.

Tuek, Herman, "Interorganizational Networks in Urban Society: Initial perspectives and comparative research," *American Sociological Review,* 35:1–18, Feb. 1970.

U.S. Department of Housing and Urban Development, "Improving the Quality of Urban Life: A Program Guide to Model Neighborhoods in Demonstration Cities," Washington, D.C., 1966.

Warner, W. Lloyd, and Paul S. Lunt, *The Social Life of a Modern Community,* Yankee City Series, Vol. 1, New Haven, Yale University Press, 1941.

Watts, L. H., et al., "The Middle-Income Negro Family Faces Urban Renewal." For the Department of Commerce and Development, Commonwealth of Mass., Boston, 1964.

Wilson, James Q., "Planning and Politics—Citizen Participation in Urban Renewal," *JAIP,* Vol. XVIX, no. 4, 1963.

Wilson, James Q. "Urban Renewal: The Record and the Controversy," Cambridge, MIT Press, 1969.

Wilson, James Q. "The Urban Unease: Community vs. City," *The Public Interest,* 12:25–39, Summer 1968, N.Y. National Affairs Inc.

Winkel, G. H., R. Malek, and P. Thiel, "The Role of Personality Differences in Judgments of Roadside Quality," *Environment an Behavior,* 1:199–223, 1969, Beverly Hills, Sage Publications, Inc.

# Chapter IV

# The Effects of the Residential Environment on Health and Behavior: A Review

Stanislav V. Kasl

## The Scope of this Review

It is the intent of this report to review the English-language literature pertinent to the general question: what is known about the effects of the residential environment on health and behavior? The emphasis will be on summarizing and integrating the empirical evidence. In addition, I shall try to place this evidence in a theoretical and methodological perspective which would best illuminate the limitations of past studies and would point to the type of research which needs to be done in the future.

In a far-ranging literature survey of this kind it is necessary to tell the reader what material will be included and what will be excluded. In general, I intend to deal with the physical aspects of the residential environment (i.e., the physical dimensions which describe housing and the neighborhood), and with the link to physical and mental health and to social functioning. Specifically *excluded* will be the following areas:

1. All of the animal literature on effects of physical environment, particularly crowding; *(1–7)* the major reason for excluding this material is that it is not clear which results, if any, can be generalized to human beings. This is especially true because many of the animal studies suggest that variables characterizing the social relations among animals mediate the effects of the physical environment. *(8)* It is, of course, possible that certain segments of the animal literature, such as that which deals with effects of sensory restriction-enrichment of the organism's early environment, *(9, 10)* will have direct applicability to humans. Thus, right now, the animal literature is best viewed as a source of hypotheses; but then, the literature on human residential environment is certainly not lacking in hypotheses, speculations, and suggestive findings.

2. The literature on the purely social environment without any obvious linkage to the physical environment: for example, marital status and various family structure variables bear a reliable relationship to health, (11, 12) but no aspect of the physical environment appears to be involved. The mere presence of other people (as spectators or co-actors) increases the individual's general arousal level, (13) and the arousal is greater if one is working with strangers rather than friends; (14) but here again there is no contribution from the physical environment. Other variations in the environment, such as type of shift at work, (15, 16) also have health consequences, but the link to the physical environment, if any, is unclear. It must be remembered, however, that these purely social-environment variables can still mediate or modify the effects of the residential environment. For example, a certain housing condition may have particularly deleterious effects on individuals living alone, or noise in an apartment building can be particularly disturbing to someone who works a nightshift.

3. The literature representing the domain of environmental biology, physiology, and psychology; this includes the experimental work on immediate effects of such aspects of the ambient environment as heat, cold, sound, light, and radiation, as well as effects of unusual environments, such as high altitude, weightlessness, acceleration, and vibration. (17–22) This literature deals primarily with immediate, short term effects under controlled laboratory conditions and its relevance to housing rests primarily with its contribution to setting housing standards. (20) It is frequently concerned with establishing limits of human tolerance and, thus, tends to be outside the usual range of variation represented by adequate-inadequate housing. The present review will also omit any specific consideration of effects of air and water pollution. This is not to deny, however, that air pollution may be a correlate of poor housing, i.e., urban areas which have poor housing may also have high air pollution.

## Introduction to the Problem

In American society today, the concern with environmental quality is an unmistakable component of our weltschmerz, and such words as "crisis" and "national mission" are liberally invoked. (23, 24) Upon closer scrutiny, however, this heightened consciousness of the inadequacy of our environment contains surprisingly little concern with human health consequences—either because the link to health is presumed to be obvious and fully established, or because the concern is with the esthetic quality of our surroundings and with man's degradation of the natural environment. In contrast, the interest in residential environment has a long history (25) characterized by a continued interest in establishing empirically a link to health and well-being.

Until recently, social scientists (especially psychologists) have shown relatively little interest in the physical environment (26, 27) and, therefore, have contributed only modestly to building the link with health and well-being. Their dominant interest is and has been in the social environment. A few small examples will suffice: a) a recent attempt to understand the human consequences of impending disasters (28) shows a total disinterest in considering any environmental variables. b) a recent comprehensive review of correlates of personal happiness (29) establishes no links to dimensions of the physical environment. c) a comprehensive review of effects of malnutrition on mental development (30) concludes that "disregard for ecology of malnutrition . . . has made it impossible to assess effects on performance on developmental tests."

Some writers have basically rejected the viewpoint of ecological determinism, especially the naive version of it which presupposed direct effects of the physical environment on man. Gans (31) talks of the failure of physical planning, while Blumenfeld (32) clearly believes that the social environment and cultural variables, not the physical environment, are the causal variables. Dubos is another author who has given increasing emphasis to the social environment at the expense of the physical environment. (33, 34) (See Abu-Lughod (35) for a historical account of the rise and fall of ecological determinism.)

However, there are many writers left who espouse the position of ecological determinism, in one form or another, and some of them have generated a large speculative literature. Psychiatrists in particular have been interested in "psychiatric architecture" and in the possibility of designing mental hospitals in a way which would mitigate some of the deleterious effects of institutionalization on inpatients. (36–41) This literature is immensely interesting and rich in intuition, insightful observations, and challenging hypotheses. In some instances, it represents a solid framework upon which to build a theory of how the physical aspects of an institutional setting can modify the behavior of a particularly vulnerable group of human beings. Needless to say, this literature is quite devoid of research findings in support of the many propositions. The same kind of psychiatric orientation applied to designing whole cities has been less successful; for example, Alexander (42) reduces the problems of mental health to one of "intimate contacts" between people and then goes on to speculate which types of housing characteristics will optimize intimate contact. Such approach is a good example of what has been labelled as naive ecological determinism.

Close on the heels of the speculative literature are the publications which deal with standards and recommendations for the residential environment. The World Health Organization and the American

Public Health Association are the two organizations which have been active in this field. (*43–46*) These recommendations are probably the best that can be offered at the moment, even though they do seem to suffer from a lack of input from social scientists and from users. They are a mixture of a) extrapolations from research data (from epidemiology and public health, from environmental biology and physiology, from engineering, and occasionally from housing and health studies); b) consensus of experts (i.e., the committee which wrote them) regarding good practice; c) standards pulled out of thin air; and d) quasi-guidelines where some undefined word, such as "adequate," carries the whole burden of the recommendation. For our purposes, these standards and recommendations, when juxtaposed to a comprehensive review of the effects of the residential environment, become a useful guideline for needed future research.

### Previous Reviews and the Organization of the Present Report

The number of previous reviews and annotated bibliographies (*25, 26, 47–60*) testifies to the great interest in the effects of the residential environment. All of these reviews, of course, do not examine the same literature, are not equally comprehensive, critical, and probing, and are variously out of date. What one learns from these reviews can be summarized as follows:

1. The authors exhibit highly varying degrees of conviction that the evidence they reviewed establishes a causal link between housing and health and behavior.

2. All appear to be prepared to accept the force of purely logical arguments in lieu of empirical evidence; that is, certain processes linking housing conditions and health are believed to be so obvious and so well understood that empirical evidence is unnecessary, viz. peeling lead paint and lead poisoning, or presence of rats and rat bites. One article (*60*) puts it quite admirably: "By deductive reasoning, a strong relationship between housing and health can be established." The trouble is that there is no one list of the processes which one may consider beyond need for empirical confirmation.

3. As a variation on the previous point, the reviewers are also willing to accept the proposition that "extremely poor" housing, not frequently found in the United States, does affect health and behavior perceptibly. The trouble with this position is that a) "extremely poor" remains undefined, and that b) one still needs to determine, empirically, the point on the dimension where, in different cultures and societies, housing becomes "extremely poor" so that it has obvious health consequences.

68

4. Most authors are aware of the difficulty of drawing causal inferences from evidence which is overwhelmingly correlational and in which a whole host of inter-related variables are at play.

5. Many reviewers point to the need for analyzing and specifying the components of substandard housing and for tracing separately for these components the effects on specific aspects of health and behavior.

6. One author (25) argues for a stronger historical perspective on certain associations between housing and health; that is, an association such as that between poor housing and turberculosis may not be replicated at a later point in time because of possible changes in the nature and distribution of the disease, in medical care, and in components of poor housing.

The present report is concerned with the effects of the physical aspects of the residential environment on physical and mental health and on social functioning. Residential environment refers to the living unit, the immediate surroundings, and some related community services and facilities. Specific components of the residential environment which are of interest include: space within the living unit and division of living space, hidden spaces within building, indoor and outdoor recreation areas, sanitary facilities and water supply, weather protection and heat and noise insulation, neighborhood circulation patterns, neighborhood facilities and services, proximity of living unit to sources of noise and fumes, such as industries and airport, and so on. However, despite this listing of components of the residential environment, we shall look primarily at global contrasts between "good" and "poor" housing, because this is what the overwhelming majority of studies have done.

The report is organized around the following topics:

(1) urban ecology: studies of contrasting areas of city; (2) neighborhood studies of social interaction; (3) studies of correlates of certain physical parameters of housing; (4) effects of voluntary rehousing; (5) effects of involuntary relocation, including institutionalization; (6) studies of housing needs and satisfactions, of housing attitudes, preferences, and perceptions; (7) effects of variations in the proximate environment on short-term behavior; (8) theoretical and methodological commentary; (9) conclusions and recommendations.

## Urban Ecology

The basic strategy of these studies is quite simple and consists of utilizing two sources of data: a) census-type data on characteristics of individuals and of their housing, aggregated over areas of city such as census tracts; b) institution or agency data about the frequency and distribution of some disease or social pathology. The data analysis is then oriented toward isolating the differentiating characteristics of census tracts which yield high vs. low rates of the disease or pathology. (There are some variations on and embellishments of this design which shall be noted below.) The design is simple, and the study is fairly inexpensive, but the price in terms of interpretability of results, as we shall see, is a steep one.

Studies dealing with physical health variables permit the following summary:

1. Census tracts characterized by greater preponderance of overcrowded living conditions (persons per room) have yielded a higher number of: hospital-treated cases of pneumococcus infection, (61) tuberculosis, (62–66) chronic conditions and cases of disability, (67) and diverse pathologies, such as suicide, infant mortality, mental disorders, and VD cases, (65, 66) However, two other studies have failed to establish the expected association between crowding and tuberculosis (68) or cases of rheumatic fever. (69)

2. The index of overcrowding is, of course, related to other indicators of inadequate housing. (62, 64) An attempt to disentangle (by means of partial correlations, computed on census tract statistics) correlates of dilapidated housing from correlates of overcrowding (65) suggests that the former is more strongly associated with TB cases and suicide, while the latter shows stronger associations with general and infant mortality and VD cases. Similarly, an attempt to distinguish crowding (persons per room) from density (population per net residential acre) suggests (66) that density is more strongly related of the two to a variety of dependent variables, such as general and infant mortality, VD cases, tuberculosis, mental hospital admissions, juvenile delinquency, and illegitimacy, with suicide as the only exception.

3. Greater prevalence of respiratory disease (winter morning cough) was found among mothers and children who lived in higher density areas of London; among fathers, smoking and social class were related to cough but not home residence. (70)

4. In a study of hospital admissions of children from a slum and a good residential area of Copenhagen, (71) the admission rates for slum children were about twice the rates for the good residential area. The differences were especially great for younger children (under three) and for upper respiratory and gastro-intestinal disorders. An analysis of mortality rates and home visits by physicians confirmed the rate differentials of the two residential areas.

5. Occasionally, a study yields a particularly striking illustration of the greater importance of the social over the residential environment. Rates of tuberculosis among people living alone as lodgers were found to be especially high, even as the study failed to demonstrate a clear gradient with overcrowding. (68) (To be sure, this finding is merely another confirmation of the association between morbidity and marital

70

status. (11, 12) A study of the distribution of tuberculosis cases in Seattle (72) revealed the expected higher rates in poor areas of the city for Whites only. Among Blacks, highest rates were found in the wealthier areas where the Blacks, however, are in a minority.

Studies dealing with mental health variables permit the following summary:

1. Areas of the city characterized by poor housing or low rental values and high rates of diverse correlated indices of "disorganization" (percentage of people living alone, percentage of multiple family dwellings, low normal family index, and so on) have higher rates of hospitalization for psychosis. (73–80) Those studies which concern themselves with specific diagnostic categories suggest that the above association holds for schizophrenia, (73, 74, 76, 80) cerebral arteriosclerotic and senile psychosis, (75) but not for manic-depressive psychosis; (74, 76, 80) however, this generalization does not always hold. (79) There are also some studies which did not find the expected association between schizophrenia and rental values or quality of housing. (81–83)

2. The concentric hypothesis (i.e., higher rates of psychosis the closer one gets to the downtown business-factory-hotel areas) was of great interest in the earlier studies, (74–76, 79) but presumably it is time-bound and will not hold whenever the downtown district or the city as a whole have undergone certain fairly radical changes (e.g., many high-rise and high-cost apartments in the downtown district). Such evolution of a city would also affect the relative strength of the associations of pathology rates with density vs. crowding, studied by Schmitt. (66)

3. The above findings are primarily based on first admissions to state mental institutions. (Private inpatients are often included, (74) but they are a very small proportion of the total cases studied.) However, one study which conducted a thorough search of all psychiatric facilities (73) still obtained the expected rate differential in schizophrenia between good and poor areas of the city. A study of rejection rates for mental health reasons among some 60,000 Army selectees (84) replicated on a non-hospitalized population the association with socioeconomic level of a community.

4. A number of studies have again demonstrated the importance of social environment as it interacts with the effects of the residential environment. Two studies (85, 86) suggest that schizophrenics living with their families show a roughly random distribution throughout the city, whereas schizophrenics living alone show more of the expected association with quality of housing and poor city areas. And several studies (74, 78, 80, 82, 83, 87) have provided good support for the "fit" hypothesis: that persons with a certain characteristic, who are living in an area where the characteristic is less common, will have higher rates of hospitalization for mental illness than people with that characteristic who are living in areas where the characteristic is more common. The char-

71

acteristics investigated have been race, (74, 78, 80) ethnic origin, (80, 82, 83) and a number of demographic variables such as age, occupation, and place of birth. (87) (Holmes' findings (72) regarding tuberculosis in Seattle also fit this pattern.)

Studies of juvenile delinquency (88–92) generally agree with the above picture drawn for mental illness: juvenile delinquency rates are higher in areas of high crowding and density, deteriorated housing and low rental values, proximity to industrial land usage, and racial heterogeneity. Chicago data for the period from 1927 to 1961 show that neighborhoods which have been part of the "Black Belt" for 30 years have declining rates while neighborhoods which have most recently become Black show increasing rates over the same period. The association between higher rates and greater proportion of foreign born population, found in the earlier studies, is no longer obtained in the more recent investigations. (93)

## Methodological and Theoretical Comments

How much have we learned about the effects of the residential environment by examining this urban ecology literature? The answer to this question has to be a discouraging "very little." In order to see how we arrive at this judgment, let us discuss briefly the shortcomings under two categories: those which can be corrected with better (albeit more expensive and more time consuming) methodology, and those which are inherent in the whole ecological approach.

One area in which improvement is possible is the operationalization of the dependent variable. There is no need to dwell on such obvious points as: (a) police and courts are not an unbiased source of juvenile delinquency data; (b) not all persons with a given physical or mental illness or handicap end up either being treated in a particular setting (inpatients in state hospitals) or being treated at all; (c) diagnostic information, particularly in the mental health area, has uncertain reliability and validity. Some of the remedies which can or have been used are: (a) multiple operationalism, using measures which, while none is completely adequate by itself, do not share the same biases and, thus, can cumulatively yield a trustworthy picture when they show similar results; (b) use of household surveys (67, 68) which do not introduce the self-selection bias inherent in the process of entering some form of treatment or coming to the attention of some agency; (c) a more thorough search for the cases of a particular pathology which one is studying, and a more rigorous review of quality of diagnostic information. (73)

There is an unfortunate tendency to believe that if one has obtained differential results, either with different subpopulations or with different diagnoses, one has a valid finding because whatever bias there is in one's measures must be a general one. In fact, the biases may be quite subtle and complicated. For example, it has been suggested (*94*) that city areas which differ on amount of ethnic or racial homogeneity may also differ on the degree of agreement about what constitutes abnormal behavior or on the tendency to reject the mentally ill. Or, to give another example: the determination of race or ethnic background may be done accurately on hospitalized cases, but census data may be systematically underestimating that racial or ethnic characteristic which is in a minority in that area of the city. In computing the rates of hospitalized cases for these areas, one gets an inflated estimate which is interpreted as a true difference. This could account for some of the findings reported above. (*72, 74, 78, 80, 82, 83*)

Another area in which improvement of the studies is possible is in the statistical treatment of the data—specifically, in a stronger commitment to multivariate techniques, but often simply carrying out additional analyses which control for a specific variable. One study (*95*) is a particularly good illustration of the complexity of results obtained when one analyzes psychiatric hospitalizations by sex, diagnosis, and private vs. public hospital, and relates them to several clusters of ecological dimensions (in this case, "socio-economic affluence," "young marrieds," "social isolation," and "social disequilibrium"). In general, what is desperately needed is to begin to disentangle the variables describing the residential environment from those which describe the social environment. For example, in the Alameda County health survey, (*67, 96*) the contrast between the poverty and non-poverty areas not only involves differences in housing but also in purely social variables, such as incomplete family index and divorced-separated—variables known to have health implications; (*11, 12*) And the only statistical control carried out in that study is totally insufficient, viz., the splitting of respondents into those who list their income as "adequate" vs. "inadequate" and calling it controlling for income.

Another inadequacy of statistical analysis resides in the nature of ecological correlations, (*97*) e.g., using the city tract or ward as the unit of analysis and then correlating pairs of averages or aggregate values. The most frequent problem with ecological correlations is that they grossly inflate the amount of association that exists between two variables, had these been computed on individuals. Under such circumstances, it is much preferable to examine the slope of the relationship and its steepness. Incidentally, working with slope should sensitize the researcher to the problem of non-linear relationships. For example, Brett and Benjamin (*68*) simply report their results as an absence of a gradient in tuberculosis morbidity with crowding. In fact, the relationship they obtained (when controlling for social class) appears to have both linear and non-linear components and the least crowded households do have the lowest morbidity.

However, there is a limit to which a sophisticated multivariate analysis can compensate for inherent limitations of design. Teasing out causal inferences from correlational data is a hazardous business (98–100) and many assumptions have to be imposed first. Thus, a hard look at the ecological studies reveals that they tell us only one thing with certainty: the geographical concentration of the visible cases of a certain pathology. This is useful information if one is going to build, for example, a mental health center and wants to minimize the travel time of the future clients.

The ecological studies also demonstrate that there is an intercorrelated set of variables, generally referred to as poverty, which can be used to characterize either individuals or areas of the city, and that when one selects either people or areas on the basis of one variable, the other variables come tumbling along. The correlates of poverty are many: race, age, education, work status, family structure, housing, nutrition, medical care, habits, attitudes, predispositions, and so on. All of this leads to most severe problems of interpretation. For example, the ecological data on juvenile delinquency have been interpreted in support of the disorganization-lack-of-soil-control hypothesis, the anomie hypothesis, and the culture conflict or delinquent sub-culture hypothesis. Similarly, the ecological data on mental illness have been interpreted (101, 102) within such diverse frameworks as social isolation, mobility, cultural change of cultural conflict, diverse social stresses, psychological frustration, self-selective in- and out-migration, and various "biases" inherent in the social class and cultural correlates of differential detection, diagnosing, and treating of persons with mental health problems. In short, when a large number of interrelated variables are at play, numerous interpretations are tenable.

Perhaps the most significant criticism which can be made of the ecological studies is that there is a general failure a) to state clearly what is the hypothesis which is being tested, b) to consider the various available research designs, and c) to show how and why the ecological approach is the most suitable one for dealing with the problem. For example, some studies appear to be testing the hypothesis that mental illness is more prevalent among the poor or the lower socio-economic classes. If this is the case, then a population survey (103) or an enumeration of treated cases in conjunction with a general population sample (104) seem to be the more suitable designs. Even a thoughtful investigator like Dunham (73) fails to make explicit the relationship between his specific hypotheses and the design he has chosen; and as Dunham's interpretations become progressively more complicated (muddled) and further removed from the evidence presented, the reader feels that the investigator has failed to draw the implications of the various features of the design.

It would seem that, in the long run, most investigations are seeking to identify factors which would be of etiological significance to some disease or pathology. These factors are presumably either characteristics of the person or of the environment in which the person lives (or of the interaction between the two), and the design should be such as to permit an evaluation of the role of these factors in the total etiological picture. If an ecological study uses person characteristics, aggregates them over areas of the city, and then treats them as environmental variables, we have a research design which is inherently ambiguous. For example, if one chooses areas of the city which are very high and very low on adult crime rates, and then discovers that the mental illness rates are correspondingly high and low, is one looking at an association between crime and mental illness in individuals, or is it because presence of crime creates a stressful environment which is pathogenic to the non-criminals? And, when selecting areas of the city along one dimension introduces a multiplicity of differences along correlated dimensions, then the ambiguity of the design is quickly multiplied. Beyond this, there are other sources of ambiguity, such as a) not having enough information about the movement of the population into and out of the areas, and b) the use of an average value to characterize all individuals living in a certain city area when that average still hides a good deal of heterogeneity of individual values for that area.

Finally, we might note that a most useful (and most rare) addition to the ecological approach is to collect, *in conjunction with* the health data and the area information, also data on the individuals' perceptions of their environment. Thus, one study (*105*) has collected blood pressure data on individual respondents, their subjective perceptions of their neighborhood, and objective information about the high and low "stress" areas.

### A Note on Rural-Urban Differences

A contrast of urban vs. rural places of residence is a natural extension of the urban ecology approach and as such, presents similar problems of interpretation. That is to say, the contrast contains in it not only differences in residential environment (known and unknown), but also in a host of other factors, such as education, occupation, physical activity, diet, availability of services, and so on, as well as some less obvious ones, such as interpersonal contacts, (*106*) and attitudes, values, and beliefs about medical services. (*107*) The data from the National Health Survey about rural-urban differences in general health characteristics, (*108*) specific indices of morbidity, (*109*) and specific conditions, (*110*) have, of course, high practical value for national medical planning, but otherwise most information about rural-urban health differences is inherently ambiguous from a theoretical or etiological

75

viewpoint. Consequently, below we shall only sketch briefly some of the findings which have been obtained.

Many studies (*111–115*) have generally shown lower rates of mortality, morbidity, and mental hospital admissions for persons living in rural areas. In addition, there is some evidence that rural death rate goes up as the proportion of rural area which is non-farm goes up. (*115*) Ecological analyses of counties on a state-wide basis (*113, 116, 117*) have replicated some of the correlates of poor housing, crowding, and social disorganization found in the urban ecological studies.

Frequently, the findings are more complicated and reveal the influence of social factors and the factors involved in migration from rural to urban settings. For example, studies of coronary heart disease in a rural state (North Dakota) (*112, 118, 119*) show higher rates for such groups as: a) sons of American-born fathers in urban occupations, b) white-collar workers of rural background, and c) those showing high occupational or geographically mobility. In general, the transition from rural to urban settings has been interpreted as representing cultural mobility (*118*) or cultural change, (*120, 121*) which presumably leads to cultural conflict, uncertainty about appropriate behavior, and severe demands for acculturalization, which, in turn, appear to have significant health consequences. (*120–125*) These data are also consistent with the observations that rapidly growing communities or suburbs will show a greater incidence of emotional disorders among women (*126*) and children, (*127*) higher rates of hospitalization for depressive disorder and of suicide, (*128*) and a different pattern of psychosomatic illnesses. (*129*) One may also recall here the previously discussed findings (*72, 74, 78, 80, 82, 83, 87*) regarding lower rates of physical and mental illness for individuals whose racial or ethnic characteristics are the same as for the dominant majority of individuals living in that area.

In short, the health studies dealing with the rural-urban continuum cannot tell us anything precise about the effects of the residential environment. This is not only because the rural-urban contrast is too global and involves too many variables which cannot be pinned down, but also because the picture is further muddied by factors associated with selective migration and by presumed health consequences of cultural change.

## Neighborhood Studies of Social Interaction

The literature which we shall be examining next deals with two broad issues: a) the nature of the slums and the life of the slum dwellers, and b) physical parameters (primarily distance) in social interaction. And, as before, we shall also be concerned with the role of social

76

factors which mediate the effects of the physical aspects of the neighborhood. The focus of this section is the neighborhood, a unit of analysis which we shall partly treat as a link between the urban ecology studies already examined and the studies of effects of housing and rehousing, to be examined below.

The traditional description of the slum areas of the city in the earlier urban ecology literature has been in terms of a number of interrelated variables reflecting poor housing, high rates of crime-delinquency-disease, and a high proportion of broken families and individuals living alone. The label most frequently applied to this cluster of variables was "social disorganization," a concept which in turn was used to account for the high rates of some pathology. However, studies of the slum community (130, 131) began to show that the slums were actually well organized, with a good internal structure—"a hierarchy of personal relations based upon a system of reciprocal obligations" (131). Evidence began to accumulate, showing that most slum dwellers are not newcomers or transients, (132) that they like their neighborhood much better than dwellers in public housing, (133) and that there is a strong sense of local spatial identity which is based on extensive networks of interpersonal contacts and overlapping role relationships, primarily within the family-kinship group and the street corner friendship group. (134, 135) In fact, some of the deficiencies attributed to large metropolitan areas, such as their "illegibility" and their lack of visible identity, (136) did not seem to apply to the slums.

In short, a different picture of the slums emerged: (a) The slums are not "disorganized," and the slum dwellers do not necessarily suffer from anomie. (b) The slum is a residential area in which a vast and interlocking set of social networks is localized. (c) The physical area has considerable meaning as an extension of home and is the focus of many positive feelings, including a sense of belonging. (d) Residential mobility is fairly low and the residents do not view themselves as living in a slum.

However, it is not clear how much validity and generalizability this ethnographic description of the slum communities has. It is clearly a sympathetic one, perhaps a bit nostalgic, and has served the good purpose of undermining some earlier preconceptions about slums. It has also been part of a useful argument against thoughtless, indiscriminate urban renewal. But better research techniques are needed (e.g., probability samples of households instead of the investigator's participant observation in the community) and a great variety of slums in different cities have to be studied before we gain a more accurate picture. For example, a survey of slum dwellers in Puerto Rico (137) revealed that, when asked about why they want to stay, reasons such as owning a house and good location were much more frequent than a feeling of belonging or liking neighbors. And the more recent studies have once

77

again begun to emphasize some of the obvious negative aspects of slums. Rainwater, *(138)* for example, discusses the very evident housing needs of the slum dwellers (enough space, absence of noxious and dangerous elements inside the house and in the outside environs, availability of minimum community services) and the great many sources of danger from both human and non-human sources which are present; (for a similar account of perceptions of neighborhood by dwellers of slums, see Harburg*(105)*).

Another important development in the literature on slums and slum dwellers has been to discard the implicit assumption that slum dwellers are a homogeneous group and to begin to develop a typology of slum dwellers. *(139–141)* Thus, Gans *(139)* talks about the "cosmopolites," the unmarried or childless, the "ethnic villagers," the "deprived," the "trapped," and the downwardly mobile; while Seeley *(141)* uses such categories as temporary and permanent "necessitarians" and temporary and permanent "opportunists." Thus far, such categories have evolved informally and good operational definitions are still lacking. However, there should be little doubt that in a study of effects of living in a slum, or effects of being relocated from one, some such typology will be needed for a better understanding of differences in impact.

In the long run, all of these developments have served to undermine the investigators' easy confidence in being able to detect and trace the consequences of the physical aspects of slum dwellings. Thus, the social disorganization hypothesis can no longer be applied uncritically; instead, one must determine the types of social controls which are actually present in the slums, and how they may lead to behaviors (crime and delinquency) which are considered deviant by the dominant society. Similarly, the social isolation hypothesis as an explanation of high rates of schizophrenia in poverty areas of the city can no longer be accepted uncritically, since it is no longer self-evident either that such isolation is indeed highly prevalent in those areas, nor that that form of isolation (as opposed to isolation which comes from rejection by significant others *(142)*) is truly of etiological significance in schizophrenia.

Let us now turn to studies which deal with the role of physical parameters of the neighborhood (primarily distance) in influencing social interaction. The first general conclusion which can be derived from this literature is that increasing physical distance is a powerful factor in reducing contact with relatives and existing friends; *(56, 143–145)* this conclusion applies to face-to-face contact as well as to telephone conversations and letters. *(143)* For example, Rosenberg *(145)* found that among a group of working class respondents, there was an average of 5 visits with close kin during the previous week, if they lived within the same block; if the distance was 6 blocks or more, the average frequency dropped to one visit during the previous week. It has also been shown *(147)* that a large proportion of marriages is between partners whose residences were close to each other. Incidentally, some authors, (35, 144) have raised the question whether the social contact which is studied in relation to proximity is friendship or merely superficial neighborliness .

Many more investigators, however, have emphasized that residential proximity affects social interaction only if there is social homogeneity among the neighbors. (35, 139, 144, 148–152) The dimensions along which homogeneity is important are: socio-economic status and its components, and variables related to the life cycle. (As we shall see later, these are also the major dimensions which influence individuals' preferences about type of housing and neighborhood.) In suburban communities, other dimensions of social homogeneity, such as values about child-rearing, leisure time interests, and general cultural preferences may also be significant in influencing social interaction. (144)

What happens when there is physical proximity but a lack of social homogeneity? Here, studies of planned communities show that propinquity alone is not sufficient to overcome the influence of socio-economic status on social interaction and friendship formation, and that obvious stratification takes place. (153–155) One author (150) has also suggested that the combination of physical proximity and social heterogeneity leads to more hostility among neighbors, but the evidence for this is not that compelling.

Of course, if we are dealing not with planned communities but the usual circumstances under which individuals make their housing choices, then spatial distance is the consequence of social distance; (156, 157) that is, studies of residential segregation show that occupational groups which are far apart in terms of conventional indicators of socio-economic status are also far apart spatially in the city.

The above discussion once again illustrates the interplay of social and physical variables. Physical proximity fosters social interaction provided there is social homogeneity. Moreover, certain groups are more dependent on proximity than others; namely, housewives with children, the old and the infirm, and those of lower social class. (144, 146, 150, 158) In addition, these studies also indicate that proximity is of greater importance in initiating contact than in maintaining friendships. Finally, a particularly complex interplay of factors is seen in the Rosenberg study: (159) in a given neighborhood, the greatest isolation from friends is experienced by older, poor men whose socio-demographic or racial characteristics are different from the dominant characteristics of the local residents of the neighborhood. Rosenberg calls this phenomenon "neighborhood contextual dissonance;" we have previously seen that this phenomenon is related to higher rates of physical and mental illness. (72, 74, 78, 80, 82, 83, 87)

Finally, we want to consider briefly the factor of distances from residence to neighborhood facilities. Because the proximity of services, such as shopping facilities and medical services, is of special importance to the elderly, (160, 161) much of the literature concentrates on them. Among the elderly, satisfaction with housing is more prominently dependent upon satisfaction with various aspects of the neighborhood rather than the residential unit, (160, 162) and distance to facilities is the most important aspect. At the moment, we know more about what managers of publicly supported housing projects think is important to the elderly (163) than what the elderly themselves say is important to them. However, there is no doubt that distance to grocery and to some form of transportation have an influence on the frequency and type of shopping, which in turn affect the adequacy of nutrition among the aged. (164) Similarly, the decline in church attendance among the elderly—even as their religious feelings and attitudes grow stronger— is largely due to problems of accessibility of the church. (165, 166) Schooler's survey work with the elderly, (167, 168) utilizing structured interviews, has identified through factor analysis a number of dimensions of the environment, of which distance to facilities and perceived convience of location of facilities appear as two related factors. (See Schooler's summary in first part of his Chapter IX below). Moreover, he has shown that these environmental variables have certain complex consequences: for example, the association between the amount of neighboring and visiting, and the degree of morale and happiness among elderly men depends on the relative distance from such services as transportation, the library, and major shopping centers. Thus, once again we find evidence for strong interaction between the physical-environmental and social factors.

## Correlates of Physical Parameters of Housing

In this section, we shall be reviewing studies which in one way or another have attempted to link some aspect of housing to physical and mental health and to behavior. The focal unit of these studies is the building or the apartment complex, not, as in the previous work, the neighborhood or the city census tract. However, there will be some overlap with the work already reviewed, because we shall still be interested in such associations as between poor housing and health, or between propinquity and social interaction.

The results based on the National Health Survey data (169–171) can be summarized as follows:

1. Households characterized by high crowding (persons per habitable room) had a) higher rates of the common communicable diseases of childhood, with the cases of these diseases also appearing at a relatively younger age, b) more "secondary" attacks of tuberculosis (given the presence of a "primary" case of tuberculosis in the household), c) higher

adult illness rates due to acute but not chronic conditions, with pneumonia and tuberculosis showing especially strong association; further analyses revealed that the association between crowding and disability due to illness was the strongest among those on relief or with very low income.

2. Absence of private (inside) flush toilets was associated with higher rates of disability from digestive diseases such as diarrhea or typhoid.

3. Disabling home accidents, especially for men, were more common in housing with low rental value. Other studies, specifically concerned with diarrheal diseases, (172–176) have repeatedly established a relationship between higher rates of disease and aspects of inadequate housing, such as lack of proper sanitary facilities and/or limited water supply.

It should be obvious that these correlational studies share certain weaknesses of design with the work reviewed earlier under the urban ecology heading. For example, even though the report analyzes a relationship between one particular aspect of housing (e.g., crowding) and health, selecting households on this one variable also pre-selects them on a whole host of other variables which relate to other aspects of poor housing, as well as to such socio-demographic and behavioral variables as education, income, employment status, intact family, personal hygiene, housekeeping efficiency, medical care, and so on. Studies of the health of the elderly in relation to the housing environment (177) suffer from even greater difficulties of interpretation since in that segment of the population, poor health can influence changes in housing and since there is a selective attrition due to the institutionalization of the elderly with severe disability or very poor health.

It might also be noted that aside from the problem of interpretation of the associations, we have also the issue of the magnitude of these relationships. For example, the data from the National Health Survey (171) show that the percentages of individuals experiencing a disabling illness for one week or more (age adjusted) go from 14.8% to 15.7% to 17.8% for the three ordered categories of degree of crowding. The previously mentioned Alameda County Health Survey (67) also showed small differences between the poverty and non-poverty areas; e.g., 46% vs. 38% for presence of one or more chronic conditions. It is, of course, possible that more refined analyses could reveal stronger associations.

There exists also studies which examine the health consequences of some more limited variations in the physical dimensions of housing, rather than the more typical global comparisons of adequate vs. inadequate housing. Negative findings were obtained in three studies which related: (a) living in one- vs. two- vs. three-apartment tenement houses to such morbidity indices as hospital admissions, visits to doctors, and doctors calling at home; (178) (b) living in high vs. low rise apartments and visits to surgery or home calls for wives and children of British soldiers; (179) (c) living in open bay vs. closed bay Air Force barracks and incidence of some common respiratory diseases. (180) The one study which did obtain significant differences (181) compared two groups of families of British soldiers stationed in Germany: those living in flats and those living in houses. Women and children living in flats had considerably higher rates of visits to physicians, especially for respiratory conditions and what the physicians labelled as "neurotic" complaints. No differences were obtained on rates of hospitalization or of accidents. Since the largest differences in rates were obtained for mild, common complaints, there is good reason to believe that the dependent variable reflected illness behavior (182) much more closely than true morbidity.

The last study (181) is worth an additional comment because it represents a truly excellent non-experimental research design. The two groups of families were comparable on all the significant dimensions—husband's occupational status, stage of life cycle, adequacy of medical care—except the one under study, flats vs. houses. Complete medical data were available on all the subjects because they had no access to other sources of medical care. And the study excluded those families who lived in one of the two types of dwelling by request rather than by chance. The moral here is that good non-experimental designs which permit strong causal inferences are feasible, provided investigators are sufficiently diligent in searching for naturally equivalent groups who came to live in contrasting residential environments more by chance than choice.

A number of writers have been specifically concerned with effects of housing on children and child development. Some reports are clinical case histories (183) which emphasize the deleterious effects of crowding on privacy, consistency of child care, and competition between parents and grandparents. Other reports are reviews of the literature (26, 58) which emphasize the lack of control parents have over their children when they live in crowded conditions or in high rise apartments. This particular conclusion, however, appears to be more an intuitive observation than a summary of research findings. And it would certainly be difficult to disentangle effects of housing from social class differences in child rearing practices. The empirical studies which have been done in this area permit the following conclusions:

1. The negative relationship between amount of crowding and total school achievement is quite small when one controls for social class and race. (184) A more telling conclusion comes from a study (185) which found that physical crowding and lack of privacy were not an important influence on school achievement; rather, it was how the space at home was used, i.e., setting aside times when a particular room was devoted only to quiet pursuits.

82

2. Even when the study fails to control for other variables, the negative association between adequacy of housing and school progress is small (*186*) (gamma = −.20, as computed from data presented by the author).

3. A more satisfactory study of effects of housing compared low rent public housing pupils with controls living in slums. (*187*) The two groups were initially comparable on age, race, IQ, size of family, family stability, and occupation of head of family. The results revealed that the public housing sample was somewhat superior on a standardized IQ test, on grades in reading and arithmetic, and on teachers' ratings of anti-social behavior. Interestingly, there were no differences in performance on standardized reading and arithmetic tests, and the slum sample appeared superior on physical growth and development.

4. Children of pre-school age living on upper floors of high rise buildings stay in open fresh air for considerably shorter periods of time and are delayed in motoric development. (*188*)

In one study with a controlled research design, using ex post facto data, 83 families which came before community case work agencies or courts with family problems and conflicts (e.g., between parents and child, among siblings, or between parents), were compared to a control sample of 83 families (paired for household size, age and sex distribution, and group-matched for nationality, occupation, rent, and mobility), who had not sought outside help for such problems. It was found that, with the exception of one factor which is a mixture of physical design and socio-cultural characteristics, both samples were living in housing with about the same characteristics of standardness-substandardness, as measured by the APHA Appraisal Method for Measuring the Quality of Housing. The exception was that the "experimental" group had experienced significant and meaningful negative differences from the control in any measure of density in the dwelling or the neighborhood. The density characteristics found significant were total space in the dwelling, number of rooms dividing it, amount of space heated, total space used in common, and the three elements in the environmental index of the neighborhood concerning the number of interacting individuals, distance to park, and the residential versus mixed land-use of street. This pilot study in an urban Massachusetts area generated three hypotheses for further research:

1. "A physical characteristic of housing can be an element . . . related to social disorganization only if it is a factor in a density ratio."

2. "Social density, definable in terms of social or cultural roles simultaneously acting in given physical space," beyond some threshold contributes to conflicts and stress.

3. This "over-density presented by usage of housing or neighborhood space may aggravate or accelerate, not cause or motivate, any tendency to disorganization in a personality or group."

It was noted that, if the first hypothesis is supported by later research, "it would mean that certain physical elements (of environment), having little or no symbolic value, may operate as parts of social action systems in two distinct relational contexts, distance and density. In regard to the physical distance context, it was noted that studies of S. A. Stouffer, R. K. Merton and L. Festinger indicate that the time-distance from one's dwelling bears an inverse relationship to one's use of a neighborhood facility. "The other context would be density in terms of the number of people and their goals (or activities) operating in given physical space at a given time." This study suggests that physical over-density of persons per unit or dwelling space is not as relevant to health and disorganization as social or role over-density, i.e., activity over-crowding, which relates to cultural use of space. (189)

That suggestion seems to be borne out by excellently probing interviews in three surveys reported from Hong Kong in which, compared to the Massachusetts study, a combination of much greater physical density with markedly less density of social roles or cultural activities in the dwelling appeared to have no adverse relation to health and inter-family relationships, with the following exceptions. Relational problems or emotional strain were found in respect to each of the following: households containing non-kin members, families living on upper floors of high-rise apartments, families where parents lost knowledge of where-abouts and control of children by encouraging them to leave the dwelling after eating or sleeping, and (in forty-nine percent of married households), total discouragement of friendship practices among neighbors and friends." (189a)

Let us now turn to studies which are concerned with effects of housing on social interaction. As in the previous section on neighborhood studies of social interaction, here, the major concern of studies is with the effects of physical proximity. There are several reports which are specifically concerned with inter-racial housing and the consequences for interaction and attitudes. (190–193) In general, these studies agree that physical proximity between White and Negro residents leads to more contact, both casual and intimate, and to more positive attitudes toward Negroes, and fewer negative sterotypes about them, among the Whites. (Apparently, the Negro residents were not asked about their perceptions of Whites). However, a comparison of the self-concepts among Negro tenants living in low income housing, some in integrated sections and some in segregated sections, failed to reveal any effects of integration. (193)

These studies were not longitudinal investigations in which families were assigned randomly to integrated housing. Thus, it is possible that initially favorable attitudes toward Negroes were antecedent to the Whites' desire to live in integrated housing and to their intentions to engage in inter-racial activities. Two of the studies (190, 192) present some data which tend to refute this possibility, but the design doesn't permit a convincing rejection of this alternative. It is also interesting to note that the authors of both studies acknowledge the possibility that their findings need not be generalizable to the typical, community-wide housing—partly because of the unmeasured effects of the prestige of the housing authority which, in setting up the inter-racial housing, appeared to legitimize and support inter-racial contact. This possibility is supported by the results of a community study of residential contact and attitudes toward Negroes, (194) which obtained some rather complex relationships. Prejudice of white residents living in white neighborhoods was curvilinearly related to distance from the integrated residential area, with the least prejudice found among those living the closest and the farthest away. But an indirect, more subtle measure of prejudice and concern with the racial issue revealed the highest concern among those living closest to the integrated area. And a survey of Kansas City residents (195) suggested that Whites are more threatened by residential proximity of Negroes than by personal-social closeness.

When one is dealing with a highly homogeneous population, then residential proximity is a powerful determinant of social contacts and friendship formation. (196) The authors of this well-known study of married student housing at MIT also note that aside from physical distance, "functional distance" also influences friendship formation; that is, those aspects of the physical layout of the buildings and of the facilities therein which generate passive contact between neighbors also increase the likelihood of friendship. In another study of a homogeneous population, (197) recruits on an Air Force base, it was found that in long, open barracks, the recruits knew names of more people than in partitioned barracks, but in the latter they had more friends or "buddies." Inasmuch as assignment to barracks was pretty much random, this difference may be safely attributed to the physical variation in housing. The authors speculate that the closed barracks generated greater cohesiveness within the cubicles.

Among the aged, spatial proximity is an important determinant of social interaction, (198) especially if the elderly individual is less competent and reports low levels of well-being. (199) The reduction in competence heightens the elderly person's dependence on external conditions. In a study of Cleveland apartment buildings which varied in the proportion of older tenants living in each one, Rosow (200) found that the working class elderly person, in contrast to the middle class one, exhibits greater dependency on spatial proximity for friendships. As a result, he is more sensitive to the variation in the age composition of the residents of the apartment building in which he lives: the greater the density of age peers, the more friends he has. Those who are also more sensitive to such age peer density are women, unattached individuals, the very old, and those middle class individuals who have recently experienced some "loss" such as retirement, widowhood, or illness. In short, these studies of the elderly again show the interplay of the physical environment factors and the social factors in influencing behavior.

### Effects of Voluntary Rehousing

Most of the studies which have been examined thus far represented inadequate research designs which made it very difficult to pinpoint the effects, if any, of the residential environment. However, the study of people moving from one residential environment to another represents a "natural experiment" which potentially can yield much superior study designs. The ideal here is a longitudinal investigation in which data are secured before the move and on several occasions after the move; moreover, a control group is available and the allocation of subjects to the control or the rehoused group is done with a minimum of self-selection bias.

As we shall see below, not many studies approach this ideal. The weakest ones collect only after-the-move data on rehoused subjects; some studies add to this retrospective accounts about the subjects' situation before the move. Better studies seek comparison groups of respondents who were not rehoused, or they collect data on the respondents prior to the move. However, even when the research design approaches the practical ideal, it retains one major limitation: the rehousing is a change not only in the residential environment, but also in a possibly large number of known and unknown factors as well. Schorr, (58) for example, points out that moves to better housing for poor people are frequently accompanied by: segregation, unfamiliar surroundings and unknown new requirements, inadequate schools and police service, rigid and unfriendly management, and so on. A related issue is that rehousing represents to many individuals a major life change which, as the recent developments in psychosomatic medicine suggest, can be stressful and can have definite health consequences. (201–207)

The studies in this section deal with rehousing which to all appearances was voluntary and sought by the respondents, while the next section deals with the material relating to involuntary relocation, mostly of elderly subjects. Insofar as most studies in this field do not make this distinction, or ask the subjects about this aspect of the move, the classification of an occasional study may be unclear regarding this dimension.

The classical study of the effects of rehousing on health is that of Wilner and his collaborators. (59) In spite of certain inevitable shortcomings of design, this study remains a model for other investigators to follow. Briefly, some 300 rehoused families and some 300 control families, both obtained from the files of the Baltimore Housing Authority, were seen approximately 10 times over a period of 3 years, starting when the families to be rehoused were still living in their old residences. The two groups were young, black families and they were initially comparable on major demographic and some health characteristics. However, as the study progressed, some of the families made spontaneous moves of their own, which necessitated their removal from the study, thereby also destroying the comparability of the two groups. Specifically, those rehoused families moving back to poor slum housing and those controls moving on their own to better public housing were removed. These may easily be two processes of selective attrition both of which favor the rehoused group over the control group in terms of some general dimension of social adjustment-efficacy. For the rehoused families, the major aspects of improved housing included: less crowding, better heating and refrigeration, running hot and cold water, screens, garbage disposal and absence of rodent infestation.

The major findings of the Wilner study may be summarized as follows:

1. On a number of morbidity and disability indices, the rehoused group proved to be somewhat healthier than the controls, but only for the period of follow-up covering 16 to 36 months after the move. For the period 12–14 months after rehousing, there were either no differences, or the controls were somewhat healthier, especially in comparisons involving young males. The young males (under 20) were also the ones who showed the biggest benefits in the later follow-up period, while older respondents (over 35) seemed to show no health benefits at all. The control group had a somewhat higher adult mortality ráte, but there were no differences in perinatal mortality or in rates of hospitalization. Overall, the health effects of rehousing were rather small, applied largely to the younger individuals, and were not manifest till some 16 months after the move.

2. In the area of personal and family relations, no differences were found in common family activities, in parental interest in children's activities, in family quarrels, and in assistance to the housewife. The only significant difference was that control families reported more difficulty over the children spending too much time away from home.

3. There appeared to be more neighborly activity (casual contact, helping out) among the rehoused families. However, they also complained more about being farther away from facilities and relatives. The rehoused families felt better about the neighborhood as a place to live than did the controls, but they were less likely to call it their "home."

4. Various measures reflecting the psychological state of the respondents (mood, nervousness, general morale, self-esteem, general anxiety) failed to differentiate the two groups.

5. The rehoused group were more likely to "feel better off in life than 5 years ago," but only for housing-related reasons. The rehousing had no effect on the parents' occupational and educational aspirations for the children, on the husbands' job aspirations and on various self-promotive activities of the adults.

6. On measures of the children's school performance, no differences were found on IQ tests, or arithmetic and reading achievement tests. However, the rehoused children did show better school attendance and were more likely to be promoted at the regular pace.

There are a few other reports specifically concerned with the physical health consequences of rehousing. (208–213) Rehoused families, as compared with those remaining in the slums, experienced lower infant mortality in two studies (209, 211) and a gradual decrease over time in a third one. (212) Two studies (210, 212) also demonstrated a lower incidence of tuberculosis among rehoused families; further analysis of results, however, revealed that race was a much more powerful determinant of tuberculosis rates than rehousing status: (212) rehoused Negro families had five times as high rates as rehoused White families. There is also some evidence that infectious and respiratory diseases are higher among the rehoused families, (210, 212, 213) especially in the period right after the move. In one of these studies, (213) rehousing meant a considerable increase in crowding (people/room) and density (people/acre).

In the above studies, rehoused families are compared with controls who have remained in the slums. At best, the two groups are comparable on superficial demographic variables, and there is a strong suspicion that the rehoused group is usually a seriously biased sample of the slum residents. (214) If the rehoused and control groups are both obtained from a list of applicants for rehousing, then the implicit and explicit policy of the housing authority may introduce other biases. There is a tendency in the British studies to give priority to families who have special problems and needs, including medical problems, while in the American studies there is some tendency to select out the potentially "good" tenants. (212) Another difficulty in interpreting the results is caused by the fact that rehoused families generally spend more on housing than before the move. (57, 211, 215, 216) Occasionally, the family budget is so tight that expenditures for food are reduced and the family diet suffers: this is apparently the reason for the higher mortality rates found among the rehoused families, as compared with the controls. (211)

There is another group of studies which has examined the effects of rehousing on mental health and related social-psychological variables.

88

Inasmuch as few of these studies use the type of design seen in the Wilner study, (59) the above reservations regarding research design apply to this work as well. The British studies, (217–227) which deal with rehousing onto new housing estates, can be summarized as follows:

1. There is no agreement on the mental health effects of rehousing— (a) one study (217) reports no differences as seen in data obtained from interviews, general practitioners' records, and hospital records; (b) another study (220) reports higher rates of mental health problems in the housing estate sample, using admissions to mental hospital, general practitioners' consultation rates, and self-reports of complaints; (c) a third study (226) finds the rehoused population better off by some standards (in-patient hospitalizations), no different by others (out-patient psychiatric hospital referrals, reports of nervous symptoms), and sicker by still another (psychiatric conditions treated by general practitioners). The last difference is interpreted by the authors as a greater readiness to consult a physician rather than a "true" difference in mental health.

2. There is strong agreement that the move to housing estate represents a greater physical distance to relatives and old friends, and a sizable reduction in social interaction with them. (218, 221–223, 225, 227) Some authors describe the move as a transition from a closed network of relationships (all friends and kin know each other) to an open network (not all of the contacts are interconnected). The consequences of this breaking of old social ties are many: (a) reduced possibility of mutual helping out among relatives; (227) (b) a more flexible division of labor at home; (222) (c) more neighboring and mutual help from new neighbors, (221, 222) even though some of the contact may be quite superficial; (218) (d) spending more time at home (226) and belonging to a greater number of (non-church-related) associations. (222)

3. There is also strong evidence that families on housing estates are more satisfied with the new dwelling but less satisfied with the housing estate neighborhood and its lack of amenities, especially right after they have made the move. (217, 218, 221, 226)

4. There is some evidence of a higher rate of juvenile delinquency and of child guidance clinic consultations among families living on a housing estate. (219) However, this effect is distinctly temporary and the elevation disappears within 4–5 years of the move. Interestingly, the same study also reports more outdoor play among the housing estate children, (221) and conflict within families appears to be somewhat reduced.(218)

5. There is no acceptable evidence that moving to the housing estate increased the wives' loneliness, except in a very temporary way. (225) This goes contrary to the earlier informal observations about the British housing estates, but the authors of this well designed study (225) show that even though loneliness was correlated with dissatisfaction with

neighbors, the residential area, and the home, the loneliness was not produced by the rehousing per se. And a cross-cultural study (228) has shown that loneliness is much more of an issue for English than for American women.

The above British studies show a mixed picture of points on which they agree and other points on which there is disagreement. The disagreement may be attributed to: (a) differences in the length of the period of observation after the move, since when the period of observation is sufficiently long, some of the adverse effects of rehousing are shown to be temporary and reversible; (b) the study of different types of housing estates, e.g., those which are planned (226) vs. those which are unplanned (220) (purely dormitory suburbs); (c) the extent to which families to be rehoused are given priority on the basis of known and unknown problems and needs; (d) the nature of the different measures used and the nature of the "control" group from which normative data are provided.

Among the American studies of rehousing, the work of Chapin (229, 230) is frequently quoted in support for all sorts of claims of beneficial effects of rehousing. In fact, when he matched the rehoused families with controls still residing in the slums (waiting list applicants) on a number of important demographic variables, he was unable to show any differences in morale or general adjustment in a one year follow-up. However, the rehoused families did show a larger gain in social participation, in quality of home furnishings, and showed a reduction in "use overcrowding" (subjecting the living room to different uses). Another of the early American studies (231, 232) has shown a sizeable reduction in juvenile delinquency (as determined from court records) as a result of rehousing in a public housing project. However, since the determination of the pre-rehousing delinquency rates is somewhat in question, the result should be viewed as suggestive only; it is also in disagreement with a previously discussed study, (212) which found no differences.

The elderly, as a group, are less mobile, less likely to plan or desire to move, and are less successful in anticipating their mobility behavior; (233) the elderly who are especially unwilling to move out of their neighborhood are those who have lived there a long time and who have many friends there. (234) Nevertheless, a study of voluntary rehousing of the elderly into a new public housing facility showed some striking benefits of the move: (235–237) (a) greater life satisfaction, morale, and better feelings about life accomplishments; (b) more positive evaluation of health; (c) increased membership in social groups and greater enjoyment of activities with others; (d) decrease in "lost" time and time spent sleeping; (e) decrease in services they felt they needed. Even though the study has certain obvious defects (no control group; acceptance of applicants who were better adjusted, more alert, in especially poor housing), the presumptive evidence is that no spontaneous changes would have taken place without the rehousing. Studies of elderly relocating into retirement communities (238, 239) have been cross-sectional studies and any differences observed on the elderly— whether among the different types of these specialized settings, (239) or between these settings and the general elderly community (238)— can be just as easily attributed to the self-selection process as to effects of the environment. Thus, in one study (239) the activities and morale of the elderly living in different retirement housing sites are compared. However, since the individuals recruited into these different settings are so vastly different on social class and marital status, one cannot learn anything about the differential effects of living in these settings. Similar disclaimers are appropriate about the finding that aged migrants to retirement communities have higher morale than those selecting regular, age integrated communities. (238)

The American literature on housing moves to the suburbs (35, 240–247) is also relevant to our concern here with effects of voluntary rehousing. However, many of the studies utilize a particularly weak design: retrospective interviews with only those who moved to the suburbs. Thus, their findings, summarized below, must be seen as suggestive only.

1. Many of the changes which take place after the move to the suburb are what Gans (242, 243) calls "intended" changes, i.e., the reasons for which the move to the suburb was made in the first place. These include: greater satisfaction with housing, especially with space, increased social life and visiting with neighbors, better morale, and reduction in boredom and loneliness. These intended changes are particularly strong on previous city dwellers who lived in an apartment or were renters.

2. There seem to be no effects of the move on mental health, marital happiness, or family life.

3. Among the possible "unintended" changes, only greater organizational activity was observed, and this presumably had to do with the fact that the suburban community was a new one. (242) Otherwise, one observes no increase in involvement in local organizations and institutions. (246)

4. The easy sociability and the rapid and intense intimacy which has been observed appears to be limited to the early, pioneering phase of a suburb and does not hold for more established suburban communities; (35, 247) moreover, it is limited to middle class suburbs with a good deal of social homogeneity. It does not hold for working class suburbs (240) or for lower class housewives living in middle class neighborhoods. (244)

In general, then, the conclusion has been made that the suburban residential environment per se has little influence: it does not alter the life style of working class individuals so that it comes to resemble that of the middle class, (240) and the changes which take place after the move are part and parcel of the family's overall intentions, their desired and aspired change in way of life. Gans (241) summarizes the situation as follows: "In short, the community itself does not shape people's ways of life as significantly as has been proposed by ecological and planning theory. The major behavior patterns are determined, rather by the period of the life-cycle, and the opportunities and aspirations associated with class position." It is interesting to note that a study of rehousing of slum dwellers into housing projects (137) comes essentially to the same conclusions: the planned change in housing is embedded in the family's overall aspirations to change their way of life.

## Effects of Involuntary Relocation and Institutionalization

In this section we wish to consider two types of changes in the residential environment: (a) enforced change in residence, primarily associated with urban renewal or highway construction, and (b) the change from community living to institutional living, involving primarily the elderly, and some work on institutional transfer. As in the previous section, the main orientation here is to see if the study of change in the residential environment will reveal something about its importance and its effects. However, in contrast to the previous section, the emphasis will be more on the dislocation resulting from the enforced move and less on the change in the quality of housing which, in these studies, is not always an improvement.

A good deal of the relocation literature is not directly concerned with the psychological and health consequences of relocation. Rather, such reports deal primarily with other issues: numbers of persons affected by relocation in different parts of the country, the economic circumstances of the relocated persons, selected demographic characteristics of the relocatees, their housing preferences, the living conditions of the residence and the characteristics of the neighborhood from which relocation took place, and so on. Some of the reports are impressionistic, narrative accounts (248) while others are criticisms of current relocation practices, (249, 250) where the criticism is based on policy considerations, general humanistic concerns, as well as data about effects of relocation. Slum residents who are relocated generally pay higher rent without necessarily experiencing better housing. (215, 249, 251) sometimes they scatter throughout the city, (252) but more often they move to adjacent areas where similar housing is available. (215, 251) Since such housing is usually substandard, the relocatees experience additional moves later.

The largest impact of relocation is due to the uprooting of existing social networks, as is well demonstrated in the study of relocation of

West End Boston. (*249, 253, 254*) Fried reports that even two years after relocation, over 40% of the sample gave evidence of fairly severe grief reaction. Such a grief reaction was especially likely among those who had a stronger pre-relocation commitment to the area, who knew a greater part of the neighborhood, who had a great number of close friends in the area, and who had positive feelings about their neighbors. The grief reaction, and the associated variables, were also predictive of poor adjustment-adaptation to the new neighborhood. In addition, poor adjustment was likely if the respondents: were low on educational and occupational status and first generation American, had a poor knowledge of Boston other than West End, and had had no plans to move out of West End. A five year follow-up study of relocation in Washington (*252*) showed that 26% of the respondents had made no new friends in the 5 years in the new neighborhood, and even though 50% of them clearly liked their new homes better, only 30% indicated that they had been happy to move.

The literature concerned specifically with relocation of elderly persons has been summarized by Niebanck (*163, 255, 256*) and the following conclusions appear defensible. The relocated elderly are generally those who have been less mobile and who have lived in the old neighborhood longer than the average person. For the elderly, the move frequently represents an added financial hardship because their economic circumstances are already quite precarious. The old neighborhood which they are forced to leave has two major advantages for which the better housing conditions of the new location cannot adequately compensate: the extensive friendship ties and the convenience to many facilities (grocery, drug store, church, transportation, etc.). The social ties to the old neighborhood are a particularly strong impediment, and the stronger the ties, the more dissatisfied are they with the new neighborhood (*234*) and the more severe is their grief reaction. (*253*) Those who are able to maintain old contacts with friends from the old neighborhood show the least emotional distress. The loss of friends creates not only loneliness but also a certain amount of insecurity, inasmuch as the elderly depend partly upon their friends for help in case of some emergency. (*257*) It is also worth emphasizing that among all age groups, the elderly appear to be the most vulnerable to the adverse effects of the involuntary relocation: Key, (*258*) for example, found more intense depression, sadness, and negative feelings among the older persons who were forced to move because of urban renewal or highway construction.

There appear to be no prospective studies and only one retrospective survey in which the psychological effects of involuntary relocation on the elderly were systematically studied and a previously established attitude and adjustment scale was used. (*259*) In this study, 48 subjects aged 55 and older who had been relocated because of highway construction during the previous 5 years were compared with 268 subjects who were selected on a random basis from the total community. The relocated persons scored consistently less adjusted and more dissatisfied on most of the sub-scales of the "Activities and Attitude Inventory." (260) These are striking findings of an apparently long lasting effect of relocation. However, since this is not a longitudinal study, such differences could also be the result of a selection process which failed to yield comparable groups of relocatees and controls. No data on the comparability of the two groups on socio-economic status are presented and it is doubtful, in fact, that a random sampling of all areas of the community would have yielded a group comparable to those who lived in the residential section through which a highway was built.

Let us now turn to some evidence concerning effects of the change from community living to institutional living. Prominent among the relevant studies are the numerous reports of high mortality rates of aged subjects within the first year (or some shorter period) of hospitalization or institutionalization in a state hospital, nursing home, or old age home. (261–268) These studies also suggest that particularly high mortality rates will be found among men, the very old, and those in poor physical health (e.g., focal lesions of the central nervous system). Especially high rates are found in state hospitals, while old age homes have the lowest rates. (264) Since these data appear to have a widespread generality, (268) it seems safe to accept the high mortality rates as a fact. How this fact should be interpreted is another matter altogether. Since it is typically assumed that institutionalization represents a profound environmental change which is stressful, (269) the high mortality rates are frequently taken as evidence of the serious health consequences such environmental changes may have on the elderly. Logical analysis, however, reveals that two other variables could be operating: (a) self-selection, i.e., individuals who are in a seriously debilitated or incapacitated state are most frequently the ones who get admitted; (b) adverse effects of the institutional environment, i.e., it is not the environmental *change* as such, but the exposure to some aspect of the institutional environment (poor diet, infections, poor medical care, sensory deprivation, etc.) which raises the mortality rates. The first alternative is clearly the more plausible one and as long as we cannot estimate the extent to which this variable could be operating, we must acknowledge that it could "explain away" *all* of the phenomenon of excess mortality.

Another attack on this problem is represented by the design in which mortality of subjects on a waiting list (accepted into an institution but not yet admitted) is compared with the mortality after admission. There are two studies (263, 270) which utilize this design: one shows a somewhat higher waiting list mortality (263) while another shows a slightly lower one. (270) (The latter study contains an elementary error in computing the annual death rate and, as a result, the author claims to have demonstrated a strikingly lower wating list mortality rate.)

It needs to be pointed out that while the comparison of waiting-list and post-admission mortality rates rules out self-selection, it brings in another problem: the waiting period may be one of stressful anticipation and a finding of no difference may mean either that anticipation and institutionalization are equally stressful or that the high post-admission mortality rates are due to self-selection factors. A number of recent studies suggest that anticipating such events as examinations, (271) underwater demolition training, (272) and job termination (273, 274) can be quite stressful.

Some suggestive results about effects of environmental change (predominantly institutionalization) are reported by Blenker. (275) In an experiment designed to test the effects of social work and public health nursing services for non-institutionalized aged, participants were randomly assigned to three service programs, ranging from minimal (providing information and direction) to maximal (intensive program of direct service). At a sixth month follow-up, the death rate in the maximal program group was the highest and in the minimal program, the lowest. The explanation for this unexpected finding appears to reside in the fact that frequently the maximal service was directed toward securing the necessary care in settings other than the person's own home. That is, in order to provide "better" medical care, participants in the maximal service were often uprooted from their familiar surroundings. It must be noted that this study, while strong in research design (random assignment to conditions), does not have large enough numbers to permit any firm conclusions about the differential mortality rates.

There is also some evidence that among the elderly who are institutionalized, those who had had no choice but to be placed in an institution, have higher mortality rates after admission than those for whom other alternatives were also available. (276) However, it is not clear to what extent initial differences in health status can account for the difference in mortality rates.

The most convincing data concerning the possible health effects of environmental change on the elderly came from two studies in which aged subjects were relocated from one institution to another and where the mortality rates before and after relocation, or between relocatees and controls, are compared. (277, 278) Both studies find that transfer to another institution is associated with an increase in mortality. A third study (279) arrives at a similar conclusion, but the numbers of cases are too small to be more than suggestive. Additional analyses of the data from the Aldrich-Mendkoff study (280) reveal that: (a) patients whose adjustment to the institution prior to news of relocation was characterized as "satisfactory" or "angry, demanding" were much more likely to survive than those whose adjustment was "neurotic, depressed" or "psychotic;" (b) patients whose adjustment to the news of relocation was judged to be "philosophical, angry, anxious, or regression" were much more likely to survive than those whose adjustment was "depression, denial, or psychotic."

There is also evidence that the way the relocation process is managed may influence the mortality rates. Jasnau (281) has shown that patients who are mass-moved within the hospital with little or no preparation will show an increased death rate after relocation while those who receive individualized attention (casework service, psychological support) show a lower than expected death rate following the move. Unfortunately, these results are not fully conclusive because it is not clear that the way the patients were assigned to the individualized or mass transfer procedures was without bias. Similarly interesting data are reported by Novick: (282) the relocation program involving some 125 chronically disabled aged residents was extremely carefully worked out and detailed attention was paid to such issues as resident's fear of unknown, preservation of familiar relationships, retention of familiar belongings, and so on. Under such an excellently managed relocation program, the post-relocation death rate was found to be actually lower than the rate at the old hospital for the previous year.

There is only one study (283) where the stress reaction following relocation from one site to another was also assessed at the level of physiological functioning, in this case plasma levels of cortisol. The results indicated that men, but not women, had elevated plasma cortisol levels some 1–2 weeks after relocation. Moreover, the amount of stress reaction was of prognostic significance for subsequent morbidity and mortality status. Men and psychotic patients had higher mortality rates than women and normal aged after the relocation.

Another study (284) showed that when a rather select group of physically healthy and mentally unimpaired aged women are relocated from one home for the aged to another, then those showing negative changes after relocation (death or serious physical illness or severe psychological deterioration) are the women who before relocation had a very negative evaluation of their past life and who saw the future in bleak terms. Another longitudinal investigation (285) looked at reactions to nursing home placement; however, because of a very brief observation period, one week after placement, no significant changes on diverse ratings of patient behavior were observed.

A large proportion of studies of effects of institutionalization are in reality cross-sectional surveys in which institutionalized elderly are contrasted with those living in the community. In such studies, it is not possible to disentangle: (a) self-selection from effects of the institution; (b) effects of moving into the institution from effects of living in it; and

c) differential survival from effects of the institution. Consequently, findings such as that institutionalized elderly are more concerned with the past and less with the future, (286) perform more poorly on memory and perceptual functioning tests, (287) give more self-derogatory responses, (288) show more constricted human figure drawings, (289) and report lower moral and life satisfaction (290)—cannot be simply attributed to the effects of institutionalization. Much of this literature has been recently reviewed and evaluated by Lieberman. (291)

Somewhat more sophisticated studies of institutionalization have, in their efforts to isolate the effects of the institutional environment, included in their design (in addition to a group of community residents) either a group of applicants waiting to be institutionalized or a group of elderly just placed in the institution. (292–295) Some of these studies (292, 293) certainly throw into doubt some differences previously attributed to institutionalization. But beyond that, they still yield ambiguous data and further illustrate the difficulties of trying to apply a cross-sectional approach to a problem which basically demands a longitudinal design if it is to yield relatively unambiguous data. For example, what does it mean that the waiting list subjects are higher on anxiety, helplessness, and depression than both the community group and the institutionalized aged, but that the latter two groups are not different from each other? What are the relative contributions of self-selection, the anticipation effect, and short- and long-term selective attrition (mortality) in producing this result?

The studies reviewed in this section represent, in their totality, rather convincing evidence that involuntary change in the residential environment can have adverse effects on the physical and mental health of the individuals involved, especially if they are a more vulnerable segment of the population, such as the elderly. But the evidence appears equally convincing that these adverse effects cannot be directly attributed to the changes in the physical environment, but rather to the concomitant and consequent changes in the social environment. That is, the involuntary physical relocation has adverse consequences because it precipitates a severe disruption of the existing social networks and relationships, i.e., a profound change in the social environment. And individuals who are particularly well embedded in these social networks and dependent upon them, appear to suffer the most adverse consequences. However, when the intimate link between physical relocation and social disruption is broken—as in the well-managed institutional transfer of the aged described by Novick (282)—no serious health consequences are evident. The literature on effects of institutionalization is certainly consistent with the above viewpoint. However, because of certain methodological difficulties, most of these studies do not necessarily support only a single interpretation. And in any case, it is not clear to what extent the presumed institutional effects are due to the physical dimensions of the environment, as opposed to the "institutional totality," (296) the institutional regimen permeating the social environment of an institution.

## Studies of Housing Needs and Satisfactions, Housing Attitudes, Preferences, and Perceptions

The studies which have been reviewed so far dealt directly, but in various ways, with the question: What are the effects of the residential environment on health and behavior? In this section we turn to studies which, though still relevant to the central question, no longer deal with it directly. That is, knowing about housing preferences and satisfactions alone tells us little about the physical and mental health consequences of the residential environment. However, a better understanding of this area should lead to a clearer picture of other issues, such as the dynamics of residential mobility. And since there is already a separate literature on the correlates and consequences of mobility (123, 297–299) (see also the data from the previous two sections), we will thus be in a better position to establish some probable consequences of housing preferences and satisfactions via the link to mobility. In short, one intent of this section is to describe some of the links in the overall association between the residential environment and health and behavior.

Another reason for our interest in these studies stems from a fundamental meta-theoretical orientation, namely that we must distinguish between: (a) the objective environment, describable in the physicalistic language of the physical sciences and measurable, ultimately, in cgs units (centimeters-grams-seconds), and (b) the perceived environment, which is the way the individual perceives (as well misperceives and does not "see") the objective environment and which is measurable along psychological dimensions. This distinction between objective and subjective environment is central to Lewinian field theory (300) and some of its implications for the study of effects of the environment have been discussed elsewhere. (301) And unless one is committed to a simplistic ecological determinism, the distinction appears essential if one is to understand the effects (the average effects as well as the variability of effects) of the residential environment on health and behavior.

The measurement of housing values, preferences, and satisfactions is fraught with many difficulties, one of which is the question of the behavioral significance of such measures. In the review which follows, we shall specifically *avoid* making the following assumptions:

1. That a statement of a certain housing preference or value automatically implies that the respondent is dissatisfied if his actual housing situation is discrepant from the preference.

98

2. That planners and architects should necessarily be guided by users' values and preferences and should seek to maximize them.

3. That dissatisfaction has self-evident consequences for mental and physical health.

Studies of sources of satisfactions and complaints (302–308) suggest that satisfaction with housing is clearly related to size of dwelling and amount of space available, and that crowding and lack of privacy are important sources of dissatisfaction. Complaints about meals, hygiene, sleeping, housework, child care, and leisure are all associated with crowding. Social class of the respondent is clearly an important variable modifying users' preferences and satisfactions. (309) Class differences affect specific preferences, such as whether the family eats in the kitchen or the living room when dining room is missing. (310) But they also influence major orientations, such as the far-reaching differences in needs and concerns of slum dwellers as compared with working class individuals. (138) In general, it has been concluded (305) that higher social groups take for granted the amenities which the lower classes are aspiring to possess. The only areas of preference where stage of life cycle and lifestyle override social class influences are in the desires of people to move from single family homes to multiple dwellings or to the center of the city, and in the perception that their (normal-sized) urban lot is too large for them. (311)

In general, the nature of the dwelling is a more important source of satisfactions and dissatisfactions than is the neighborhood location, (307) though the situation appears reversed for elderly subjects (160, 162) and does not hold in all studies. (312) Social characteristics of neighbors appear to be a chief determinant of satisfaction with neighborhood. (307) Beyond that, an ideal neighborhood is described as spacious, beautiful, good for children, exclusive, having country-like character and being close to nature (in that order of importance), and neighborhood facilities listed as important include a religious building, grocery, bus stop, elementary school, and shopping center. (313) Housing preferences are also influenced by such diverse variables as consciousness of one's socio-economic standing, one's instrumental value orientation, and whether or not one's personal friends live far away. (312)

In discussing these studies, it is a useful reminder to note that in a broader perspective on sources of personal satisfaction and happiness, satisfaction with one's residential environment doesn't compare in importance with such other sources as family relationship, job satisfaction, and social adjustment. (314)

There is also a sizable literature on the housing needs and preferences of elderly subjects. Some 80% of the aged, whether married or widowed, maintain independent households, and fully 84% of the elderly who have living children live less than an hour away from the nearest child. *(290)* Studies of living preferences among the elderly agree quite well that the elderly prefer what has been called "independent propinquity," *(315)* "supported independence," *(316)* and "intimacy par distance." *(317)* That is, they desire to live alone but near their children and relatives. *(163, 257, 318, 319)* Thus, the living preferences and the actual living arrangements of the elderly are reasonably congruent with each other as well as with the expectations others seem to have for the elderly. *(320)* However, given the fact that lower income elderly are more likely to live in rooming houses or in the houses of relatives, *(321)* one may assume that the congruence between preferences and actual living arrangements is probably lower for the poorer elderly. Smith *(321)* also found that unattached men, more than unattached women or elderly couples, were willing to accept rooming house arrangements in lieu of independent housekeeping. The wish for privacy is quite strong among the elderly, especially those who consider themselves in good health, *(322)* and they do not relish the idea of entering a residential home, especially middle and upper class elderly with living children. *(323)* Finally, as was indicated above, satisfaction with the neighborhood is of greater importance to the elderly than satisfaction with housing per se; *(160, 162, 324)* and the aspect of neighborhood which is of greatest concern to the elderly is nearness to various facilities. *(160, 163, 325)*

The literature on the subjective perception of the residential environment is, at the moment, not extensive enough to permit any kind of understanding of the relationship between the objective residential environment and the subjective perceptions of it, and the variations in the latter. Moreover, a lot of the environmental perception literature is concerned with such topics as perception of various aspects of the geography, *(326)* with "imageability" of the city *(327)* the (qualities of the city which give it a high probability of evoking a strong image), judgments of roadside quality, *(328)* dimensions involved in the perception of an urban shopping center *(329)* or of houses and interiors of houses, *(330)* and variables critical to the definition of a neighborhood. *(331)* Even though this literature is intrinsically interesting, it does not deal with those dimensions of the residential environment which have previously been linked—perhaps suggestively rather than convincingly—with health and behavioral consequences. Thus, it is not yet possible to build a causal chain which links the environment and health and involves the perceptions of the environment as well. Clearly, we need more of the kinds of studies in which both the objective and the perceived environments are assessed. *(105, 332)*

In closing this section, it is useful to emphasize the limitations of the various measures of housing preferences and satisfactions. Riemer *(333)* lists the following: (a) housing attitudes are related to the housing conditions with which the respondent is familiar; (b) preferences are not absolute and permanent; (c) as some needs are satisfied, other needs become paramount; (d) housing attitudes are not based on full information; (e) housing attitudes and satisfactions are more volatile after rehousing. To these problems one could add others, perhaps more technical ones in nature, such as the issue of intransitivity of a set of preferences, or the difficulty of not knowing whether one is dealing with "ideal" preferences or realistically aspired goals. In spite of these problems, there can be no doubt that the issues covered in this section are important ones and that a better understanding of the perceived environment (Lewin's "life space" (300) is needed if we are to understand better the effects of the built environment, in general, and special problems, such as "non-conforming" usage, (56) in particular.

### Effects of Variations in the Proximate Physical Environment on Short Term Behavior

In the previous section, it was argued that our understanding of the association between the residential environment and health can be clarified by considering one kind of an intervening link or process, that which involves perceptions, attitudes, preferences, and satisfactions. But there are other links which concern us as well. In effect, we are trying to reconstruct the causal chain from the phyiscal environment to the perceived environment to mediating social-psychological factors (the social context) to proximate behavioral and physiological reactions to distal (lasting) outcomes in physical and mental health. In this section we wish to consider what has sometimes been designated as "proximate environment": (334) the immediate physical environment as it impinges on the individual at a given moment. By examining this area, we wish to learn something about the ways, the mechanisms, whereby the physical environment can influence behavior. The level of observation and analysis is clearly more microscopic than in the previous sections. (Barker's (335) term, "behavior setting," could also be used here, but Barker is not specifically dealing just with the physical environment, but rather with the whole problem of studying molar human behavior *in situ*.)

Much of this literature deals with man's use of space and with his immediate interaction with such aspects of his surroundings, as the arrangement of a room's furniture. (336–356) These studies are both naturalistic observations and modest experimental manipulations. The work is difficult to summarize, but the following are representative findings:

1. Activities of patients in mental hospitals have a characteristic, stable distribution in space, which is related to such factors as the patient's position in a dominance hierarchy, his possession of a territory,

101

whether or not he has friends, the number of persons assigned to the room, and so on. Verbal interaction between patients can be increased by manipulating the furniture and the decor.

2. In leaderless discussion groups, seating arrangements of persons around a table affect the choice of individual with whom one is likely to interact, but do not influence the eventual leadership ratings. In discussion groups with designated leaders, the leaders prefer the end positions of a rectangular table and the other members then sit close by; if the leader doesn't occupy the head position, other members sit opposite or across from him but not alongside him. In normal conversation, people prefer to sit across from one another rather than side by side unless the distance is too great for comfortable conversation (over 5 feet). People at corner positions of a table interact more than those seated opposite or alongside each other. When asked to sit down and discuss a topic, schizophrenic patients pick more distant seating arrangements than normal subjects. The seating choices of readers seeking privacy in public reading areas are quite different from choices made by individuals who will engage in a conversation. (Much of this work has been influenced by Hall's work (341) on personal, social, and public space, and by related ideas, such as the "body-buffer zone." (342))

3. Seating proximity in classrooms and partitioned (vs. open) offices in office buildings promote friendship formation. Productivity and behavior of office workers can be altered by changes in the physical surroundings. Different designs of nursing units in hospitals can influence patient care, nurse satisfaction, and absenteeism.

In addition to the above work, other studies have been concerned with: (a) the effects of color on behavior and performance; (357–359) (b) the effects of surroundings upon problem solving efficiency (360) and the effects of changes in environmental conditions upon intellectual task performance; (361, 362) (c) the effects of esthetic surroundings on mood, discomfort, and perceptions. (363–365) And there are also some downright silly studies, such as the effects of windowless classrooms on students' drawings of a school, (366) or effects of temperature and crowdedness of a room on subjects' ratings of liking-disliking a hypothetical person. (367)

Relevant to the topic of this section are also the studies which deal with the effects of restricted sensory environment and sensory deprivation. (368–377) The literature on this topic is quite extensive, but also frequently confusing and not always very consistent. The writers in this area are still trying to disentangle the various possible components of the phenomenon under study: reduction in sensory stimulation, social isolation, and physical confinement. In addition, there is a particularly vexing problem which has to do with the artificiality of the experimental-laboratory setup, with the creation of an experimental set in the subjects (the creation of explicit and implicit expectations in the subjects, the "experimental demand" characteristics of the way the experiment is setup and run (378)), and the self-selection involved in the type of subjects who volunteer for this kind of a study. The results of these studies do not lead to a coherent picture and a distinction between short-term and long-term effects is obviously necessary. Personality variables, such as field dependence, also seem to play a role. In short, it is difficult to infer from these studies the probable effects of living in a residential environment which is so impoverished as to resemble sensory deprivation. Spitz's famous study of hospitalism (374) involved not only the highly restricted physical environment of the foundling home, but also a lack of human contact between the infants and some maternal figure, and it is this latter variable which Spitz selects in explaining the developmental retardation and higher mortality of the foundling home children. In general, the reviews of the developmental literature (369, 372) are unable to separate out the effects of sensory and perceptual deprivation from the effects of maternal and social deprivation, and the role of the restricted physical environment thus remains ambiguous.

There are also some experimental studies and naturalistic observations of groups of individuals living in isolated settings such as a fallout shelter, an Arctic base, or a submerged submarine. (379–387) The findings generally demonstrate a higher overall frequency of certain symptoms, such as sleep disturbance, depression, irritability, fatigue, and boredom, but no changes in anxiety. Also observed were increases in territorial behavior (consistent and mutually exclusive uses of particular chairs or beds or tables) and in time spent alone. There is no doubt that the individuals who join these isolated groups are self-selected as well as carefully screened. For example, marine engineers working in relatively isolated situations consider good interpersonal relations with peers as a particularly important aspect of job satisfaction. (385) Individuals who adjust more poorly to such isolated work environments come from an urban background, are of higher socioeconomic status, and have gained independence from their family of origin very early or very late. (380)

These studies of isolated settings are interesting, but it is difficult to see how this kind of an environment should be conceptualized and what the specific role of the physical environment may be. Haythorn and Altman (384) list the ingredients of isolation as: limited freedom of movement, reduced variety of stimulation, and reduced access to valued stimuli, especially social stimuli. Thus, the physical aspects, such as crowded and confined space, are interwoven with the social aspects, such as lack of variety of activities or absence of individuals of the opposite sex. It is also interesting to note that different types of isolated environments appear to produce different symptoms: in prolonged marine submergence headaches are frequently mentioned and quality of sleep improves after the first few weeks, (386) while on an Antarctic base sleep disturbances increase with time but headaches are rarely mentioned. (381)

The studies reviewed in this section were introduced with the hope that they will provide a more microscopic level of observation which may teach us something about the mechanisms, the specific ways in which the residential physical environment affects behavior. This appears to have been a false hope inasmuch as these studies are difficult to fit in with the general housing and health literature examined previously. We now know something about seating arrangements of individuals seeking privacy in a library (352) or the seating of members of a discussion group in relation to a leader, (350) and we also know that two-person interaction on a geriatric ward can be increased by manipulating the furniture arrangement and the decor. (354) But this still leaves us in the dark about how different members of a family seek privacy in their home or apartment, what are the different ways (short and long term) of coping with lack of privacy, and what are the trade-offs and consequences. Nor do we know how the various arrangements of rooms or of furniture affect social interaction in the family, its amount, and its quality. In short, what is needed are studies done in the setting in which we are most interested, the residential environment. Studies done in the social scientist's laboratory, or in selected public places, or in institutions have limited generalizability because in those settings, the individuals have a minimum opportunity to alter the built environment, only to react to it. And the observation period is generally so brief that one can talk only about short-term reactions, not a long-term accommodation.

## Methodological and Theoretical Comments

In this section, we want to comment briefly on the methodological and theoretical implications of the work which has been under review. Many such comments have been made along the way and we shall therefore limit ourselves to the highlights.

The major methodological difficulty encountered in these studies is our inability to disentangle the many variables which could be operating in an association between an environmental variable and some outcome. Primarily, we need to disentangle: (a) individual components of housing from each other, (b) aspects of poor housing from other aspects of poverty, and (c) aspects of the physical environment from aspects of the social environment. Large scale, cross-sectional surveys or ecological studies of city census tracts are the most ambiguous ones in this respect. There seems little point in continuing to do such studies, unless we have a special reason, such as: (a) to determine the magnitude of an association, no matter what its interpretation, or to show that an association exists with a previously unsuspected variable; (b) to provide basic data for health care planning; or (c) to establish a historical trend, at this level of analysis, by replicating specific old studies. Beyond such specific reasons, we are better off looking for special design opportunities which offer us natural built-in controls.

We must be more opportunistic in locating and using populations which differ on some aspect of housing but are unusually comparable in other respects. The Fanning study, (181) discussed previously, is a good example of such an approach. This research opportunism is especially likely to be successful, if we are prepared to use a longitudinal design and are on the lookout for "natural experiments" in order to design studies around them. By natural experiments we mean those planned and predictable changes in the residential environment which take place because of diverse efforts such as urban renewal, highway construction, public housing, high rise housing, new planned communities, and so on. Especially valuable are those opportunities in which the new residential environment is not completely uniform, but rather where the builder has introduced some variations in design. If the groups of clients which move in are comparable, then the effects of such variation can be easily assessed. (Campbell (388) has recently dealt with the issue of strategies for using an experimental approach to social reform and planned change.)

There are other methodological issues which have been noted throughout this review. They dealt with such points as: (a) the need for better multivariate analysis of data, including formal attempts at causal analysis and path analysis, (98–100) (b) the need to dimensionalize the residential environment by using such techniques as factor analysis and cluster analysis, (c) a greater commitment to obtaining control subjects who are as comparable as possible to the study population, and (d) collecting outcome data which are not biased by various social and institutional practices. These are traditional issues of methodology and there is no need to dwell on them in detail.

However, there is one other area of recommendations regarding the design of future studies which we want to discuss, and it has to do with the type of data which need to be collected. This is an issue which is really methodological as well as conceptual and meta-theoretical, since it reflects the interplay between the set of questions which the investigator is asking and the research design he generates in order to answer the questions. A design may be fully adequate in that it answers the questions raised by the investigator, but the study may be inadequate because not all the important questions were asked. Below, we shall consider some of the general questions which have been raised, but were poorly answered or left unanswered. Then we shall propose a schema which should be of some use in organizing the questions to be asked.

In attempting to understand the way the residential environment affects health and behavior, a number of important questions have been raised. How do we conceptualize and dimensionalize the environment and the way it operates to influence behavior? (*245, 389–392*) What aspects of the physical residential environment in particular can influence behavior? (*58, 391*) How can we understand "nonconforming" usage, (*56*) or the distinction between "potential" environment (the way it was built) and "effective" environment (the way it is used)? (*243*) How do we separate out the physical factors from the social factors in the overall way the residential environment affects people? (*393*) What are the goals which planners and builders are trying to achieve and how do the various aspects of the built environment promote or hinder such goals? (*394–396*) What are the needs of individuals vis a vis the residential environment? (*54, 397–399*) What is the best way to understand the congruence or fit between the characteristics of the person and of the specific environment in which he is living? (*26, 400–402*)

These are some of the questions which have been raised as investigators probed beyond the simple fact of some association between an environmental variable and a health or behavioral outcome. These questions call both for new theoretical formulations as well as additional empirical evidence. Below, we shall sketch out a framework within which such problems can be attacked more systematically. This framework, which is an elaboration and modification of a previously suggested field-theoretical approach to the study of the effects of the environment, (*301, 403, 404*) certainly does not provide either the empirical data or the detail of the needed theoretical reformulation. It is merely a skeleton which has the following objectives: (a) it should be a comprehensive guide for inclusion of variables for study and a potential reminder of what variables may be neglected or forgotten; (b) it should allow the various disciplines to include the variables they consider important; (c) it should be a rough guide for the type of data analysis to be performed and the kinds of interpretations of results which are intended.

Figure 1 is a summary statement of the proposed framework and the major classes of variables which need to be considered. The actual listing of the variables within each class is for illustrative purposes only and is not intended to suggest that these are the crucial ones. The basic notion of the diagram is that there is a direction of influence from left to right, and that at any one juncture the conditioning variables may modify the mediating processes or the outcome. That is, if there is a causal influence from the physical environment to physical and mental health and social functioning, then the process can best be understood if one also takes into consideration the objective social en-

**FIGURE 1.—A Diagrammatic Presentation of Major Classes of Variables in the Study of Effects of the Residential Environment on Health and Behavior**

**Conditioning Variables in the Person**

| Demographic | Cultural-Subcultural | Stable Personality |
|---|---|---|
| Age, Sex, Race | Religion, Religiosity | Ego strength |
| Marital Status | Ethnic-Racial Origin | Flexible-Rigidity |
| Education | Extended Family Kin Contact | Coping Styles |
| Occupation | Values about deviant behavior | Self-Identity |
| Income | | Habit Patterns, Needs |
| Stage of Life Cycle | | |

**Objective Environment**

**Physical Environment**

Characteristics of
Dwelling Unit
Distance to Facilities
Characteristics of
Neighborhood

**Social Environment**

Availability of
Relatives, Friends
Demographic Similar-
ity to Others in
Neighborhood
Presence of Crime,
Addiction in
Neighborhood

**Subjective (Perceived) Environment**

Perceived Crowding
and Privacy
Perceived Convenience
to Facilities
Perceived Pollution in
Neighborhood
Perceived Closeness
to Kin, Friends
Perceived Similarity
to Neighbors
Perceived Dangers in
Neighborhood

**Behavioral Reactions**

Daily Patterns of
Living
Behavioral Adaptions
Coping Behaviors
Interpersonal Behavior
Leisure-Time Activities

**Mediating Processes**

**Biochemical and Physiological**

Blood Pressure
Pulse Rate
Lipids
Glucose
Clotting Time
Plasma Cortisol

**Affective**

Anxiety-Tension
Depression
Anger-Irritation
Morale
Satisfaction-
Complaints

**Outcome-Variables**

Disease States
Illness and Sick-
Role Behavior
Social Deviance
Social Effectiveness
and Competence
Addictions

vironment (the social setting), the individual's perceptions or interpretations of his environment, and the mediating processes which include physiological, affective, and behavioral reactions. Moreover, a number of characteristics of the person should be examined in order to see how the overall process may be modified by them.

The diagram, of course, is a very limited statement of the overall problem. For example, it excludes a broader context within which the whole process may be taking place, such as community structure variables. A more complete representation would also include the time dimension and an endless array of feedback loops to portray how changes in the "outcome" variables can affect the "independent" variable, the residential environment. Also not represented are such complexities as sequences of reactions, or the distinction between short- and long-term effects.

The integrating concept behind the diagram is the notion of a person-environment fit (P-E fit). In order to apply this notion, the environmental variables have to be seen from still another perspective, i.e., dimensions which are environmental supplies vs. dimensions which are environmental demands, and dimensions which enable or facilitate certain activities vs. dimensions which are restrictive or interfering with such activities. Coordinated to these distinctons about the environment are distinctions about the person: characteristics which represent the person's requirements or needs vs. his skills and abilities. Derived measures of the degree of P-E fit are then possible, provided one has measured the environment (objective and perceived) and the person along dimensions which are in some sense commensurate. For example, it should then be possible to juxtapose the degree of manipulability and flexibility which exists in a particular environment with the increasingly limited skills and abilities of the elderly. (402) Changes in the residential environment may be described as changes in P-E fit, thereby perhaps illuminating some of the consequences of such moves. Furthermore, the P-E fit paradigm should be useful in understanding the ways in which individuals cope with various types of poor P-E fit, e.g., altering some aspect of the physical environment, improving their skills, changing their subjective perceptions of the environment, and so on.

## Conclusions and Recommendations

The reader of this review may feel that he has been inexorably led through a myriad of studies to the overwhelming conclusion that "there is no evidence of any direct effects of the residential environment on health and behavior." This would certainly be an unintended and unfortunate consequence of this review, especially if it also meant a simplistic dethroning of the physical environment and enthroning of the purely social environment. Instead, the reader should recognize that our state of ignorance in this field is not that simple and that there exists a definite typology of ". . . there is no evidence that . . ." statements. Regarding the influence from residential environment to health and behavior, one may be concluding that "there is no evidence" because:

1. The matter hasn't been studied yet;
2. Only poor studies have examined the matter, and the results can't be trusted;
3. The results of various studies are all over the place and, in effect, "cancel" each other out;
4. The association can be trusted, but a causal interpretation is unclear;
5. A causal relation exists but it is powerfully mediated or influenced by social-psychological or individual difference variables;
6. Good studies agree that no association exists.

The great majority of studies reviewed appear to fall into categories 3, 4, and 5—in short, there is a lot of accumulated evidence on which to build.

It would be equally unfortunate if the reader were to conclude that only studies which are as comprehensive as Figure 1 are worth doing. Figure 1 is merely a schema which invites the reader to view the issue of effects of residential environment on health and behavior from a certain perspective. Moreover, it is intended as a reminder for the investigator planning a research design to consider the potential relevance for his own study of the different classes of variables which are listed there.

It is true, however, that given the plethora of suggestive but inconclusive findings, we are badly in need of better designed studies. Specifically, such a study should be strong in one or more of the following respects: (a) it permits before-after comparisons and, even better, permits a distinction between short-term and long-term changes; (b) it permits some handle on the problem of self-selection, i.e., the lack of initial equivalence between the group of individuals who are exposed to some residential environment (which is under study) and those who are not; (c) it devotes some effort to studying the intervening behavioral processes through which the effects of the residential environment can be traced, particularly the proximal reactions to the residential environment and the actual usage to which it is subjected; (d) it includes a consideration of selected social-psychological variables, such as those which characterize the social support system and the interactions of the individuals, or those which characterize the socio-demographic similarity between the individual and his neighbors. In addition to these design issues, there is also a great need for investigators to be sensitive to the total social milieu or setting in which the problem they are investigating is embedded. For example, moves to better housing for poor people may represent not only the intended change in residential environment, but also such unintended changes as: increased social segregation, greater unfamiliarity with rules and regulations, greater social distance between tenants and management, and so on.

There would seem to be three compromise research design strategies which combine feasibility with a certain amount of promise of advancing our state of knowledge. The first is a cross-sectional design which compares individuals living in residential environments which differ from each other in some significant aspect, such as high rise vs. low rise. However, the crucial stipulation here is that the individuals living in these different residential environments be unusually comparable in all important respects (e.g., socio-economic status, racial-ethnic background, stage of life cycle, etc.) and that, moreover, the way they came to live in one kind of a residential environment or another had little to do with their own choices and preferences. Admittedly, the opportunities for carrying out such a study will not occur frequently, but they do exist (viz the Fanning study (*181*)). For example, two comparable communities may have built similar low cost public housing which differ in some important respect, such as location in the center of one community and at the outskirts of the other. If the housing draws on similar clients and if the clients differ basically only in that they were born and raised in one community or the other, then we have a good compromise design which can yield some useful information.

The second kind of design is best conceived at the point where the planner and the builder are contemplating the introduction of some variation in design within one housing development complex. For example, the selective introduction of indoor nursery-like facilities in some but not all of the buildings in the complex can lead to a good study of the effects of such a facility on child development, on mothers' life satisfaction and leisure activities (especially social interaction with other tenants), and on the development of a sense of cohesion and community among neighbors which, in turn, may lead to group action, such as the setting up of a true day care center. However, such a study must be planned from the start, since it requires near random assignment of tenants to the housing and since, in general, it calls for great sensitivity in anticipating the various unexpected consequences of such a differential in facilities.

The third approach is represented by the strategy of designing longitudinal studies around "natural experiments," i.e., changes in the residential environment which are planned and predictable, especially those which involve some governmental action which calls for program evaluation. These "natural experiments" could involve such events as: institutional transfer of the elderly, urban renewal and re-housing of residents, introduction (or closing down) of some commercial or recreational facility in a neighborhood, and building low income housing in high income suburban neighborhoods. In these kinds of studies, self-selection may remain a problem, but they are very useful because they allow before-after comparisons and because they can provide valuable evaluation data on consequences of programs to which a governmental agency is already committed but which are subject to modifications.

In the long run, Figure 1 represents a call for a broader more interdisciplinary and more systematic attack on the problem of the effects of the residential environment on health and behavior. A single study need not encompass the whole domain represented by the diagram, but surely a program of studies is needed which would cumulatively build a picture, describing both the overall association between the residential environment and health as well as the various intervening processes. In 1948, Merton (52) criticized the "social bookkeeping" approach used by most of the housing studies, and he summarized the housing literature as follows: "The social psychology of housing has a short, inglorious past and, I believe, a long productive future." A quarter of a century later, the promising future is still there, the past is a bit longer and a bit less inglorious, and the need for re-thinking and re-directing our future efforts as great as ever.

## References

1. Calhoun JB: Population density and social pathology. *Sci Amer* 206:139–146, 1962.
2. Calhoun JB: A 'behavioral sink,' in Bliss EL (ed.) : *Roots of Behavior*. New York, Harper, 1962, pp. 295–315.
3. Chance MRA, MacKintosh JA: The effects of caging, in *Symposium Report, Royal Veterinary Laboratory*. London, FJ Milner & Sons, 1962, pp. 59–64.
4. Christian JJ: The potential role of the adrenal cortex as affected by social rank and population density on experimental epidemics. *Amer J Epidemiol* 87: 255–264, 1968.
5. Ratcliffe HL, Cronin MTI: Changing frequency of arteriosclerosis in mammals and birds at the Philadelphia Zoological Garden. *Circulation* 18: 41–52, 1958.
6. Snyder RL: Reproduction and population pressures, in Stellar E, Sprague J (eds) : *Progress in Physiological Psychology*. New York, Academic Press, 1968, pp. 119–160.
7. Thiessen DD: Population density and behavior: A review of theoretical and physiological contributions. *Texas Rep Biol Med* 22: 266–314, 1964.
8. Cassel J: Physical illness in response to stress, in Levine S, Scotch NA (eds) : *Social Stress*. Chicago, Aldine, 1970, pp. 189–209.
9. Cooper RM, Zubek JP: Effects of enriched and restricted early environments on the learning ability of bright and dull rats. *Canad J Psychol* 12: 159–164, 1958.
10. Rosenzweig MR: Environmental complexity, cerebral change, and behavior. *Amer Psychologist* 21: 321–332, 1966.
11. Chen E, Cobb S: Family structure in relation to health and disease. *J Chron Dis* 12: 545-567, 1960.
12. LaHorgue Z: Morbidity and marital status. *J Chron Dis* 12: 476–498, 1960.
13. Zajonc RB: *Social Psychology: An Experimental Approach*. Belmont, Calif., Wadsworth, 1966.

111

14. Back KW, Bogdonoff MD: Plasma lipid responses to leadership, conformity, and deviation, in Leiderman PH, Shapiro D (eds) : *Psychobiological Approaches to Social Behavior*. Stanford, Stanford University Press, 1964, pp. 24–42.
15. Mott PE, Mann FC, McLoughlin Q, Warwick DP: *Shift Work*. Ann Arbor, University of Michigan Press, 1965.
16. Thiis-Evensen E: Shiftwork and health. *Industr Med Surg 27:* 493–497, 1958.
17. Altman PL, Dittner DS (eds) : *Environmental Biology*. Bethesda, Md., Federation of American Societies for Experimental Biology, 1966.
18. Broadbent DE: *Perception and Communication*. New York, Pergamon Press, 1958, Ch. 5.
19. Burns NM, Chambers RM, Hendler E (eds) : *Unusual Environments and Human Behavior*. New York, Free Press of Glencoe, 1963.
20. Goromosov MS: The physiological basis of health standards for dwellings. *WHO: Public Health Papers* No. 33: 1–99, 1968.
21. Plutchik R: The effect of high intensity intermittent sound on performance, feeling, and physiology. *Psychol Bull 56:* 133–151, 1959.
22. Rohles FH Jr: Environmental psychology: A bucket of worms. *Psychology Today 1:* No. 2, 54–63, 1967.
23. The Editors of Fortune: *The Environment: A National Mission for the Seventies*. New York, Perennial Library, Harper & Row, 1970.
24. Helfrich HW Jr (ed.) : *The Environmental Crisis*. New Haven, Yale University Press, 1970.
25. Martin AE: Environment, housing, and health. *Urban Studies 4:* 1–21, 1967.
26. Michelson W: *Man and His Urban Environment: A Sociological Approach*. Reading, Mass., Addison-Wesley, 1970.
27. Winkel GH: The nervous affair between behavior scientists and designers. *Psychology Today 3:* No. 10, 31–35, 74, 1970.
28. Grosser GH, Wechsler H, Greenblatt M (eds) : *The Threat of Impending Disaster*. Cambridge, MIT Press, 1964.
29. Wilson W: Correlates of avowed happiness. *Psychol Bull 67:* 294–306, 1967.
30. Pollitt E: Ecology, malnutrition, and mental development. *Psychosom Med 31:* 193–200, 1969.
31. Gans HJ: Social and physical planning for the elimination of urban poverty, in Rosenberg B, Gerver I, Howton FW (eds) : *Mass Society in Crisis*. New York, Macmillan, 1964, pp. 629–644.
32. Blumenfeld H: Criteria for judging the quality of the urban environment, in Schmandt HJ, Bloomberg W Jr (eds) : *The Quality of Urban Life*. Beverly Hills, Cal., Sage Publications, Inc., 1969, Vol. 3, pp. 137–163.
33. Dubos R: Promises and hazards of man's adaptability, in Jarrett H (ed.) : *Environmental Quality in a Growing Economy*. Baltimore, The Johns Hopkins Press, 1966, pp. 23–39.
34. Dubos R: *So Human an Animal*. New York, Scribner's, 1968.
35. Abu-Lughod J: The city is dead—long live the city. Some thoughts on urbanity, in Fava SF (ed.) : *Urbanism in World Perspective*. New York, T.V. Crowell Co., 1968, pp. 155–165.
36. Baker A, Davies RL, Sivadon P: Psychiatric services and architecture. *WHO: Public Health Papers* No. 1, 1959.
37. Good LR, Siegel SM, Bay AP: *Therapy by Design: Implications of Architecture for Human Behavior*. Springfield, Ill., CC Thomas, 1965.
38. Goshen CE: A review of psychiatric architecture and the principles of design, in Goshen CE (ed.) : *Psychiatric Architecture*. Washington, D.C., The American Psychiatric Association, 1959.
39. Osmond H: Function as the basis of psychiatric ward design. *Mental Hospital (Archit. Suppl.) 8:* 23–29, 1957.

112

40. Searles HF: *The Nonhuman Environment in Normal Development and in Schizophrenia.* New York, International Universities Press, 1960.
41. Stainbrook E: Architects not only design hospitals; they also design patient behavior. *Modern Hospital* 106: 100, 1966.
42. Alexander C: The city as a mechanism for sustaining human contact, in Ewald. WR Jr (ed.) : *Environment for Man.* Bloomington: Indiana University Press, 1967, pp. 60–102.
43. American Public Health Association, Program Area Committee on Housing and Health. 1968: Basic health principles of housing and its environment. *Amer J Public Health 59:* 841–853, 1969.
44. Senn CL: Planning of housing programmes, in Housing programmes: the role of public health agencies. *WHO: Public Health Papers* No. 25, 1964.
45. World Health Organization: Environmental health aspects of metropolitan planning and development. *Wld Health Org Techn Rep Ser No. 297,* 1965.
46. World Health Organization: Appraisal of the hygienic quality of housing and its environment. *Wld Health Org Techn Rep Ser No. 353,* 1967.
47. Barr CW: *Housing-Health Relationships: An annotated Bibliography.* Monticello, Ill., Council of Planning Librarians, Exchange Bibliography No. 82, 1969.
48. Dalla Valle JM: Some factors which affect the relationship between housing and health. *Public Health Rep 52:* 989–998, 1937.
49. Gilbertson WE, Mood EW: Housing, the residential environment and health: A re-evaluation. *Amer J Public Health 54:* 2009–2013, 1964.
50. Griffin WV, Mauritzen JH, Kasmer JV: The psychological aspects of the architectural environment: A review. *Amer J Psychiat 125:* 1057–1062, 1959.
51. Heyman M: Space and behavior. *Landscape 13:* 4–10, 1964.
52. Merton RK: The social psychology of housing, in Dennis W (ed.) : *Current Trends in Social Psychology.* Pittsburgh, University of Pittsburgh Press, 1948, pp. 163–217.
53. Pan American Health Organization: Environmental determinants of community well-being. *WHO Sci Publ No. 123:* 1965.
54. Pond MA: How does housing affect health? *Public Health Rep 61:* 665–672, 1946.
55. Pond MA: The influence of housing on health. *Marriage and Family Living 9:* 154–159, 1957.
56. Rosow I: The social effects of the physical environment. *J Amer Inst Planners 27:* 127–133, 1961.
57. Schorr AL: *Slums and Social Insecurity.* Washington, D.C., HEW, Social Security Administration Research Report No. 1, 1963.
58. Schorr AL: Housing the poor, in Bloomberg W Jr, Schmandt HJ (ed) : *Urban Poverty.* Beverly Hills, Cal., Sage Publications, Inc., 1968, pp. 201–236.
59. Wilner DM, Walkley RP, Pinkerton TC, Tayback M: *The Housing Environment and Family Life.* Baltimore, The Johns Hopkins Press, 1962.
60. World Health Organization: Expert committee on the public health aspects of housing. *Wld Health Org Techn Rep Ser No. 225:* 1961 p. 13.
61. Benjamin JE, Ruegsegger JW, Senior FA: The influence of overcrowding on the incidence of pneumonia. *Ohio State Med J 36:* 1275–1281, 1940.
62. McMillan JS: Examination of the association between housing conditions and pulmonary tuberculosis in Glasgow. *Brit J Prev Soc Med 11:* 142–151, 1957.
63. Stein L: A study of respiratory tuberculosis in relation to housing conditions in Edinburgh. *Brit J Soc Med 4:* 143–169, 1950.
64. Stein L: Glasgow tuberculosis and housing. *Tubercle 35:* 195–203, 1954.
65. Schmitt RC: Housing and health on Oahu. *Amer J Public Health 45:* 1538–1540, 1955.

113

66. Schmitt RC: Density, health, and social disorganization. *J Amer Institute Planners 32:* 38-40, 1966.

67. Hochstim JR: Health and ways of living, in Kessler II, Levin ML (eds) : *The Community as an Epidemiologic Laboratory.* Baltimore, The Johns Hopkins Press, 1970, pp. 149–175.

68. Brett GZ, Benjamin B: Housing and tuberculosis in a mass radiography survey. *Brit J Prev Soc Med 11:* 7–8 ,1957.

69. Coulter JE: Rheumatic fever and streptococcal illness in two communities in New York State. *Milbank Mem Fund Quart 30:* 341–358, 1952.

70. Colley JRT, Holland WW: Social and environmental factors in respiratory disease *Arch Envir Health 14:* 157–161, 1967.

71. Christensen V: Child morbidity in a good and bad residential area. *Danish Med Bull 3:* 93–98, 1956.

72. Holmes TH: Multidiscipline studies of tuberculosis, in Sparer PJ (ed) : *Personality, Stress, and Tuberculosis.* New York, International Universities Press, 1956.

73. Dunham HW: *Community and Schizophrenia.* Detroit, Wayne State University Press, 1965.

74. Faris REL, Dunham HW: *Mental Disorders in Urban Areas.* Chicago, The University of Chicago Press, 1939.

75. Gruenberg EM: Community conditions and psychoses of the elderly. *Amer J Psychiat 110:* 888–896, 1954.

76. Hare EH: Mental illness and social conditions in Bristol. *J Ment Sci 102:* 349–357, 1956.

77. Jaco EG: Social stress and mental illness in the community, in Sussman MB (ed) : *Community Structure and Analysis.* New York, TY Crowell Co, 1959, pp. 388–409.

78. Klee GD, Spiro E, Bahn AK, Gorwitz K: An ecological analysis of diagnosed mental illness in Baltimore, in Monroe RR, Klee GD, Brody EB (ed) : *Psychiatric Epidemiology and Mental Health Planning.* Washington, D.C., Psychiatric Research Report No. 22, American Psychiatric Association, 1967.

79. Schroeder CW: Mental disorders in cities. *Amer J Sociol 48:* 40–47, 1942.

80. Weinberg SK: Urban areas and hospitalized psychotics, in Weinberg SK (ed) : *The Sociology of Mental Disorders.* Chicago, Aldine, 1967, pp. 22–26.

81. Clausen JA, Kohn ML: The relation of schizophrenia to the social structure of a small city, in Pasamanick B (ed) : *Epidemiology of Mental Disorder.* Washington, D.C., American Association for the Advancement of Science, Publication No. 60, 1959.

82. Mintz NL, Schwartz DT: Urban ecology and psychosis: Community factors in the incidence of schizophrenia and manic-depression among Italians in greater Boston. *Int J Soc Psychiat 10:* 101–118, 1964.

83. Schwartz DT, Mintz NL: Ecology and psychosis among Italians in 27 Boston communities. *Social Problems 10:* 371–374, 1963.

84. Hyde RW, Kingsley LV: Studies in medical sociology. I. The relation of mental disorders to the community socioeconomic level. *New Engl J Med 231:* 543–548, 1944.

85. Gerard DL, Houston LG: Family setting and the social ecology of schizophrenia. *Psychiat Quart 27:* 90–101, 1953.

86. Hare EH: Family setting and the urban distribution of schizophrenia. *J Ment Sci 102:* 753–760, 1956.

87. Wechsler H, Pugh TF: Fit of individual and community characteristics and rates of psychiatric hospitalization. *Amer J Sociol 73:* 331–338, 1967.

88. Gordon RA: Issues in the ecological study of delinquency. *Amer Sociol Rev 32:* 927–944, 1967.

114

89. Harlan H, Wherry J: Delinquency and housing. *Social Forces 27:* 58–61, 1948.
90. Landner B: *Towards an Understanding of Juvenile Delinquency.* New York, Columbia University Press, 1954.
91. Schmitt RC: Density, delinquency, and crime in Honolulu. *Sociol and Soc Res 41:* 274–276, 1957.
92. Shaw CR, McKay HD: *Juvenile Delinquency and Urban Areas.* Chicago, The University of Chicago Press, Revised edition, 1969.
93. Short JF Jr: Introduction to the revised edition, in Shaw CR, McKay HD: *Juvenile Delinquency and Urban Areas.* Chicago, The University of Chicago Press, 1969, revised edition, pp. xxv-liv.
94. Linsky AS: Community homogeneity and exclusion of the mentally ill: Rejection versus consensus about deviance. *J Health Soc Behav 11:* 304–311, 1970.
95. Bloom BL: An ecological analysis of psychiatric hospitalizations. *Multivariate Behav Res 3:* 423–463, 1968.
96. Hochstim JR, Athanasopoulos DA, Larkins JH: Poverty area under the microscope. *Amer J Public Health 58:* 1815–1827, 1968.
97. Robinson WS: Ecological correlations and the behavior of individuals. *Amer Sociol Rev 15:* 351–357, 1950.
98. Blalock HM Jr: *Causal Inferences in Nonexperimental Research.* Chapel Hill, University of North Carolina Press, 1961.
99. Blalock H MJr: Theory building and causal inferences, in Blalock HM Jr, Blalock AB (eds) : *Methodology in Social Research.* New York, McGraw-Hill, 1968, pp. 155–198.
100. Boudon R: A new look at correlational analysis, in Blalock HM Jr, Blalock AB (eds) : *Methodology in Social Research.* New York, McGraw-Hill, 1968, pp. 199–235.
101. Clausen JA, Kohn ML: The ecological approach of social psychiatry. *Amer J Sociol 60:* 140–149, 1954.
102. Dunham HW: Epidemiology of psychiatric disorders as a contribution to medical ecology. *Arch Gen Psychiat 14:* 1–19, 1966.
103. Srole L, Langner TS, Michael ST, Opler MK, Rennie TAC: *Mental Health in the Metropolis.* New York, McGraw-Hill, 1962.
104. Hollingshead AB, Redlich FC: *Social Class and Mental Illness.* New York, Wiley, 1958.
105. Harburg E, Schull WJ, Erfurt JC, Schork MA: A family set method for estimating heredity and stress. I. A pilot survey of blood pressure among Negroes in high and low stress areas, Detroit, 1966–1967. *J Chron Dis 23:* 69–81, 1970.
106. Reiss AJ Jr: Rural-urban and status differences in interpersonal contacts. *Amer J Sociol 65:* 182–195, 1959.
107. Steinman D: Health in rural poverty: some lessons in theory and from experience. *Amer J Public Health 60:* 1813–1823, 1970.
108. National Center for Health Statistics: *Health Characteristics by Geographic Region, Large Metropolitan Areas, and Other Places of Residence. United States, July 1963–June 1965.* Washington, D.C., U.S.P.H.S., Series 10, No. 36, 1967.
109. National Center for Health Statistics: *Disability Days. United States, July 1963–June 1964.* Washington, D.C., U.S.P.H.S., Series 10, No. 24, 1965.
110. National Center for Health Statistics: *Characteristics of Persons with Diabetes. United States, July 1964–June 1965.* Washington, D.C., U.S.P.H.S., Series 10, No. 40, 1967.
111. Kjelsberg M, Stamler J: Epidemiologic studies on cardiovascular-renal diseases. II. Analysis of mortality by age-race-sex-place of residence, including urban-rural comparisons. *J Chron Dis 12:* 456–463, 1960.

112. Syme LS, Hyman MM, Enterline PE: Some social and cultural factors associated with the occurrence of coronary heart disease. *J Chron Dis 17:* 277–289, 1964.
113. Thompson JF: Some observations on the geographic distribution of premature births and perinatal deaths in Indiana. *Amer J Obs and Gyn 101:* 43–51, 1968.
114. Wanklin MJ, Fleming DF, Buck CW, Hobbs GE: Factors influencing the rate of first admission to mental hospital. *J Nerv Ment Dis 121:* 103–116, 1955.
115. Wiehl DG: Mortality and socio-economic factors. *Milbank Mem Fund Quart 26:* 335–365, 1948.
116. Neser WB, Tyroler HA, Cassel JC: Social disorganization and stroke mortality in the black population of North Carolina. *Amer J Epidemiol 93:* 166–175, 1971.
117. Vail DJ, Lucero RJ, Boen JR: The relationship between socioeconomic variables and major mental illness in the counties of a midwestern state. *Community Mental Health J 2:* 211–212, 1966.
118. Syme SL, Hyman MM, Enterline PE: Cultural mobility and the occurrence of coronary heart disease. *J Health and Human Behavior 6:* 178–189, 1965.
119. Wardwell WI, Hyman M, Bahnson CB: Stress and coronary heart disease in three field studies. *J Chron Dis 17:* 73–84, 1964.
120. Cassel J, Tyroler HA: Epidemiologic studies of culture change. I. Health status and recency of industrialization. *Arch Environ Health 3:* 25–33, 1961.
121. Tyroler HA, Cassel J: Health consequences of culture change. II. The effect of urbanization on coronary heart mortality in rural residents. *J Chron Dis 17:* 167–177, 1964.
122. Abramson JH: Observations on the health of adolescent girls in relation to cultural change. *Psychosom Med 23:* 156–165, 1961.
123. Fried M: Effects of social change on mental health. *Amer J Orthopsychiat 34:* 3–28, 1964.
124. Hoobler S, Tejada C, Guzman M, Pardo A: Influence of nutrition and "acculturation" on the blood pressure levels and changes with age in the Highland Guatemalan Indian. *Circulation 32:* Suppl II, 116, 1965.
125. Scotch NA: Sociocultural factors in the epidemiology of Zulu hypertension. *Amer J Public Health 53:* 1205–1213, 1963.
126. Gordon RE, Gordon KK: Social psychiatry of a mobile suburb. *Int J Soc Psychiat 6:* 89–100, 1960.
127. Gordon RE, Gordon KK: Emotional disorders of children in a rapidly growing suburb. *Int J Soc Psychiat 4:* 85–97, 1958.
128. Wechsler H: Community growth, depressive disorders, and suicide. *Amer J Sociol 67:* 9–16, 1961.
129. Gordon RE, Gordon KK: Psychosomatic problems in a rapidly growing suburb. *JAMA 170:* 1757–1764, 1959.
130. Gans HJ: *The Urban Villagers.* Glencoe, Ill., The Free Press, 1962.
131. Whyte WF: *Street Corner Society: The Social Structure of an Italian Slum.* Chicago, University of Chicago Press, 1943.
132. Marris P: A report on urban renewal in the United States, in Duhl LJ (ed.): *The Urban Condition.* New York, Basic Books, 1963, pp. 113–134.
133. Hollingshead AB, Rogler LH: Attitudes towards slums and public housing in Puerto Rico, in Duhl LJ (ed.): *The Urban Condition.* New York, Basic Books, 1963, pp. 229–245.
134. Fried M, Gleicher P: Some sources of residential satisfaction in an urban slum. *J Amer Institute Planners 27:* 305–315, 1961.
135. Ryan EJ: Personal identity in an urban slum, in Duhl LJ (ed.): *The Urban Condition.* New York, Basic Books, 1963, pp. 135–150.
136. Lynch K: The city as environment, in Scientific American: *Cities.* New York, Knopf, 1965, pp. 192–201.

137. Back KW: *Slums, Projects, and People*. Durham, N.C., Duke University Press, 1962.
138. Rainwater L: Fear and the house-as-haven in the lower class. *J Amer Institute of Planners 32:* 23–31, 1966.
139. Gans HJ: Urbanism and suburbanism as ways of life; a re-evaluation of definitions, in Rose AM (ed.) : *Human Behavior and Social Processes*. Boston, Houghton Mifflin, 1962, pp. 625–648.
140. Salzman DM: Redevelopment effectiveness contingent on understanding slum occupants. *J Housing 13:* No. 8, 289–296, 298, 1956.
141. Seeley JR: The slum: Its nature, use, and users. *J Amer Institute Planners 25:* 7–14, 1959.
142. Weinberg SK: The relevance of the forms of isolation to schizophrenia. *Int J Social Psychiat 13:* 33–41, 1966.
143. Adams BN: *Kinship in an Urban Setting*. Chicago, Markham Publishing Co, 1968.
144. Gans HJ: Planning and social life: Friendship and neighbor relations in suburban communities. *J Amer Institute Planners 27:* 134–140, 1961.
145. Rosenberg GS: *Poverty, Aging, and Social Isolation*. Washington, D.C. Bureau of Social Science Research, Inc., 1967.
146. Rosow I: Housing and local ties of the aged, in Neugarten BL (ed.) : *Middle Age and Aging*. Chicago, University of Chicago Press, 1968, pp. 382–389.
147. Kennedy R: Premarital residential propinquity. *Amer J Sociol 48:* 580–584, 1943.
148. Caplow T, Forman R: Neighborhood interaction in a homogeneous community. *Amer Sociol Rev 15:* 357–366, 1950.
149. Durant R: *Watling*. London, King, 1939.
150. Keller S: *The Urban Neighborhood: A Sociological Perspective*. New York, Random House, 1968.
151. Mitchell GD, Lupton T: The Liverpool estate, in *Neighborhood and Community*. Liverpool, Liverpool University Press, 1954.
152. Willmott P: *The Evolution of a Community*. London, Routledge & Kegan Paul, 1963.
153. Bultena GL: The relationship of occupational status to friendship ties in three planned retirement communities. *J Gerontol 24:* 461–464, 1969.
154. Form WH: Status stratification in a planned community. *Amer Sociol Rev 10:* 605–613, 1945.
155. Form WH: Stratification in low and middle income housing areas. *J Social Issues 7:* No. 1–2, 109–131, 1951.
156. Duncan OD, Duncan B: Residential distribution and occupational stratification, in Hatt PK, Reiss AJ Jr (eds) : *Cities and Society*. Glencoe, Ill., The Free Press, 1957, pp. 283–296.
157. Feldman AS, Tilly C: The interaction of social and physical space. *Amer Sociol Rev 25:* 877–884, 1960.
158. Smith J, Form WH, Stone GP: Local intimacy in a middle-sized city. *Amer J Sociol 60:* 276–284, 1954.
159. Rosenberg GS: Age, poverty, and isolation from friends in the urban working class. *J Gerontol 23:* 533–538, 1968.
160. Hamovitch MB, Peterson JE: Housing needs and satisfaction of the elderly. *The Gerontologist 9:* 30–32, 1969.
161. Lawton MP: Supportive services in the context of the housing environment. *The Gerontologist 9:* 15–19, 1969.
162. Carp FM: Housing a minority group elderly. *The Gerontologist 9:* 20–24, 1969.
163. Niebanck PL, Pope JB: *The Elderly in Older Urban Areas*. Philadelphia, Institute for Environmental Studies, University of Pennsylvania, 1965.

164. Howell SC, Loeb MB: Nutrition and aging: A monograph for practitioners. *The Gerontologist 9:* No. 3, Pt II, 7–122, 1969.
165. Gray RM, Moberg DO: *The Church and the Older Person.* Grand Rapids, Eerdmans, 1962.
166. Moberg DO: Religiosity in old age, in Neugarten BL (ed.) *Middle Age and Aging,* Chicago, University of Chicago Press, 1968, pp. 497–508.
167. Schooler KK: The relationship between social interaction and morale of the elderly as a function of environmental characteristics. *The Gerontologist 9:* No. 1, 25–29, 1969.
168. Schooler KK: On the relation between characteristics of residential environment, social behavior, and the emotional and physical health of the elderly in the United States. Paper presented at the 8th International Congress of Gerontology, Washington, D.C., 1969.
169. Britten RH: New light on the relation of housing to health. *Amer J Public Health 32:* 193–199, 1942.
170. Britten RH, Altman I: Illness and accidents among persons living under different housing conditions. *Public Health Rep 56:* 609–640, 1941.
171. Britten RH, Brown JE, Altman I: Certain characteristics of urban housing and their relation to illness and accidents: Summary of findings of the National Health Survey. *Milbank Mem Fund Quart 18:* No. 1, 91–113, 1940.
172. Beck MD, Muñoz JA, Scrimshaw NS: Studies on diarrheal diseases in Central America. I. Preliminary findings on cultural surveys of normal population groups in Guatemala. *Amer J Trop Med and Hygiene 6:* 62–71, 1957.
173. Bruch HA, Ascoli W, Scrimshaw NS, Gordon JE: Studies of diarrheal disease in Guatemalan villages. V. Environmental factors in the origin and transmission of acute diarrheal disease in four Guatemalan villages. *Amer J Trop Med and Hygiene 12:* 567–579, 1963.
174. Kourany M, Vásquez MA: Housing and certain socioenvironmental factors and prevalence of enteropathogenic bacteria among infants with diarrheal disease in Panama. *Amer J Trop Med and Hygiene 18:* 936–941, 1969.
175. Schliessmann DJ, Atchley FO, Wilcomb MJ, Welch SF: Relation of environmental factors to the occurrence of enteric disease in areas of eastern Kentucky. *Public Health Service Monogr. No. 54.* 1958.
176. Watt J, Hollister AC Jr, Beck MD, Hemphill EC: Diarrheal diseases in Fresno County, California. *Amer J Public Health 43:* 728–741, 1953.
177. Hobson W, Pemberton J: *The Health of the Elderly at Home.* London, Butterworth, 1955.
178. Lunn JE: A Study of Glasgow families living in one-apartment, two-apartment, and three-apartment tenement houses. *Scot Med J 6:* 125–129, 1961.
179. Power JGP: Health aspects of vertical living in Hong Kong. *Community Health 1:* 316–320, 1970.
180. Bernstein SH: Observations on the effects of housing on the incidence and spread of common respiratory diseases among Air Force recruits. *Amer J Hygiene 65:* 162–171, 1957.
181. Fanning DM: Families in flats. *Brit Med J 4:* 382–386, 1967.
182. Kasl SV, Cobb S: Health behavior, illness behavior and sick role behavior. *Arch Environ Health 12:* 246–266, and 531–541, 1966.
183. Grootenboer EA: The relation of housing to behavior disorder. *Amer J Psychiat 119:* 469–472, 1962.
184. Tulkin SR: Race, class, family, and school achievement. *J Pers Social Psychol 9:* 31–37, 1968.
185. Michelson W: The physical environment as a mediating factor in school achievement. Presented at the Annual Meeting of the Canadian Sociology & Anthropology Association, Calgary, Alberta, 1968.

186. Keller M: Progress in school of children in a sample of families in the Eastern Health District of Baltimore, Maryland. *Millbank Memorial Fund Quart 31:* 391–410, 1953.
187. Jackson WS: Housing and pupil growth and development. *J Educ Sociol 28:* 370–380, 1955.
188. Havránek J: Investigation of housing quality in Czechoslovakia. Paper presented at the Conference on the Influence of the Urban and Working Environment on the Health and Behavior of Modern Man. Prague, Charles University, October 1969.
189. Loring WC Jr: Housing characteristics and social disorganization. *Social Problems 3:* 160–168, 1956. (Note error on p. 162, in first paragraph of second column: a "not" was omitted between "were" and "matched" in 13th line.)
189a. Mitchell, RE: "Some Social Implications of High Density Housing," *American Sociological Review, 36:* 27 & 28, 1971.
190. Deutsch M. Collins ME: *Interracial Housing: A Psychological Evaluation of a Social Experiment.* Minneapolis, University of Minnesota Press, 1951.
191. Jahoda M. West PS: Race relations in public housing. *J Social Issues 7:* No. 1–2, 132–139, 1951.
192. Wilner DM, Walkley RP, Cook SW: *Human Relations in Interracial Housing.* Minneapolis, University of Minnesota Press, 1955.
193. Works E: Residence in integrated and segregated housing and improvement in self-concept of Negroes. *Sociology and Social Research 46:* 294–301, 1962.
194. Kramer BM: *Residential Contact as a Determinant of Attitudes Toward Negroes.* Cambridge, Harvard University, Unpublished Dissertation, 1951.
195. Goldman M, Warshay LH, Biddle EH: Residential and personal social distance toward Negroes and non-Negroes. *Psychol Rep 10:* 421-422, 1962.
196. Festinger L, Schachter S, Back K: *Social Pressures in Informal Groups.* Stanford, Stanford University Press, 1950.
197. Blake R, Rhead CC, Wedge B, Mouton JS: Housing architecture and social interaction. *Sociometry 19:* 133–139, 1956.
198. Friedman EP: Spatial proximity and social interaction in a home for the aged. *J Gerontol 21:* 566–570, 1966.
199. Lawton MP, Simon B: The ecology of social relationships in housing for elderly. *The Gerontologist 8:* No. 2, 108–115, 1968.
200. Rosow I: *Social Integration of the Aged.* New York, The Free Press, 1967.
201. Holmes TH, Rahe RH: The social readjustment rating scale. *J Psychosom Res 10:* 213–218, 1967.
202. Jacobs MA, Spilken AZ, Norman MM, Anderson LS: Life stress and respiratory illness. *Psychosom Med 32:* 233–242, 1970.
203. Rahe RH, Arthur RJ: Life change patterns surrounding illness experience. *J Psychosom Res 11:* 341–345, 1968.
204. Rahe RH, Gunderson EK, Arthur RJ: Demographic and psychosocial factors in acute illness reporting. *J Chron Dis 23:* 245–255, 1970.
205. Rahe RH, McKean JD, Arthur RJ: A longitudinal study of life change and illness patterns. *J Psychosom Res 10:* 355–366, 1967.
206. Rahe RH, Meyer M, Smith M, Kjaer G, Holmes TH: Social stress and illness onset. *J Psychosom Res 8:* 35-44, 1964.
207. Schmale AH: Object loss, "giving up," and disease onset. An overview of research in progress. *Symposium on Medical Aspects of Stress in the Military Climate.* Washington, D.C., U.S. Government Printing Office, 1965, pp. 433–443.
208. Bhandari NP, Harold Hill: A medico-social study of rehousing. *J Royal Inst of Public Health and Hygiene 23:* 187–204, 1960.
209. Ferguson T, Pettigrew MG: A study of 718 slum families rehoused for upwards of ten years. *Glasgow Med J 35:* 183–201, 1954.

119

210. Hopper JMH: Disease, health, and housing. *Medical Officer 107:* 97–104 and 117–122, 1962.
211. M'Gonigle GCM: Poverty, nutrition, and public health. *Proc Royal Soc Med 26:* 677–687, 1933.
212. Rumney J, Shuman S: *A Study of the Social Effects of Public Housing.* Newark, N.J., Housing Authority of the City of Newark, 1944.
213. Worth RM: Urbanization and squatter resettlement as related to child health in Hong Kong. *Amer J Hygiene 78:* 338–348, 1963.
214. Brennan T: *Reshaping a City.* Glasgow, Grant, 1959.
215. Lichfield N: Relocation: The impact on housing welfare. *J Amer Institute Planners 27:* 199–203, 1961.
216. Wood E: *The Needs of People Affected by Relocation.* Philadelphia, Community Renewal Program, City of Philadelphia, Technical Report No. 17, 1965.
217. Hare EH, Shaw GK: *Mental Health on a New Housing Estate.* London, Oxford University Press, 1965.
218. Hole V: Social effects of planned rehousing. *Town Planning Rev 30:* 161–173, 1959.
219. Martin FM: The Community. Social and psychological aspects of rehousing. *The Advancement of Science 12:* 448–453, 1956.
220. Martin FM, Brotherston JHF, Chave SPW: Incidence of neurosis in a new housing estate. *Brit J Prev Soc Med 11:* 196–202, 1957.
221. Maule HG: The family. Social and psychological aspects of rehousing. *The Advancement of Science 12:* 443–448, 1956.
222. Mogey JM: Changes in family life experienced by English workers moving from slums to housing estates. *Marriage and Family Living 17:* 123–128, 1955.
223. Mogey JM: *Family and Neighborhood.* London, Oxford University Press, 1956.
224. Mogey JM, Morris RN: Causes of change in family role patterns. *Bull on Family Development.* Kansas City, Community Studies, Inc., 1, 1960.
225. Morris RN, Mogey JM: *The Sociology of Housing.* London, Routledge & Kegan Paul, 1965.
226. Taylor L, Chave S: *Mental Health and Environment.* London, Longmans, 1964.
227. Young M, Willmott P: *Family and Kinship in East London.* New York, The Free Press, 1957.
228. Bracey HE: *Neighbours.* Baton Rouge, Louisiana State University Press, 1964.
229. Chapin FS: The effect of slum clearance and rehousing on family and community relationships in Minneapolis. *Amer J Sociol 43:* 744–763, 1938.
230. Chapin FS: An experiment on the social effects of good housing. *Amer Sociol Rev 5:* 868–879, 1940.
231. Barer N: *A Study of the Effects of Improved Housing on the Physical and Social Health of a Group of Families in a Public Housing Project.* New Haven, Yale University School of Medicine, Unpublished M.P.H. essay, 1945.
232. Barer N: Delinquency before, after admission to New Haven Housing development. *J Housing 3:* 27, 1945.
233. Goldscheider C: Differential residential mobility of the older population. *J Gerontol 21:* 103–108, 1966.
234. Langford M: *Community Aspects of Housing for the Aged.* Ithaca, N.Y., Center for Housing and Environmental Studies, Cornell University, Research Report No. 5, 1962.
235. Carp FM: *A Future for the Aged.* Austin, University of Texas Press, 1966.
236. Carp FM: The impact of environment on old people. *The Gerontologist 7:* No. 2, Pt. 1, 106–108, 135, 1967.
237. Carp FM: Effects of improved housing on the lives of older people, in Neugarten BL (ed.) : *Middle Age and Aging.* Chicago, University of Chicago Press, 1968, pp. 409–416.

238. Bultena GL, Wood V: The American retirement community: Bane or blessing? *J Gerontol 24:* 209–217, 1969.

239. Sherman SR, Mangum WP Jr, Dodds S, Walkley RP, Wilner DM: Psychological effects of retirement housing. *The Gerontologist 8:* No. 3, Pt. 1, 170–175, 1968.

240. Berger B: *Working Class Suburb: A Study of Auto Workers in Suburbia.* Berkeley, University of California Press, 1960.

241. Gans HJ: Effects of the move from city to suburb, in Duhl LG (ed.) : *The Urban Condition.* New York, Basic Books, 1963, pp. 184–198.

242. Gans HJ: *The Levittowners.* New York, Pantheon Books, 1967.

243. Gans HJ: *People and Plans. Essays on Urban Problems and Solutions.* New York, Basic Books, 1968.

244. Gutman R: Population mobility in the middle class, in Duhl LJ (ed.) : *The Urban Condition.* New York, Basic Books, 1963, pp. 172–183.

245. Gutman R: A sociologist looks at housing, in Moynihan DP (ed.) : *Toward a National Urban Policy.* New York, Basic Books, 1970, pp. 119–132.

246. Hallowitz DL: The relationship between selected goals of prospective homeowners and their experiences in a new suburban housing development. *Dissert Abstr 29A:* 2435–2436, 1969.

247. Thoma L, Lindemann E: Newcomers' problems in a suburban community. *J Amer Institute of Planners 27:* 185–193, 1961.

248. Millspaugh M, Breckenfeld G: *The Human Side of Urban Renewal.* Baltimore, Fight-Blight, Inc., 1958.

249. Gans HJ: The human implications of current redevelopment and relocation planning. *J Amer Institute of Planners 25:* 15–25, 1959.

250. Gans HJ: The failure of urban renewal: A critique and some proposals. *Commentary 39:* 29–37, 1965.

251. Pozen MW, Goshin AR, Bellin LE: Evaluation of housing standards of families within four years of relocation by urban renewal. *Amer J Public Health 58:* 1256–1264, 1968.

252. Thursz D: *Where Are They Now?* Washington, D.C., Health and Welfare Council of the National Capital Area, 1966.

253. Fried M: Grieving for a lost home, in Duhl LJ (ed.) : *The Urban Condition,* New York, Basic Books, 1963, pp. 151–171.

254. Fried M: Transitional functions of working-class communities: Implications for forced relocation, in Kantor MB (ed.) : *Mobility and Mental Health.* Springfield, Ill., C.C. Thomas, 1965, pp. 123–165.

255. Niebanck PL: Knowledge gained in studies of relocation, in Carp FM, Burnette WM (eds) : *Patterns of Living and Housing of Middle Aged and Older People.* Washington, D.C., U.S.P.H.S. Publication No. 1496, 1966, pp. 107–116.

256. Niebanck PL: *Relocation in Urban Planning: From Obstacle to Opportunity.* Philadelphia, University of Pennsylvania Press, 1968.

257. Shanas E: *The Health of Older People.* Cambridge, Harvard University Press, 1962.

258. Key WH: *When People Are Forced to Move.* Topeka, The Meninger Foundation, 1967.

259. Kasteler JM, Gray RM, Carruth ML: Involuntary relocation of the elderly. *The Gerontologist 8:* 276–279, 1968.

260. Cavan R, Burgess EW, Havinghurst RJ, Goldhammer H: *Personal Adjustment in Old Age.* Chicago, Science Research Associates, 1949.

261. Camargo O, Preston GH: What happens to patients who are hospitalized for the first time when over sixty-five years of age. *Amer J Psychiat 102:* 168–173, 1945.

262. Cook LC, Dax EC, Maclay WS: The geriatric problem in mental hospitals. *Lancet 1:* 377–382, 1952.

121

263. Costello JP, Tanaka GM: Mortality and morbidity in long-term institutional care of the aged. *J Amer Geriat Soc 9:* 959–963, 1961.

264. Goldfarb AI: The evaluation of geriatric patients following treatment, in Hoch PH, Zubin J (eds) : *The Evaluation of Psychiatric Treatment.* New York, Grune and Stratton, 1964, pp. 271–308.

265. Josephy H: Analysis of mortality and causes of death in a mental hospital. *Amer J Psychiat 106:* 185–189, 1949.

266. Kay DWK, Norris V, Post F: Prognosis in psychiatric disorders of the elderly. *J Ment Sci 102:* 129–140, 1956.

267. Trier TR: A study of change among elderly psychiatric inpatients during their first year of hospitalization. *J Gerontol 23:* 354–362, 1968.

268. Whittier JR, Williams D: The coincidence and constancy of mortality figures for aged psychotic patients admitted to state hospitals. *J Nerv Ment Dis 124:* 618–620, 1956.

269. Kent EA: Role of admission stress in adaptation of older persons in institutions. *Geriatrics 18:* 133–138, 1963.

270. Lieberman MA: Relationship of mortality rates to entrance to a home for the aged. *Geriatrics 16:* 515–519, 1961.

271. Dreyfuss F, Czaczkes JW: Blood cholesterol and uric acid of healthy medical students under stress of examination. *Arch Intern Med 103:* 708–711, 1959.

272. Rahe RH, Arthur RJ: Stressful underwater demolition training: Serum urate and cholesterol variability. *JAMA 202:* 1052–1054, 1967.

273. Kasl SV, Cobb S: Blood pressure changes in men undergoing job loss: A preliminary report. *Psychosom Med 32:* 19–38, 1970.

274. Kasl SV, Cobb S, Brooks GW: Changes in serum uric acid and cholesterol levels in men undergoing job loss. *JAMA 206:* 1500–1507, 1968.

275. Blenker M: Environmental change and the aging individual. *The Gerontologist 7:* 101–105, 1967.

276. Ferrari NA: Freedom of choice. *Social Work 8:* No. 4, 105–, 1963.

277. Aldrich CK, Mendkoff E: Relocation of the aged and disabled: a mortality study. *J Amer Geriat Soc 11:* 185–194, 1963.

278. Killian EC: Effect of geriatric transfers on mortality rates. *Social Work 15:* 19–26, 1970.

279. Aleksandrowicz DR: Fire and its aftermath on a geriatric ward. *Bull Menninger Clinic 25:* 23–32, 1961.

280. Aldrich CK: Personality factors and mortality in the relocation of the aged: *The Gerontologist 4:* 92–93, 1964.

281. Jasnau KF: Individualized versus mass transfer of nonpsychotic geriatric patients from mental hospitals to nursing homes, with special reference to the death rate. *J Amer Geriat Soc 15:* 280–284, 1967.

282. Novick LJ: Easing the stress of moving day. *Hospitals 41:* No. 16, 67–74, 1967.

283. Kral VA, Grad B, Berenson J: Stress reactions resulting from the relocation of an aged population. *Canad Psychiat Assoc J 13:* 201–209, 1968.

284. Miller D, Lieberman MA: The relationship of affect state and adaptive capacity to reactions to stress. *J Gerontol 20:* 492–497, 1965.

285. Linn MW, Gurel L: Initial reactions to nursing home placement. *J Amer Geriat Soc 17:* 219–223, 1969.

286. Fink HH: The relationship of time perspective to age, institutionalization, and activity. *J Gerontol 12:* 414–417, 1957.

287. Klonoff H, Kennedy M: A comparative study of cognitive functioning in old age. *J Gerontol 21:* 239–243, 1966.

288. Pollack M, Karp E, Kahn RL, Goldfarb AI: Perception of self in institutionalized aged subjects. I. Response patterns to mirror reflection. *J Gerontol 17:* 405–408, 1962.

289. Lakin M: Formal characteristics of human figure drawings by institutionalized aged. *J Gerontol 15:* 76–78, 1960.
290. Riley MW, Foner A: *Aging and Society. Vol. I. An Inventory of Research Findings.* New York, Russel Sage Foundation, 1968.
291. Lieberman MA: Institutionalization of the aged: Effects on behavior. *J Gerontol 24:* 330–340, 1969.
292. Anderson NN: Effects of institutionalization on self-esteem. *J Gerontol 22:* 313–317, 1967.
293. Bortner RW: Test differences attributable to age, selection processes, and institutional effects. *J Gerontol 17:* 58–60, 1962.
294. Lieberman MA, Prock VN, Tobin SS: Psychological effects of institutionalization. *J Gerontol 23:* 343–353, 1968.
295. Prock VN: *Effects of Institutionalization—A Comparison of Community, Waiting List, and Institutionalized Aged Persons.* Chicago, The University of Chicago, Unpublished doctoral dissertation, 1965.
296. Bennett R, Nahemow L: Institutional totality and criteria of social adjustment in residence of the aged. *J Soc Issues 21:* No. 4, 44–78, 1965.
297. Brody EB (ed.) : *Behavior in New Environments.* Beverly Hills, Cal., Sage Publications, 1969.
298. Kantor MB: Some consequences of residential and social mobility for the adjustment of children, in Kantor MB (ed.) : *Mobility and Mental Health.* Springfield, Ill., C.C. Thomas, 1965, pp. 86–122.
299. Murphy HBM: Migration and the major mental disorders, in Kantor MB (ed.) : *Mobility and Mental Health.* Springfield, Ill., C.C. Thomas, 1965, pp. 1–29.
300. Cartwright D: Lewinian theory as a contemporary systematic framework, in Koch S (ed.) : *Psychology: A Study of a Science.* New York, McGraw-Hill, Vol. 2, 1959.
301. French JRP Jr, Kahn RL: A programmatic approach to studying the industrial environment and mental health. *J Social Issues 18:* No. 3, 1–47, 1962.
302. Chapin FS: Some housing factors related to mental hygiene. *Amer J Public Health 41:* 839–845, 1951.
303. Chapin FS: The psychology of housing. *Social Forces 30:* 11–15, 1951.
304. Cottam HR: *Housing and Attitudes Toward Housing in Rural Pennsylvania.* State College: Pennsylvania Agricultural Experiment Station, Bulletin 436, 1942.
305. Cutler V: *Personal and Family Values in the Choice of a Home.* Ithaca, N.Y., Cornell University Agricultural Experimental Station, 1947.
306. Dean J: The ghosts of home ownership. *J Social Issues 7:* No. 1–2, 59–68, 1951.
307. Foote NN, Abu-Lughod J, Foley MM, Winnick L: *Housing Choices and Housing Constraints.* New York, McGraw-Hill, 1960.
308. Riemer S: Maladjustment to the family home. *Amer Sociol Rev 10:* 642–648, 1945.
309. Keller S: Social class in physical planning. *Int Social Sci J 18:* 494–512, 1966.
310. Federal Public Housing Authority: *The Livability Problems of 1000 Families.* National Housing Agency Bulletin No. 28, Oct. 1945. (E. Coit) .
311. Michelson W: Potential candidates for the designers' paradise. *Social Forces 46:* 190–196, 1967.
312. Michelson W: An empirical analysis of urban environment preferences. *J Amer Institute of Planners 32:* 355–360, 1966.
313. Wilson RL: Livability of the city: Attitudes and urban development, in Chapin FS, Weiss SF (eds) : *Urban Growth Dynamics in a Regional Cluster of Cities.* New York, Wiley, 1962, pp. 359–399.
314. Wessman AE: *A Psychological Inquiry into Satisfaction and Happiness.* Princeton, Princeton University, Unpublished doctoral dissertation, 1956.
315. Sheldon JH: The social philosophy of old age. *Lancet 267:* 151–155, 1954.

316. Shanas E, Townsend P, Wedderburn D, Friis H, Milhøj, P, Stenhouner J: *Old People in Three Industrial Societies.* New York, Atherton Press, 1968.

317. Rosenmayr L, Kockeis E: Housing conditions and family relations of the elderly, in Carp FM, Burnett NM (eds) : *Patterns of Living and Housing of Middle-Aged and Older People.* Washington, D.C., U.S.P.H.S. Publication No. 1496, 1966, pp. 29–46.

318. Beyer GH, Woods ME: *Living and Activity Patterns of the Aged.* Ithaca, N.Y., Cornell University, Center for Housing and Environmental Studies, Research Report No. 6, 1963.

319. Kleemeier RW: Attitudes toward special settings for the aged, in Williams RH, Tibbitts C, Donahue W (eds) : *Processes of Aging.* New York, Atherton Press, Vol. II., 1963, pp. 101–121.

320. Britton JH, Mather WG, Lansing AK: Expectations for older persons in a rural community: Living arrangements and family relationships. *J Gerontol 16:* 156–162, 1961.

321. Smith WF: The housing preferences of elderly people. *J Gerontol 16:* 261–266, 1961.

322. Lawton MP, Bader J: Wish for privacy by young and old. *J Gerontol 25:* 48–54, 1970.

323. van Zonneveld RJ: Sociomedical investigations of housing for the aged. *Geriatrics 13:* 668–672, 1958.

324. Report of a special committee of the Gerontological Society: Living arrangements of the elderly: Ecology, in Havinghurst RJ (ed.) : Research and Development Goals in Social Gerontology. *The Gerontologist 9:* No. 4, Pt. II., 37–54, 1969.

325. Donahue W, Ashley EE: Housing and the social health of older people in the United States, in Katz AH, Felton JS (eds) : *Health and the Community.* New York, The Free Press, 1965, pp. 149–163.

326. Lowenthal D (ed.) : *Environmental Perception and Behavior.* Chicago, The University of Chicago, Department of Geography Research Paper No. 109, 1967.

327. Lynch K: *The Image of the City.* Cambridge, The Technology Press and Harvard University Press, 1960.

328. Winkel GH, Malek R, Thiel P: The role of personality differences in judgments of roadside quality. *Environment and Behavior 1:* 199–223, 1969.

329. Downs RM: The cognitive structure of an urban shopping center. *Environment and Behavior 2:* 13–39, 1970.

330. Canter D: An intergroup comparison of connotative dimensions in architecture. *Environment and Behavior 1:* 37–48, 1969.

331. Lee T: Urban neighborhood as a socio-spatial schema. *Human Relations 21:* 241–268, 1968.

332. Van Arsdol MD Jr, Sabagh G, Alexander F: Reality and the perception of environmental hazards. *J Health and Human Behav 5:* 144–153, 1964.

333. Riemer S: Architecture for family living. *J Social Issues 7:* No. 1–2, 140–151, 1951.

334. Sommer R: Man's proximate environment. *J Social Issues 22:* No. 4, 59–70, 1966.

335. Barker RG: *Ecological Psychology.* Stanford, Stanford University Press, 1968.

336. Bass BM, Klubeck S: Effects of seating arrangements on leaderless group discussions. *J Abnorm Social Psychol 47:* 724–727, 1952.

337. Bryne D, Bouehler JA: A note on the influence of propinquity upon acquaintanceships. *J Abnorm Social Psychol 51:* 147–148, 1955.

338. Carson DH: The interactions of man and his environment, in *SER 2: School Environments Research.* Ann Arbor, The University of Michigan, 1965, pp. 13–50.

339. Esser AH, Chamberlain AS, Chapple ED, Kline NS: Territoriality of patients on a research ward, in Wortis J (ed.) : *Recent Advances in Biological Psychiatry* 7: 36–44, 1965.

340. Gullahorn JT: Distance and friendship as factors in the gross interaction matrix. *Sociometry 15:* 123–134, 1952.

341. Hall ET: *The Hidden Dimension.* Garden City, N.Y., Doubleday, 1966.

342. Horowitz MJ, Duff DF, Stratton LO: Personal space and the body-buffer zone. *Arch Gen Psychiat 11:* 651–656, 1964.

343. Ittelson WH, Proshansky HM, Rivlin LG: Bedroom size and social interaction of the psychiatric ward. *Environment and Behavior 2:* 255–270, 1970.

344. Ittelson WH, Proshansky HM, Rivlin LG: The environmental psychology of the psychiatric ward, in Proshansky HM, Ittelson WH, Rivlin LG (eds) : *Environmental Psychology: Man and His Physical Setting.* New York, Holt, Rinehart, & Winston, 1970, pp. 419–439.

345. Proshansky HM, Ittelson WH, Rivlin LG (eds) : *Environmental Psychology: Man and His Physical Setting.* New York, Holt, Rinehart & Winston, 1970.

346. Richards CB, Dobyns HF: Topography and culture: The case of the changing cage. *Human Organiz 16:* 16–20, 1957.

347. Sommer R: Studies in personal space. *Sociometry 22:* 247–260, 1959.

348. Sommer R: The distance for comfortable conversation: A further study. *Sociometry 25:* 111–116, 1962.

349. Sommer R: Personal space. *Amer Instit Architects J 38:* 81–83, 1962.

350. Sommer R: Leadership and group geography. *Sociometry 24:* 99–110, 1961.

351. Sommer R, Gilliland GW: Design for friendship. *Canad Architect 6:* 59–61, 1961.

352. Sommer R: The ecology of privacy. *The Library Quarterly 36:* 234–248, 1966.

353. Sommer R: Small group ecology. *Psychol Bull 67:* 145–152, 1967.

354. Sommer R, Ross H: Social interaction on a geriatrics ward. *Int J Social Psychiat 4:* 128–133, 1958.

355. Steinzor B: The spatial factor in face-to-face discussion groups. *J Abnorm Social Psychol 45:* 552–555, 1950.

356. Trites DK, Galbraith FD Jr, Sturdavant M, Leckwart JF: Influence of nursing-unit design on the activities and subjective feelings of nursing personnel. *Environment and Behavior 2:* 303–334, 1970.

357. Lewinski RJ: An investigation of individual responses to chromatic illumination. *J Psychol 6:* 155–160, 1938.

358. Norman RD, Scott WA: Color and affect: A review and sematic evaluation. *J Gen Psychol 46:* 185–223, 1952.

359. Rice AH: Color: What research knows about the classroom. *Nation's Schools 52:* 1–8, 64, 1953.

360. Wong H, Brown W: Effects of surroundings upon mental work as measured by Yerkes' multiple choice method. *J Comp Psychol 3:* 319–331, 1923.

361. Abernathy EA: The effect of changed environmental conditions upon the results of college examinations. *J Psychol 10:* 293–301, 1940.

362. Bilodean JM, Schlosberg H: Similarity in stimulating conditions as a variable in retroactive inhibition. *J Exp Psychol 41:* 199–204, 1959.

363. Kasmar JV, Griffin WV, Mauritzen JH: Effect of environmental surroundings on outpatients' mood and perception of psychiatrists. *J Consult and Clin Psychol 32:* 223–226, 1968.

364. Maslow AH, Mintz NL: Effects of esthetic surroundings: I. Initial effects of three esthetic conditions upon perceiving "energy" and "well-being" in faces. *J Psychol 41:* 247–254, 1956.

365. Mintz NL: Effects of esthetic surroundings. II. Prolonged and repeated experience in a "beautiful" and an "ugly" room. *J Psychol 41:* 459–466, 1956.

125

366. Karmel LJ: Effects of windowless classroom environment on high school students. *Perceptual and Motor Skills 20:* 277–278, 1965.
367. Griffitt W, Veitch R: Hot and crowded: Influences of population density and temperature on interpersonal affective behavior. *J Pers Social Psychol 17:* 92–98, 1971.
368. Brownfield CA: Deterioration and facilitation hypotheses in sensory-deprivation research. *Psychol Bull 61:* 304–313, 1964.
369. Casler L: Perceptual deprivation in institutional settings, in Newton G, Levine S (eds): *Early Experience and Behavior.* Springfield, Ill., CC Thomas, 1968, pp. 573–626.
370. Cohen SI: Central nervous system functioning in altered sensory environments, in Appley MH, Trumbull R (eds): *Psychological Stress.* New York, Appleton-Century-Crofts, 1967, pp. 77–122.
371. Haggard EA: Isolation and personality, in Worchel P, Byrne D (eds): *Personality Change.* New York, Wiley, 1964, pp. 433–469.
372. O'Connor N: Children in restricted environments, in Newton G, Levine S (eds): *Early Experience and Behavior.* Springfield, Ill., CC Thomas, 1968, pp. 530–572.
373. Silverman AJ, Cohen SI, Shmavonian BM, Greenberg G: Psychophysiological investigations in sensory deprivation: The body-field dimension. *Psychosom Med 23:* 48–61, 1961.
374. Spitz RA: Hospitalism: *Psychoanal Study of Child 1:* 53–74, 1945.
375. Walters RH: The effects of social isolation and social interaction on learning and performance in social situations, in Glass DC (ed.): *Environmental Influences.* New York, Rockefeller University Press, 1968, pp. 155–184.
376. Zubek JP (ed.): *Sensory Deprivation.* New York, Appleton-Century-Crofts, 1969.
377. Zubek JP, Bayer L, Shephard JM: Relative effects of prolonged social isolation and confinement: Behavioral and EEG changes. *J Abnorm Psychol 74:* 625–631, 1969.
378. Orne MT, Scheibe KE: The contribution of nondeprivation factors on the production of sensory deprivation effects: the psychology of the 'panic button'. *J Abnorm Soc Psychol 68:* 3–12, 1964.
379. Altman I, Haythorn WW: The ecology of isolated groups. *Behav Sci 12:* 169–182, 1967.
380. Eilbert LR, Glaser R: Differences between well and poorly adjusted groups in an isolated environment. *J Appl Psychol 43:* 271–274, 1959.
381. Gunderson EKE: Emotional symptoms in extremely isolated groups. *Arch Gen Psychiat 9:* 362–368, 1963.
382. Hammes JA, Ahearn TR, Keith JF Jr: A chronology of two weeks' fallout shelter confinement. *J Clin Psychol 21:* 452–456, 1965.
383. Hammes JA, Osborne RT: Fallout shelter survival research. *J Clin Psychol 22:* 344–346, 1966.
384. Haythorn WW, Altman I: Personality factors in isolated environments, in Appley MH, Trumbull R (eds): *Psychological Stress.* New York, Appleton-Century-Crofts, 1967, pp. 363–399.
385. Ullrich RA: A study of the motivating and dissatisfying forces in an isolated work situation. *Dissert Abs 29A:* 1629–1630, 1968.
386. Weybrew BB: Psychological problems of prolonged marine submergence, in Burns NM, Chambers RM, Hendler E (eds): *Unusual Environments and Human Behavior.* New York, The Free Press of Glencoe, 1963, pp. 87–125.
387. Wilkins WL: Group behavior in long-term isolation, in Appley MH, Trumbull R (eds): *Psychological Stress.* New York, Appleton-Century-Crofts, 1967, pp. 278–296.
388. Campbell DT: Reforms as experiments. *Amer Psychologist 24:* 409–429, 1969.

389. Chein I: The environment as a determinant of behavior. *J Soc Psychol 38:* 115–127, 1954.
390. Gutman R: Site planning and social behavior. *J Soc Issues 22:* No. 4, 103–115, 1966.
391. Loring WC: Residential environment: Nexus of personal interactions and healthful development. *J Health and Human Behav 5:* 166–169, 1964.
392. Sherif M, Sherif CW: Varieties of social stimulus situations, in Sells SB (ed.) : *Stimulus Determinants of Behavior.* New York, Ronald Press, 1963, pp. 82–106.
393. Chapin FS: Some housing factors related to mental hygiene. *J Soc Issues 7:* No. 1–2, 164–171, 1951.
394. Carr S: The city of the mind, in Ewald WR Jr (ed.) : *Environment for Man.* Bloomington, Indiana University Press, 1967, pp. 197–226.
395. Lynch K, Rodwin L: A theory of urban form, in Gutman R, Popenoe D (eds) : *Neighborhood, City, and Metropolis.* New York, Random House, 1970, pp. 756–776.
396. World Health Organization: Environmental health aspects of metropolitan planning and development. *Wld Health Org Techn Rep Ser 297:* 1–66, 1965.
397. Riemer S: Sociological theory of home adjustment. *Amer Sociol Rev 8:* 272–278, 1943.
398. Riemer S: Sociological perspective in home planning. *Amer Sociol Rev 12:* 155–158, 1947.
399. World Health Organization: Appraisal of the hygienic quality of housing and its environment. *Wld Health Org Techn Rep Ser 353:* 1–54, 1967.
400. Carp FM: Person-situation congruence in engagement. *The Gerontologist 8:* No. 3, Pt. I, 184–188, 1968.
401. Lawton MP: Assessment, integration, and environments for older people. *The Gerontologist 10:* No. 1, 38–46, 1970.
402. Yarrow MR: Appraising environment, in Williams RH, Tibbitts C, Donahue W (eds) : *Processes of Aging.* New York, Atherton Press, 1963, Vol. I, pp. 201–222.
403. Cobb S, French JRP Jr, Kahn RL, Mann FC: An environmental approach to mental health. *Ann NY Acad Sci 107:* 596–606, 1963.
404. Cobb S, Brooks GW, Kasl SV, Connelly WE: The health of people changing jobs: A description of a longitudinal study. *Amer J Public Health 56:* 1476–1481, 1966.

# Chapter V

## The Relation of the Urban Environment to Health: Towards a Conceptual Frame and a Research Strategy

JOHN CASSEL

*Bibliographic Assistance* by LYNN WALLER

The past century has witnessed a change from a complete conviction that there is a simple and direct relationship between the urban envirorment, particularly the quality of the housing, and health status, to one of considerable uncertainty and confusion. A review of the literature since 1920 reveals some studies showing a relationship between housing and various indicators of poor health, others showing no such relationship, and yet others showing an inverse relationship. Poor housing has been related to higher overall mortality rates, (*1*) to higher infant mortality rates, (*2, 3*) to higher mortality and incidence rates of tuberculosis, (*4-11*) to the incidence of meningococcal disease, (*12*) to digestive diseases, (*8*) home accidents, (*8-13*) anemia, (*14*) and to higher hospital admission rates for contagious and nutritional disease. (*15*) In addition, beginning with the classic study of Faris in 1939, (*16*) a plethora of investigators have shown a relationship between deteriorated neighborhoods and mental disorders, particularly the major psychoses. (*17*) Finally, the relationship between slum conditions and violence, drug abuse, and alcoholism is too painfully evident at this point in history to require documentation by formal research.

In contrast to these studies, other investigators have been unable to find any correlation between quality of housing and health of the inhabitants. Brett, (*18*) McKinlay, (*19*) Mackintosh, (*20*) McMillan, (*21*) Lockhart, (*22*) and Holmes (*23*) could find no relationship between crowding in households and tuberculosis; rheumatic fever and streptococcal illness did not occur more frequently in adequate than inadequate houses, (*24*) respiratory illnesses were no more common in crowded than uncrowded conditions, (*25*) and morale and "general adjustment" were found to be no better in slum dwellers following rehousing than in those living in the original slums. (*26*) M'Gonigle's study in 1933 (27) showed an actual increase in death rates following the rehousing of a slum population from an "unhealthy area" to a municipal housing estate, and Martin et al. (28) showed an increase in neurosis in inhabitants moved from inadequate housing to a new housing estate.

In part, these conflicting findings may be due to inadequates in the research design employed in many of the studies. These include inadequate or, in some cases, the complete absence of controls; problems of selection; varying definitions employed to categorize the quality of the housing; and varying degrees of completeness and accuracy in the ascertainment of health status. In addition, few studies have attempted any longterm follow-up and if the health changes are of short duration (for example, following relocation), studies conducted at different points in time following the event might be expected to produce discrepant findings. Perhaps of greater importance is the fact that in the majority of the studies, poor housing, however measured, is so closely correlated with other environmental and personal variables that it is difficult if not impossible to determine whether it was the quality of the housing *per se* that was responsible for the relationship or the cluster of the correlated variables.

Even when strenuous attempts have been made to overcome these methodological and conceptual problems, as in the study by Wilner et al., (29) the role of housing itself as a determinant of health status remains unclear. As a result, an increasing number of investigators (30-38) are beginning to stress the point that the processes through which housing may be linked to health need to be examined, and that these processes, which may vary for different health conditions, are likely to be more complex than was originally suspected. This approach suggests that the link between housing and health may be quite indirect, and that unless the intervening processes are understood, changes in the physical structure of the housing alone may have no effect on health if such a change does not simultaneously affect these intervening factors.

## Processes Linking Housing to Health

There can be little disagreement that certain health conditions are directly determined by the physical structure of housing. The relationship of peeling lead paint to lead poisoning, of dilapidated structures to home accidents; the effects of inadequate heating, broken plumbing systems, the presence of insects and rodents, stagnant water in cellars, and inadequate waste management and disposal are perhaps self-evident and hardly need to await further research findings before action can be taken. Once the area of concern extends beyond these issues, however, the need for clarification of concepts and new research strategies be-

130

comes evident. This is particularly true insofar as infectious diseases (especially respiratory infections), the chronic diseases, and mental and behavioral disorders are concerned.

One of the more widely held and cherished notions in medicine is that the spread of infectious disease is facilitated by crowding. This assumption underlies many of the research endeavors seeking to establish a relationship between housing and health, and has been accepted as a truism by policy makers. There is little question that under certain circumstances crowding may be related to an increased incidence of communicable diseases, but as reported above, under other circumstances no such relationship has been discovered. In fact, in two relatively recent studies of tuberculosis the highest rates were not found to occur among the most crowded individuals but among the social isolates, particularly those living alone in one room without any meaningful social ties. (18, 23) A clue as to the reason for these discrepant findings comes from some of the recent formulations of the pioneer microbiologist Rene DuBos. DuBos maintains that

"The sciences concerned with microbial diseases have developed almost exclusively from the study of acute or semi-acute infections caused by virulent micro-organisms acquired through exposure to an exogenous source of infection. In contrast, the microbial diseases most common in our communities today arise from the activities of micro-organisms that are ubiquitous in the environment, persist in the body without causing obvious harm under ordinary circumstances, and exert pathological effects only when the infected person is under conditions of physiological stress. In such a type of microbial disease the event of infection is of less importance than the hidden manifestation of the smoldering infectious process and than the physiological disturbances that convert latent infection into overt symptoms and pathology." (39)

According to DuBos, then, microbial disease is not necessarily acquired through exposure to a new micro-organism. In a large number of cases clinical manifestations of disease can occur through factors which disturb the balance between the existing ubiquitous organisms and the host that is harboring them. It may well be that under conditions of crowding this balance may be disturbed, but this disturbance, then, is not simply a function of the physical crowding (that is, the closeness of contact of susceptibles to carriers of the micro-organisms) but of other processes.

In a search for the environmental factors which may affect these homeostatic mechanisms of the host and thus profoundly influence his susceptibility to disease, attention has recently refocussed on a set of factors which, though difficult to quantify, may be of crucial importance, namely *the presence of other members of the same species*. Viewed in this context, the importance of other members of the same species lies not so much in the micro-organisms they harbor as in the pattern of relationship that exists among the members.

Some of the more convincing evidence supporting the point of view that such social processes can influence health comes from animal studies. To a large extent, these have been concerned with variations in the size of the group in which the animals interact and in situations which lead to confusion over territorial control. A number of investigators have shown, for example, that as the number of animals housed together increases, with all other factors such as genetic stock, diet, temperature, and sanitation kept constant, maternal and infant mortality rates rise, the incidence of arteriosclerosis increases, resistance to a wide variety of insults, including drugs, micro-organisms, and X-rays decreases and there is an increased susceptibility to various types of neoplasia. (40–48) Lack of territorial control has been shown to lead to the development of marked and persistent hypertension in mice, to increased maternal and infant mortality rates and also to reduced resistance to bacterial infections and decreased longevity. (49)

In addition to demonstrating the health effects that follow these variations in the social milieu, further animal studies have provided clues as to the processes through which they may be produced. Changes in group membership and the quality of group relationships have been shown to be accompanied by neuroendocrine changes, particularly, but not exclusively, by changes in the pituitary and adrenal-cortical systems. (50, 51) The changes in some of these hormones such as the 17-hydroxycorticosteroids and the catecholamines, especially if prolonged, can, by markedly altering the homeostatic mechanisms of the body, decrease resistance to a wide variety of insults. Thus, the phenomenon has been well documented in a number of animal species by studies which are methodologically sound and reasonable biological explanations for the findings.

Convincing as this animal work would appear to be, the relevance to human health is as yet unproved, and considerable doubt exists as to the appropriate analogues in the human social system. As indicated above, attempts to demonstrate that increased population density and crowding are related to poorer health status in humans have been unconvincing and have led to confusing and often conflicting results. A careful review of some of these studies taken in conjunction with the animal work suggests that, for future research in this area to be profitable, we should abandon a search for the direct human counterpart to animal crowding or territorial confusion, and concentrate instead on some more general principles or hypotheses that can be derived from these data. In my view, four such principles seem worth considering.

The first of these can perhaps best be stated as an hypothesis. This would hold that a crucial process linking high population density to enhanced susceptibility to disease is not due to crowding *per se*, but the

132

result of disordered relationships that, in animals, are inevitable consequences of such crowding. These, while being manifest by a wide variety of bizarre and unusual behaviors, often have in common a failure to elicit anticipated responses to what were previously appropriate cues, and an increasing disregard of traditional obligations and rights. Thus, habitual acts of aggression (including "ritualized" aggression) or subordination on the part of one animal fail to elicit appropriate reciprocal responses on the part of another. Characteristic obligations and responsibilities become blurred, e.g., female rats cease caring for their young and male-female relationships become disturbed to a point where the equivalent of "gang rapes" have been reported in rats under conditions of high population density. This failure of various forms of behavior to acomplish the intended results (i.e., to lead to predictable responses on the part of others) leads to one of three types of responses on the part of the animals involved, the most common of which is a repetition of the behavioral acts. Such acts are of course always accompanied by profound neuroendocrine changes, and presumably their chronic repetition leads eventually to the permanent alterations in the level of the hormones and to the degree of autonomic nervous system arousal found under conditions of animal crowding. The fact that these behavioral acts are in a sense inappropriate, in that they do not modify the situations, can be expected to enhance such hormonal changes. Under these conditions it is not difficult to envisage the reasons for the increased susceptibility to environmental insults displayed by such animals.

An alternative response on the part of some animals is to withdraw from the field—to remain motionless and isolated for long hours on end. It is apparently not uncommon, for example, to observe some mice under crowded conditions crouched in most unusual places—on top of the razor-thin edge of a partition or in the bright light in the center of the enclosure—completely immobile and not interacting with any other animals. Such animals apparently do not exhibit the increased pathology demonstrated by the interacting members. (40)

The third alternative is for animals to form their own deviant groups, groups that apparently ignore the mores and codes of behavior of the larger group. Thus, "gangs" of young male rats have been observed invading nests, attacking females, etc. I am not aware of any data on the health status of these gang members, but according to this hypothesis they also should not exhibit any increase in pathology.

This hypothesis suggests that, in human populations, increased susceptibility to disease should occur when, for a variety of reasons, individuals do not receive any evidence (feedback) that their actions are leading to desirable and anticipated consequences (i.e., in situations analogous to the first category of animal responses). In particular, this would be true when these actions are designed to modify the indi-

133

vidual's relationships to the important social groups with whom he interacts. Such circumstances might occur in a variety of situations. First, it is highly probable that when individuals are unfamiliar with the cues and expectations of the society in which they live (as in the case of migrants to a new situation, or those individuals involved in a rapid change of social scene, such as the elderly in an ethnic enclave caught up in urban renewal), their actions would be unlikely to lead to the consequence they anticipate and thus, due to the chain of events suggested above, they should be more susceptible to disease than are those for whom the situation is familiar.

Some circumstantial evidence supporting this point of view exists. Scotch (52, 53) found that blood pressure levels among the Zulu who had recently migrated to a large urban center were higher than both those who had remained in their ritual tribal surroundings and those who had lived for over 10 years in the urban setting. In two independent studies, Syme (54–56) has demonstrated that occupationally and residentially mobile people have a higher prevalence of coronary heart disease than stable populations, and that those individuals displaying the greatest discontinuity between childhood and adult situations, as measured by occupation and place of residence, have higher rates than those in which less discontinuity could be determined. Tyroler and Cassel designed a study in which death rates from coronary heart disease, and from all heart disease, could be measured in groups who were themselves stable but around whom the social situation was changing in varying degrees. For this purpose they selected 45–54 year-old, white, male, rural residents in various counties of North Carolina and classified those counties by the degree of urbanization occurring in that locality. Death rates for coronary heart disease and all heart disease showed a stepwise increasing gradient with each increase in the index of urbanization of the county. (57) In a further study, Cassel and Tyroler (58) examined two groups of rural mountaineers working in a factory. The first of these was composed of individuals who were the first of their family to engage in industrial work, while the second comprised workers who were the children of previous workers in this factory. The two groups were drawn from the same mountain coves and doing the same work for the same pay. The underlying hypothesis was that the second group, by virtue of their pervious experience, would be better prepared for the expectations and demands of industrial living than the first and would thus exhibit fewer signs of ill health. Health status was measured by responses to the Cornell Medical Index and by various indices of sick absenteeism. As predicted, the first group had higher Cornell Medical Index scores (more symptoms) and higher rates of sick absenteeism (after the initial few years of service) at each age.

A second set of circumstances in which this lack of feedback might occur would be under conditions of social disorganization. This, while

134

still being far from a precise term which can be measured accurately, has proved to be a useful concept in a number of studies. In the hands of several investigators, for example, various indicators of social or familial disorganization have been related to increased rates of tuberculosis, (23) mental disorders, (59) deaths from stroke, (60) prevalence of hypertension, (61) and coronary heart disease. (54) Clearly, more work needs to be done in clarifying and quantifying this concept, but until there is recognition of what needs to be clarified or quantified, little progress can be anticipated.

A second general principle which emerges from the animal work is that not all members of a population are equally susceptible to the effects of these social processes. Systematic and regular differences have been observed with the more dominant animals showing the least effects and the subordinate ones having the most extreme responses. (62) Those differences are manifest both in the magnitude of the endocrine changes and in increased morbidity and mortality rates. Conceivably these findings may, in part, explain the high levels of blood pressure found in American Negroes who not only usually occupy a subordinate position in society, but whose lives are frequently characterized by considerable evidence of social and familial disorganization.

A third principle is concerned with the available protective factors—those devices which "buffer" or "cushion" the individual from the physiological or psychological consequences of these social processes. These would seem to be of two general categories: biological and social. The biological category would include the adaptive capacities of all living organisms—the capacity, given time, to adjust physiologically and psychologically to a wide variety of environmental circumstances. In animals, this is illustrated by the higher responses of laboratory-naive animals to given stimuli than of veteran animals, (63) and to the much lower rate of pathology in animals born and reared in crowded conditions than in animals transferred to these conditions some time after birth. (64) In humans, the finding that death rates from lung cancer in the U.S., when controlled for cigarette smoking, are considerably higher in the farm-born who migrated to cities than in lifetime urban dwellers (despite the longer exposure of the latter to atmospheric pollution), (65) would seem to be evidence of the same phenomenon.

In addition to these biological adaptive processes, various social processes have also been shown to be protective. Chief amongst these are the nature and strength of the group supports provided to the individual. In rats, for example, the efficacy with which an unanticipated series of electric shocks (given to animals previously conditioned to avoid them) can produce peptic ulcers is determined, to a large extent, by whether the animals are shocked in isolation (high ulcer rates) or in the presence of litter mates (low ulcer rates). (66) The territorial conflict which led to elevated blood pressures quoted above (49) was produced by placing mice in intercommunicating boxes. Hypertension only occurred, however, when the mice were "strangers." Populating the system with litter mates produced none of these effects. In humans, small group studies have shown that the degree of autonomic arousal (produced by requiring solutions to what in reality are insoluble tasks) is more extreme if the group is made up of strangers than when it is made up of friends. (67) As reported above, modern studies on the epidemiology of tuberculosis in the United States and Britain have shown that the disease occurs more frequently in "marginal" people, that is, those people who are deprived of meaningful social contacts. (18, 23)

If these three principles, or hypotheses, are correct, it would appear that health changes which are dependent upon the presence of other members of the same species will not be universal—not affecting all people in the same manner. A more adequate formulation would hold that such consequences will be dependent on:

(A) The importance or salience of the relationships that become disordered.

(B) The position of the individuals experiencing such disordered relationships in the status hierarchy.

(C) The degree to which the population under study has been unprepared by previous experience for this particular situation (i.e., has had insufficient time to adapt).

(D) The nature and strength of the available group supports.

The final general principle that can be derived from the animal experiments relates to the manifestations of ill health that might be anticipated under conditions of social change and disorganization. The model of disease causation provided by the germ theory has accustomed us to think in monoetiologic specific terms. Accordingly, much of the work concerned with social or psychological antecedents to disease has attempted to identify a particular situational set (usually labelled "stress" or "a stressor") which would have a specific causal relationship to some clinical entity, analogous, say, to the relationship between the typhoid bacillus and typhoid fever. Such a formulation would appear to be clearly at variance with the animal data, a striking feature of which is the wide variety of pathologic conditions that emerge following changes in the social milieu. A conclusion more in accordance with the known evidence, then, would be that such variations in group relationships, rather than having a specific etiological role, would enhance susceptibility to disease in general. The specific manifestations of disease would be a function of the genetic predisposition of the individuals and the nature of the physico-chemical or microbiologic insults they encounter. This concept of generalized susceptibility is consistent with the situation in the United States where it has recently been demonstrated that those regions of the country having the highest death rates from cardiovascular disease (age, race, sex specific) also have higher than expected death rates from all causes, including cancer and infectious diseases. (68) This illustration, of course, does not necessarily document that social processes are responsible for such an increased susceptibility, but does lend credence to the view that variations in generalized susceptibility may be a useful concept.

Somewhat more direct evidence is provided by Christenson and Hinkle in an industrial study in the U.S. in which they have shown that managers in a company who, by virtue of their family background and educational experience, were least well prepared for the demands and expectations of executive industrial life had the highest rates of *all* diseases—major as well as minor, physical as well as mental, long-term as well as short-term. (69) In the studies on tuberculosis referred to above, (23) the highest rates of disease were found in "marginal" people, that is, people who, for a variety of reasons (ethnic minorities rejected by the dominant majority, people with high sustained rates of mobility or broken family life), were deprived of meaningful social contact. A similar set of circumstances has been observed in the case of schizophrenia, multiple accidents, suicide, alcoholism, and other respiratory diseases. (70–74) While the manifestations of ill health under these circumstances are quite diverse, the individuals share in common an increased susceptibility to disease.

Presumably, then, the causes of disease may vary under different conditions. In pre-industrial societies where people live in small, tightly organized communities the exposure to highly potent disease agents may account for the major part of disease causation. Under these circumstances, variations in susceptibility due to social processes may be of relatively little importance. With increasing urbanization, populations become increasingly protected from such disease agents, but simultaneously, they are exposed to the social processes discussed above. Variations in susceptibility now assume greater importance in the etiological picture and the concomitant changes in such factors as diet, physical activity, and cigarette smoking will facilitate the emergence of new manifestations of such susceptibility.

This formulation suggests that, insofar as the urban environment is concerned, future research should concentrate on two sets of social factors which may be linked on the one hand to the physical structure of the housing and the features of the residential neighborhood, and on the other to susceptibility to a variety of pathologies and disordered behavior. These human dimensions for planning and design would include:

1. Residential and community factors:
The degree to which the physical design of the neighborhood fosters or retards social contacts and integration of individuals into the community.

The degree to which policy and political forces facilitate the individual's control over his own destiny and help eliminate ambiguities between actions and their consequences.

2. Housing factors:

The degree to which the layout of the house augments the supportive role that can be played by a well integrated cohesive family network. Here, such concepts as "use crowding" (Chapin (34)) and a "role density" (Loring (36)) may be useful.

## Towards a Research Strategy

While the ideas discussed above may form a useful approach to new research concerned with the relationship of the urban environment to health, the current situation, particularly in the inner city, is sufficiently critical that action cannot wait the decade or more necessary for observational research to document or refute these notions. Consequently, the approach of choice might well be in the form of intervention research. By this is meant that a partnership should be formed between those agencies of society charged with the task of improving the quality of the urban environment and research scientists drawn largely from academic institutions. Such a partnership would have the responsibility for introducing changes in physical aspects of housing and the residential neighborhood, and would use this entree as a means for deliberate alteration in some of these social factors as experimental variables. Thus, improvements in housing could be introduced with greater and lesser degrees of community participation, and with varying degrees of community control and decision making, with and without attempts to modify use, crowding, etc.

The parameters that should be measured and, where possible, modified to test the hypothesis described above, can perhaps be summarized best by the following four-way classification table.

### Psychosocial Factors Potentially Related to Health Status

| | LEVEL OF MEASUREMENT | |
| | SOCIAL–"STRUCTURAL" | PERCEPTUAL |
| --- | --- | --- |
| DELETERI-OUS FACTORS | Indices of Social Disorganization<br>Indices of Status (or Role) Discrepancy | Perceived Degree of Control over Environment with Special Reference to Relatitons to Significant Social Groups |
| | Degree to which Previous Experience had Adequately Prepared Individual for Current Situation | Degree to which Expectations of Significant Others for Behavior of Index Case are Conflicting or Ambiguous |
| PROTEC-TIVE FACTORS | Indices of Strength of Affiliative Networks | Perception of Reliability of Others to Help in Times of Trouble |

The research responsibility of scientists in such an organization would then be:

1. To develop instruments to measure the parameters described above (or adapt existing ones).

2. To determine whether the relationships between the Social-"Structural" and Perceptual parameters postulated in the table above do indeed exist (e.g., is there a relationship between social disorganization and degree of perceived control of the environment?).

3. To determine the relationship between these parameters and various indices of health status and/or social pathology.

4. To determine for any given locale the feasibility of either reducing the postulated deleterious processes or strengthening the protective factors, and measuring the effect of such changes on health status.

5. To provide a continuous system of surveillance and monitoring in order to document the effect of changes in the residential environment on these psychosocial parameters.

Finally, it is important to recognize that in all such endeavours the very solutions to some problems may create or make visible new orders of problems, requiring yet another set of solutions. Resolution of the problem of rat infestation, for example (especially if accompanied by intelligent community organization), could conceivably make visible the community concern for drug abuse or violence. For this reason, and because the effects of any form of intervention on health status may not be immediately discernible and may change with time, it would appear essential that these new organizations have long term commitments, both in terms of funding and organization. Thus, they would be in a position to document the consequences of their actions, both immediate and long-term, and be available to attempt solutions to new problems before these assume crisis proportions.

## References

1. Rollo H. Britten. "The Relation Between Housing and Health." *Public Health Reports*, XLIX (44) , November 2, 1934, 1301–1313.
2. A. D. H. Kaplan. "Infant Mortality as an Index of Community Welfare." *The Trained Nurse and Hospital Review*, XC (3) , March 1933, pg. 19.
3. Norman Macfayden. "Health and Garden Cities." *Public Housing Authority Handbook*, pg. 20.
4. Lilli Stein. "A Study of Respiratory Tuberculosis in Relation to Housing Conditions in Edinburgh, The Pre-war Period." *British Journal of Social Medicine.* 4:243–69, 1950.
5. Lilli Stein. "Glasgow Tuberculosis and Housing." *Tubercule.* 35:195–203, 1954.
6. A. K. Chalmers. "The House as a Contributory Factor in the Death-rate." *Proc. R. Soc. Med.,* 6:155–182, 1913.
7. R. J. Peters. "19th Ann. Conf. Nat. Ass. Prevention Tuberc." P. 163, 1933.

8. R. H. Britten. "New Light on the Relation of Housing to Health." *American Journal of Public Health*, 32:193–9, 1942.
9. Dara I. Morse. "Housing as Related to Tuberculosis." *Journal of Outdoor Life*, XXVI (5 & 6), May–June 1929.
10. S. Laidlaw. "An Investigation into the Epidemiology of Young Adult Phthisis." Glasgow: Thesis, 1933.
11. S. Laidlaw. "Increasing Incidence of Pulmonary Tuberculosis in Children in Glasgow." *Edin. Medical Journal*, 53:49–54, 1946.
12. Bernard Blum. "The Relation of Housing to the Incidence of Meningococcic Disease in an Outbreak in Oak Ridge, Tennessee." *American Journal Public Health*. 39:1571–77, 1949.
13. R. H. Britten & I. Altman. "Illness and Accidents Among Persons Living Under Different Housing Conditions: Data Based on National Health Survey." *Public Health Report*. 56:609–40, 1941.
14. I. D. Riley. "Housing Conditions on Children in Hospitals." *Glasgow Medical Journal*. 36:393–7, 1955.
15. R. M. Worth. "Urbanization and Squatter Resettlement as Related to Child Health in Hong Kong." *American Journal Hyg.* 78:338–48, Nov. 1963.
16. R. E. L. Faris. *An Ecological Study of Insanity in the City.* University of Chicago Press, 1939.
17. B. P Dohrenwend and B. S. Dohrenwend. *Social Status and Psychological Disorder.* Wiley, New York, 1969.
18. G. Z. Brett and B. Benjamin. "Housing and Tuberculosis in a Mass Radiography Survey." *Brit. J. Prev. and Soc. Med.* 11:7–9, 1957.
19. P. L. McKinlay and S. C. Truelove. "Epidemiology of Infective Hepatitis Among Allied Troups in Italy." *Brit. J. Prev. and Soc. Med.* Vol. 1:33–50, January 1947.
20. J. M. Mackintosh. "Housing and Tuberculosis." *Brit. J. Tuberculosis.* 28:67–70, 1934.
21. J. S. McMillan. "Examination of the Association Between Housing Conditions and Pulmonary Tuberculosis in Glasgow." *Brit. J. Prev. & Soc. Med.* 11:142–51, 1957.
22. R. Lockhart (1949). "Health Bulletin of the Dept. of Health for Scotland." 7. No. 4. p. 76.
23. Thomas H. Holmes. "Multidiscipline Studies of Tuberculosis." *Personality Stress and Tuberculosis.* Phineas J. Sparer (ed.) International Universities Press, 1956.
24. J. E. Coulter. "Rheumatic Fever and Streptococcal Illness in Two Communities in New York State." *Milbank Mem. Fund Quart.* 30:341–58, 1952.
25. S. H. Berstein. "Observations on the Effects of Housing on the Incidence and Spread of Common Respiratory Diseases Among Air Force Recruits." *American J. Hyg.* 65:162–71, 1957.
26. F. S. Chapin. "An Experiment on the Social Effects of Good Housing." *Am. Soc. Rev.* 5:868–79, 1940.
27. G. C. M. M'Gonigle and J. Kirby. *Poverty and Public Health,* London: Victor Gollancz Ltd., 1936.
28. F. M. Martin, J. H. F. Brotherson and S. P. W. Chave. "Incidence of Neurosis in a New Housing Estate." *Brit. J. Prev. & Soc. Med.* 11:196–202, 1957.
29. D. M. Wilner et al. *The Housing Environment and Family Life.* Baltimore, Johns Hopkins Press, 1962.
30. J. M. Dalla Valle. "Factors Which Affect the Relationship Between Housing and Health." *Publ. Hlth Reports.* 52:989–998, 1937.
31. H. Nelson. "Housing and Health." *Brit. Med. J.* 2:395–7, 1945.
32. T. Ferguson and M. G. Pettigrew. "A Study of 718 Slum Families Rehoused for Upwards of 10 Years." *Glasgow Med. J.* 35:183–201, 1951.
33. H. Strotzka. Psychohygiene und Wohnen. *Z. Osterr. Ing. u. Architekt Vereines,* 102:67–71, 1957.

34. F. S. Chapin. "The Relationship of Housing on Mental Health." *Expert Committee on the Public Health Aspects of Housing.* WHO, 1961.
35. Alvin L. Schorr. "Slums and Social Insecurity." Wash: U.S. Dept. HEW, 1963.
36. W. C. Loring. "Residential Environment: Nexus of Personal Interactions and Healthful Development." *J. Hlth and Human Behav.* 5:166-9, Winter 1964.
37. "Housing and the Health Administration." *WHO Chronicle,* 18:463-72, December 1964.
38. D. L. Foster. "A Psychiatrist Looks at Urban Renewal." *J. Nat. Med. Assoc.* 62:95-101 passim March 1970.
39. Rene Dubos. *Man Adapting.* Yale University Press, New Haven, 1965, 164-165.
40. J. B. Calhoun. "Population Density and Social Pathology." *Sci. Amer., 206,* 1962, 139.
41. H. L. Ratcliffe and M. T. I. Cronin. "Changing Frequency of Arteriosclerosis in Mammals and Birds at the Philadelphia Zoological Garden." *Circulation,* 18, 1958, 41-52.
42. E. A. Swinyard, L. D. Clark, J. T. Miyahara, and H. H. Wolf. "Studies on the Mechanism of Amphetamine Toxicity in Aggregated Mice." *J. Pharmacol. and Exptl. Therap., 132:* 1961, 97-102.
43. D. E. Davis and C. P. Read. "Effects of Behavior on Development of Resistance in Trichinosis." *Proc. Soc. Exp. Biol. Med., 99,* 1958, 269-272.
44. R. Ader and E. W. Hahn. "Effects of Social Environment on Mortality to Whole Body—X-Irradiation in the Rat." *Psychol. Rep.,* 13, 1963, 24-215.
45. R. Ader, A. Kreutner, and H. L. Jacobs. "Social Environment, Emotionality and Alloxan Diabetes in the Rat." *Psychosom. Med.,* 25, 1963, 60-68.
46. J. T. King, Y. C. P. Lee, and M. B. Vissacher. "Single Versus Multiple Cage Occupancy and Convulsion Frequency in C. H Mice." *Proc. Soc. Exp. Biol. Med., 88,* 1955, 661-663.
47. H. B. Andervont. "Influence of Environment on Mammary Cancer in Mice." *J. Nat. Cancer Inst.,* 4, 1944, 579-581.
48. J. J. Christian and H. O. Williamson. "Effect of Crowding on Experimental Granuloma Formation in Mice." *Proc. Soc. Exp. Biol. Med.,* 99, 1958, 385-387.
49. J. P. Henry, J. P. Meehan and P. M. Stephens. "The Use of Psychosocial Stimuli to Induce Prolonged Hypertension in Mice." *Psychosom. Med.,* 29, 1967, 408-432.
50. J. W. Mason. "Psychological Influences on the Pituitary-Adrenal-Cortical System." *Recent Progress in Hormone Research,* G. Pencus (ed.), *15,* 1959, 345-389.
51. J. W. Mason and J. V. Brady. "The Sensitivity of the Psychoendocrine Systems to Social and Physical Environment." In *Psychobiological Approaches to Social Behavior,* D. Shapiro (ed.), Stanford University Press, 1960.
52. N. A. Scotch. "A Preliminary Report on the Relation of Sociocultural Factors to Hypertension Among the Zulu." *Ann. New York Acad. Sci.,* 86, 1960, 1000.
53. N. A. Scotch. "Sociocultural Factors in the Epidemiology of Zulu Hypertension." *Am. J. Publ. Health, 52,* 1963, 1205-1213.
54. S. L. Syme, M. M. Hyman and P. E. Enterline. "Some Social and Cultural Factors Associated with the Occurrence of Coronary Heart Disease." *J. Chron. Dis., 17,* 1964, 277-289.
55. S. L. Syme, M. M. Hyman and P. E. Enterline. "Cultural Mobility and the Occurrence of Coronary Heart Disease." *Health and Human Behavior,* 6, 1965, 173-189.
56. S. L. Syme, N. O. Borhani and R. W. Buechley. "Cultural Mobility and Coronary Heart Disease in an Urban Area." *Am. J. Epid.,* 82, 1965, 334-346.
57. H. A. Tyroler and John Cassel. "Health Consequences of Culture Change: The Effect of Urbanization on Coronary Heart Mortality in Rural Residents of North Carolina." *J.Chron. Dis.,* 17, 1964, 167-177.

58. John Cassel and H. A. Tyroler. "Epidemiological Studies of Culture Change" I "Health Status and Recency of Industrialization." *Arch. Envir. Health,* 3, 1961, 25.

59. D. C. Leighton, J. S. Harding, D. E. Macklin, A. M. MacMillan, and A. H. Leighton. *The Character of Danger,* Basic Book, Inc., 1963.

60. William B. Neser, H. A. Tyroler, and John Cassel. "Stroke Mortality in the Black Population of North Carolina in Relation to Social Factors." Presented at the American Heart Association Meeting on Cardiovascular Epidemiology, New Orleans, March 1970.

61. Ernest Harburg, et al. "Stress and Heredity in Negro White Blood Pressure Differences." Progress Report to National Heart Institute, 1969.

62. John J. Christian. "The Potential Role of the Adrenal Cortex as Affected by Social Rank and Population Density on Experimental Epidemics." *Am. J. Epid.,* 87, 1968, 255–264.

63. J. W. Mason, J. V. Brady, E. Polish, et al. "Concurrent Measurement of 17-Hydroxycorticosteroids and Pepsinogen Levels During Prolonged Emotional Stress in the Monkey." *Psychosom. Med.,* 21, 1959, 432.

64. Alexander Kessler. "Interplay between Social Ecology and Physiology, Genetics, and Population Dynamics of Mice." Doctoral Dissertation. 1966.

65. William Haenzel, Donald B. Loveland, and Monroe G. Sirken. "Lung-Cancer Mortality as Related to Residence and Smoking Histories." *J. Nat. Cancer Inst.,* 28, 1962, 947–1001.

66. John J. Conger, et al. "The Role of Social Experience in the Production of Gastric Ulcers in Hooded Rats Placed in a Conflict Situation." *J. Abnorm. and Soc. Psych.,* 57, 1958, 216.

67. Morton D. Bogdanoff, Kurt Back, Robert Klein, E. H. Estes, and Claude Nichols. "The Physiologic Response to Conformity Pressure in Man." *Ann. Int. Med.,* 57, 1962.

68. S. L. Syme. Personal Communication.

69. William N. Christenson and Lawrence E. Hinkle, Jr. "Differences in Illness and Prognostic Signs in Two Groups of Young Men." *J.A.M.A.,* 177, 1961, 247–253.

70. Warren H. Durham. "Social Structures and Mental Disorders: Complete Hypotheses of Explanation." *Milbank Mem. Fund Quart.,* 39, 1961, 259–310.

71. Elliot G. Mishler and Norman A. Scotch. "Sociocultural Factors in the Epidemiology of Schizophrenia. A Review." *Psychiatry,* 26, 1963, 315–351.

72. W. A. Tillman and G. E. Hobbs. "Social Background of Accident-Free and Accident Repeaters." *Am. J. Psychiat.,* 106, 1949, 321.

73. Emile Durkheim. *Suicide.* The Free Press, 1957.

74. Thomas H. Holmes. Personal Communication.

# Chapter VI

# The Assessment of the Built-Environment for Safety: Research and Practice

Robert Geddes

and

Robert Gutman

With the assistance of Constance Lieder,
Brendan Murphy, Barbara Westergaard,
Dorothy Whiteman, and Ellen Wolfe

## PART I Environmental Assessment

## A. Introduction and Definition of Environmental Assessment

This report presents the findings of the study made by the Princeton-Rutgers Environmental Assessment Group (EAG) for the project sponsored by the U.S. Bureau of Community Environmental Management.

The investigation has been concerned with several issues simultaneously:

1. To review the role of the design professions in assessing the quality of the environmental products which they help to construct, and to consider their future role as assessors. This subject is discussed in Section B.

2. To examine several critical conceptual and methodological problems which previous research indicates are important in research on environmental assessment. For this purpose, a general survey of environmental assessment research was undertaken. An examination was made of the published literature dealing with a wide range of environmental types and with different standards and criteria in terms of which environments have been evaluated. The findings of this general survey appear in Section C.

143

3. To examine in detail the conceptual and methodological problems which arise in assessing the safety of residential environments. Special concern was given to this subject because of the discovery, during the preliminary stages of the study, that residential safety was one of the most clearly articulated and best developed areas in which environmental research up to now has been conducted. We thought that it would be possible to utilize this investigation as a model for considering the issues raised in the study of social and psychological criteria. The results of our survey of research on residential safety are presented in Part II A.

4. To test our conclusions about relevant concepts and research techniques for assessing environmental quality by making a case study of a specific built environment. Radburn, New Jersey, was selected for investigation. Rather than conducting an evaluation of Radburn's quality our effort was directed to defining the empirical measures and exploring the available data sources by means of which such an assessment could be carried out in Radburn or in a similar setting. The outcome of this exploration is discussed in Part II B.

In this inquiry, we have limited ourselves to studies which attempt to measure the adequacy of the built environment in terms of certain standards centered around what constitutes an adequate setting for the social and behavioral aspects of human life. Several aspects of this working definition should be made explicit:

1. Our interest has been in the built environment; three-dimensional, man-made artifacts which are large enough to enclose, shelter, or house human activities. These artifacts are what we ordinarily think of as rooms, buildings, campuses, housing projects, gardens, and urban settlements. Several different scales of built environments are involved here and we have been interested in the widest range, including at one extreme the arrangement of furniture and, at the other extreme, the metropolitan region.

2. Environments can be evaluated according to a large number of criteria: their economic cost, their durability, the political feasibility of their construction, or, as in the case of our inquiry, in terms of their adequacy in meeting the psychological and social needs of the people who inhabit or use them. This focus is sometimes referred to as the behavioral assessment of the environment.

3. We have taken it as a guiding principle that environmental assessment studies must assume certain standards against which the adequacy of a particular environment can be measured. In some studies these standards are discussed at length; in others they are simply used without discussion. Although it is often important in environmental assessment studies to be aware of the intentions of the designer and builders, these intentions cannot by themselves be assumed to constitute an adequate

144

statement of appropriate standards. The rationale for these intentions has to be considered independently.

4. Our focus is on determining the quality of the environment rather than on understanding the relative importance of the built environment in comparison to other types of environments, for example, the social environment, in producing certain social or behavioral effects. We regard the latter type of inquiry as providing much of the scientific knowledge which eventually must go into the determination of environmental quality. In this sense, environmental assessment research is a form of applied science which derives its theory and technique from fundamental studies on man-environment relations.

## B. State of Environmental Assessment and Practice

The study of the literature dealing with environmental assessment revealed that there is no well-developed, systematic body of knowledge presently available for evaluating the human quality of buildings or communities. In our review (in Parts III and IV), we have indicated some of the factors responsible for this situation and identified some of the issues which deserve more intensive scrutiny.

Our review also indicates that even the knowledge that does exist is not being applied by the individuals and groups who are responsible for building and designing the environment. There is no single profession or social institution that has produced significant evidence of its capacity or willingness to undertake this responsibility as an ongoing activity. In short, there is no existing institutional framework for the practice of environmental assessment.

### 1. Design Practice:

At the present time, within the design professions, there is no clearly defined attitude toward environmental assessment. Isolated articles and reports do deal with it and it is even discussed at conferences on architecture, urban planning, and engineering, yet environmental assessment does not form part of the recognized professional service.

It should be noted that *The Architect's Handbook of Professional Practice,* a publication of the American Institute of Architects (AIA) *(1),* makes no mention of environmental assessment.

It is significant, too, that standard texts of the design profession, which one might expect to deal with environmental assessment, do not attend to it. These include *Principles and Practice of Urban Planning,* edited by William I. Goodman and Eric C. Freund; *(44) Creating the Human Environment,* a report of the AIA by Gerald M. McCue, William R. Ewald, Jr., and the Midwest Research Institute; *(78)* and *Comprehensive Architectural Services: General Principles and Practice,* edited by William Dudley Hunt, Jr. *(60)* The only book found which deals with the issue of environmental assessment is *Emerging Methods in Environmental Design and Planning,* edited by Gary T. Moore.(*87*) It clearly states that environmental assessment is essential to the design profession. Another report, prepared by Robert L. Geddes and Bernard P. Spring, dealing with education in the design professions, states that evaluation is a necessary part of the design process. (*41*)

### 2. Assessment Standards:

Standards exist in the design professions as a means of regulation, ostensibly to safeguard the public welfare. These standards or codes govern the behavior of materials, but only indirectly relate to human beings. It is clear from an examination of the following three sets of codes that, with few exceptions, technical concerns take precedence over human ones.

The three codes studied were: the *American Society for Testing and Materials* (ASTM) ; (*5*) the *American National Standards Institute's Catalog* (formerly the U.S.A. Standards Institute); (*3*) and the *National Building Code.* (*2*)

The ASTM states that, "standards comprise those specifications and methods of test that have been formally adopted by the Society, requiring a letter ballot approved by the entire membership." At no point in its foreword does it mention the words "social organization" or "behavior."

The *American National Standards Institute Catalog* contains safety standards, but most of its space is devoted to technical areas.

The *National Building Code* is the most socially concerned of these three major codes. Part of its stated purpose is "to provide for safety, health, and public welfare . . ." Yet, after its opening statement it deals no further with the interaction of human behavior with the environment.

Performance codes have developed recently as an alternative to more rigid specifications, which tend to stifle innovation. Two examples of this trend are the *School Construction Development Project* (SCSD), (*34*) a report from Educational Facilities Laboratories, and the *University Residential Building System* (URBS), (*17*) a project of the University of California.

The SCSD project literature reports that the performance specifications are of a technical nature. The performance specifications of the URBS project do discuss the space allotment for students, but the specifications are addressed for the most part to the performance of materials. As in the prescriptive standards, the effects on human behavior are not dealt with directly.

### 3. Newer Developments:

Although environmental assessment is not yet accepted as a part of the design professions, nor as a separate discipline, it is the subject of a growing number of interdisciplinary activities.

146

This recent concern is probably encouraged by three facts. First, the volume and scale of present and anticipated building activity has sensitized the design profession to the need for assessment. Pressures of rapidly increasing population and expanding urbanization call for larger scale development than has previously been attempted. Large-scale development makes designers accountable for more aspects of the entire built environment than in smaller scale developments.

Second, an increasing interest in scientific predictions of the future, and in planning in general, has called attention to the need for criteria by which to assess "alternative futures." Third, there is more of an awareness at the collective or governmental level of the impact of the environment on human life. This awareness is translated into government and private programs, research grants, and administrative requirements.

Illustrations of the growing concern about environmental assessment are found in four areas: federal government activity, academic programs, professional periodicals, and conferences.

The federal government, through the Bureau of Public Roads, has conducted and sponsored research on the impact of highways and expressways upon surrounding communities. A Bureau of Public Roads publication, *Highways and Economic and Social Change,* reports on one hundred such studies, (113) the first of which was recorded as early as 1929. Although primarily concerned with before-and-after studies of changes in land use and property values and of effects on business, utilities, and public services, they also included studies of user costs and benefits. While these reports may have been relatively unsophisticated when dealing with social and behavioral aspects of the man-environment relationship, they have won general acceptance among highway designers as a necessary component of their work. Since 1962, impact studies have been made in anticipation of highway design. The work of the Highway Research Board has broadened to include social and community considerations. (118)

There is other evidence of federal activity. A study recently prepared by the National Academy of Engineering for the National Science Foundation recommended that research be applied to social needs in construction and transportation. Acknowledging that no way is known to analyze the behavior of buildings or technology over time, the study urged that adequate techniques for testing these systems be developed. (110) The National Environmental Policy Act requires that all federally supported construction projects contain a statement detailing their impact on the environment. It is hoped that the concept of environment may be broadened to include the social and behavioral aspects of the man-environment relationship. Urban renewal projects, for example, must now give more consideration to their impact on relocation, community participation, and neighborhood considerations.

Other government projects at the community level are also under increased pressure to consider their behavioral effects. Also, it is encouraging that the government is presently undertaking research in environmental assessment, as noted in the section on residential safety.

In recent years, interdisciplinary graduate programs and research centers which consider aspects of the man-environment relationship have begun to be developed. Some of these are outgrowths of urban studies centers which had begun as interdisciplinary programs. Others are extensions of the more traditional professional schools of architecture, landscape architecture, and planning. A few have arisen from the fields of psychology, law, and public administration. Several of the programs and centers are listed in the Appendix to this chapter, and many more may develop as research funds increase.

While several of the established scholarly and professional journals in fields such as psychology, sociology, and political science, have published special issues on aspects of behavior and the environment, a number of periodicals have been established recently to deal specifically with these concerns. Some are newsletters and reports from academic or research institutions, some are commercial or professional journals, and a few are more scholarly publications reporting only rigorous research. All are interdisciplinary, and all presently have small circulation. In addition to these interdisciplinary journals, noted in the Appendix to this chapter the regular professional journals publish articles on behavior and the environment. The British *Architects' Journal*, (7) in particular, reports regularly on building evaluation.

There is a growth in the number of conferences being held to discuss environmental assessment. The Environmental Design Research Association conferences, which are intended to be annual events and which have met twice already, are especially noteworthy for the relatively high quality of presentation. The EDRA itself was established to facilitate multidiscipline collaboration, to promote communication between designers and scientists, and to interest scientists in the problem-solving techniques of designers.

Despite the increased activity, all of these efforts are unrelated, and no organization of information or services exists to coordinate the available knowledge of environmental assessment and to facilitate future research.

### 4. Possible Institutional Developments in the Future:

It is not yet possible to identify with certainty the probable location of continuing responsibility for environmental assessment. It is, however, possible to speculate on several ways in which the practice might be institutionalized in the near future. These potential institutional frameworks are as follows:

a. The practice of environmental assessment might be achieved by increasing the contractual scope of architects' services so as to provide continuing supervision for the *use* of the building during its initial years of habitation. This new service would, in some ways, be an extension of the architect's responsibility for supervising the construction of a building and, in some ways, be like his responsibility for programming the needs for new building. It should be emphasized that the concept of environmental assessment as part of the practice of architecture is not evident in any of the official documents of the American Institute of Architects.

b. The practice of environmental assessment might be broadly based in one or more of the environmental design professions as a whole, or in the Interprofessional Council on Environmental Design (ICED). In this case, the profession would assume the responsibility to be self-monitoring. The professionally supported research units would develop methodological standards and collect information which could be made available to others.

c. Industrial organizations, home-building firms, and other large scale consumers of design and construction services are other possible sources of initiative in this area. They would either establish environmental assessment units within their own organizations or would help to generate service firms which, like market analysis groups, would be available to conduct evaluation studies for a wide range of clients.

d. The practice of environmental assessment might be established by requiring that it be part of the on-going program of all federally sponsored and supported programs. Environmental assessment might be required of all agencies such as hospitals, housing authorities, boards of education, etc., which apply for additional funding. In this way the agency would have to undertake environmental assessment before continuing its program.

e. The practice of environmental assessment might become the responsibility of a governmental bureau, established expressly for that purpose. The bureau would serve as a continuing source of information and methodology for environmental assessment. It might work on a contract basis for agencies and other groups seeking environmental assessment of their physical environment. Precedents for the establishment of governmental bureaus have been set by the National Swedish Institute for Building Research, the Danish National Institute of Building Research, and Britain's Building Research Station. (65) In addition, Great Britain's Ministry of Housing and Local Government has sponsored studies of housing occupied by the elderly which resulted in a unique building and assessment program for flatlets for the aged. (46)

f. The practice of environmental assessment might find an institutional base in research units of universities, where the practice could be closely related to the teaching and research functions of the physical planning and design disciplines. The research units would be available for continuing research, and for contract research on particular assessments.

It is not possible to select among these possibilities at this time. It would be very helpful if all of them were in operation. Unfortunately, the practice of environmental assessment has not yet found its institutional framework, despite the evident need for it in a more rational design process.

## C. Research on the Relationship Between Environment and Behavior

Design professionals may be reluctant to have their work independently assessed. But equally important to the lack of greater understanding and evaluation of the relationship between the built environment and behavior are the fundamental difficulties of research in this area.

The difficulties arise because research of this type is necessarily interdisciplinary. Furthermore, there is no established or mutually agreed upon classification or definition for either the built environment or behavior. Each discipline tends to focus on the behavioral effects traditional to its field. Environmental properties are seldom treated comprehensively or described with enough precision to allow empirical measurement.

All too often there is not even a clear distinction between physical form and the behavior of users. In fact, our design of built-forms implicitly includes behavioral expectations which rarely are described independently. Consider for example a 500-seat auditorium, which implies both a size and a usage; a six-lane expressway, describing width and expected traffic volume.

In this Section, three principal areas within this field of research are treated. First, a definition and a classification of environmental properties are offered, together with examples of research in each category and suggestions for empirical measures. Second, a classification system for behavior is offered, and the behavioral biases of several disciplines are described. Finally, research strategies are described, together with illustrations. This is intended to provide the beginnings of a consistent scheme for designing research on the quality of the built-environment.

### 1. Environmental Properties

#### a. Requirements of an Environmental Classification:

A major effort in our study has been to establish a useful classification system for the environment. The requirements for such a general codification are as follows:

First, the word "environment" here must be qualified to refer to the "built" or physical, man-made environment—that which is capable of

150

being designed, built, altered, reproduced, or adapted by man. This is to distinguish it from an ecological concept of the environment, and to restrict it to that which is the normal concern of designers—the architects, planners, engineers, developers, etc.

Second, the man-made environment is to be considered the independent variable in research design. For designers, this is what they deal with and manipulate; for behavioral scientists, it can be a method of organizing information. A universal classification system of the environmental variable would still leave individual disciplines free to develop their own classification for dependent variables.

Third, the classification system chosen should be useful for organizing the existing information in the field.

Fourth, the classification system should be *operational*—capable of producing unambiguous measures; *replicable*—usable by anyone unerringly; *economical*—grouping and reducing reality to salient characteristics; and *relevant*—useful to designers who encode knowledge into building the environment and researchers who may decode it to advance their disciplines.

Fifth, the classification system should be one that is likely to define and select those features of the environment which it is reasonable to assume influence social action and behavior. There is no single classification scheme for the environment which is likely to be equally productive for all kinds of environmental assessment research. Our purpose in the following classification is to deliberately borrow concepts and definitions developed by other disciplines and traditions and to incorporate them into a scheme whose principal aim is to improve our understanding of the behavioral effects of the environment.

Finally, we are aware that the development of a classification scheme indicating the properties relevant to behavior necessarily is based on theoretical ideas about how and why the environment and man affect each other. We have not tried here to make these ideas explicit.

*b. Classification Relevant to Social Behavior:*

The classification scheme consists of forty-eight categories of environments, based on the conjunction of eight "properties" of environments and six levels of environmental scale.

(1) *environmental scale*

(a) *building:* the individual structure, the boundaries of whose functions are roughly equivalent to a social institution. (Sometimes the same word is used as a name for the structure and a label for the institution: school-school, church-church, etc.)

(b) *site plan:* the arrangement of a building in relation to its immediate neighbors, including the space between them. Ordinarily thought of in connection with dwelling environments, the scale applies also to other building types, including small apartment-office units in central cities, shopping centers, college campuses, educational parks, etc. (76)

(c) *neighborhood layout:* the arrangement of many individual buildings, including the spaces between them. This scalar image usually is applied to dwelling units, but it can also be used for other types of environments, such as airports, center city developments, and so on. (25)

(d) *local community:* the physical environment which is congruent with the boundaries of important political jurisdictions, such as boroughs, towns, and cities. It includes a wide range of building types. (23, 61)

(e) *region:* the environment whose boundaries are defined by a system of recurrent social interaction among residents, and a web of interdependent economic relationships. Usually a region is made up of a dominant central city and its suburbs. (31)

(f) *macro-region:* the environment of a large super-complex of interdependent smaller regions, perhaps similar to the megalopolitan developments in the Northeastern United States.

(2) *environmental properties*

There are eight properties of the physical environment which, in our judgment, have some significance for behavior. They are:

(a) *spatial organization*
(b) *circulation and movement systems*
(c) *communication systems*
(d) *ambient properties*
(e) *visual properties*
(f) *amenities*
(g) *symbolic properties*
(h) *architectonic properties*

These properties are analytical or conceptual features of built environments, operating at all scales. Some circulation systems or ambient properties may also be identifiable objects or physical states in their own right. (39, 57) In describing the present state of research with respect to the influence of each property, an important consideration will be the degree to which the studies deal with each of the six levels of environment scale. In this way, we will be able to discuss both dimensions of the classification scheme at the same time.

(3) *research in relation to the classification*

(a) *spatial organization:* the location of facilities and structures, often represented by concepts indicating degree of dispersion, of concentration, clustering, proximity, etc.

This property of the environment has been the traditional concern of sociological ecologists, location economists, land planners, and regional scientists. As a consequence, the empirical research has been conducted largely from an economic perspective to consider:

the impact of regional organization on economic growth, (52) the process through which locational decisions are made, (95) and the constraints, both political and structural, which affect these decisions. To the degree that a concern for behavioral and social effects is reflected in the literature, this concern has been principally with the site plan and neighborhood scale. (37, 68) This reflects the persistent anxiety in the United States over maintaining strong local community ties in an otherwise amorphous, dynamic mass society. (28, 35) Most of the research concludes that the spatial organization of the site plan, housing development, or neighborhood is less powerful in determining social interaction patterns than the cultural values, the social practices, and the class composition of the residents. (36, 61, 70, 71)

There has been relatively little empirical study of the consequences of alternative spatial organizations at the scale of individual buildings. The absence of such a literature is in marked contrast to English and Scandinavian building research. However, there is some evidence of change, particularly with regard to institutional building types, such as hospitals, (77) libraries, (48, 104) and offices. (53) Empirical measures that describe spatial organization include the percentage of area devoted to various land uses, population densities, land values, rental rates, vacancy rates, and measures of floor area coverage, open space ratios, and building coverage. Within a building, measures include square footages and space usage, such as the percent of area given to equipment, service, circulation, etc.

(b) *circulation and movement systems:* this category of environmental properties includes two subcategories: one is made up of the objects used for transporting people and goods, such as cars and trains, along with the infrastructure which supports them, such as rails and highways; the other subcategory includes the spaces in buildings or urban forms that regulate the flow of people and goods, including corridors, stairways, portals, public open spaces, and alleyways.

The study of transportation systems, and their influence on the economic development of a region and on land-use patterns, is a highly developed field of study. Like the research on spatial organization, it has tended to focus on economic effects. For example, one does not find in the United States much of the kind of concern that is so evident in various French discussions of the way in which transportation inefficiency contributes to worker fatigue, and the costs imposed on health and family solidarity. A curious development is now taking place, however, which probably will generate American research of this type: in response to the indignation of the black population over the way in which freeway systems have reduced the stock of inexpensive center city housing, the Highway Research Board is soliciting research contracts that will deal with the effect of road transportation on neighborhood integration.

At smaller scales, such as the individual building or the building complex, research on circulation systems is developing, but slowly. One can point to isolated studies of large institutional environments, such as universities or airports. Unfortunately, most of these studies are undertaken by private firms for specific clients; they do not enter the scientific literature. (26)

Measures that describe a circulation system are miles or lanes of highways, public transit traffic volume, schedules and numbers of stops, automobile traffic volume, degree of traffic separation, number of parking facilities, number of terminals, and miles of walkways. Within a building, the circulation system includes the lobbies, stairways, elevators, corridors, aisles, etc.

(c) *communication systems:* the properties of the environment that give users information and ideas. This category includes mechanical devices such as telephones, computer hookups, and television, as well as features that allow for direct interaction and exchange such as picture windows in houses, screened apertures in hospitals, paths in site plans, etc.

These properties can exist in different forms even in environments with similar spatial organizations. With the exception of one important book about the impact of communication systems on urban growth, (81) research has dealt mainly with the smaller scales of housing layouts and site plans. (27)

Two points should be mentioned in this context. First, communication properties have relatively little influence on the effects that have been studied up to now. (8) For example, it appears that communication systems are not major determinants of a sense of community, (19) although it might turn out that they strongly affect household efficiency. Second, although a particular environmental property may not be as important as some cultural or social factor in determining a behavioral outcome, whatever importance it has must be taken into account by the environmental designer in proposing a building or design scheme. (49)

Actually, many measures of communication features in the environment are overlooked in the literature. These include direct information givers like number and location of signs, traffic signals, information and tourist centers; communication equipment like telephones, televisions, loud speakers; and direction and privacy indicators like paths, fences, hedges, and lobbies. The frequency and type of such things are indications of communication possibilities which are "built" into the environment.

(d) *ambient properties:* the features of the environment which are critical for maintaining the physiological and psychological functioning of the human organism. These features include properties such as quality and level of illumination, heating and air conditioning, ventilation, and humidity levels.

There has been more research interest among Americans in these properties of the environment than in any of the others listed in our scheme. Many effects have been under study for a century or more. The first interest in ambient properties apparently stemmed from the public health and sanitation movements and was associated with nineteenth century ideas about contamination, quarantine, and the influence of climate on disease. This venerable tradition has proven enormously influential on environmental design, and is largely responsible for the fact that the standards for light, heat, and space are generally higher in the United States than in other countries. (*4*)

Despite the excellence of this research, it must be realized that it has dealt principally with physical health. The significance of ambient conditions in influencing mental health or eliminating social pathology is still an open question. (*99, 106*) Except at extreme levels of sensory deprivation, the effect of ambient conditions on family instability, delinquency, and school and work performance, appears to be very limited, (*105 122*)

Perhaps the most interesting thrust of recent American research on the effects of ambient properties is the greater attention being shown to their role on the regional scale in studies of the social costs of air, water, and noise pollution. Measures of ambience include number of utility and sanitary facilities, the amount of air and water pollution, decibels of sound; and within buildings, the degree of heating and air conditioning, expanse of windows, and the amount of plumbing, electricity, etc.

(e) *visual properties:* the appearance of the environment as it is perceived by users and by the general public. These properties include color, shape, light, and other visual modalities. Beginning with Vitruvius, architects have regarded the creation and manipulation of these properties as one of the principal tasks of their profession. It was not until experimental psychology developed in Germany in the nineteenth century that these properties were regarded as accessible to empirical study. The research tradition dealing with perception has progressed through two stages, at least as it applies to environmental phenomena. In the first stage, interest was concentrated on ascertaining the objectivity of visual properties: to what extent were they intrinsic to environmental form, and to what extent a product of the user's experience. (*9, 111*) More recently, during the second stage, investigations have been concerned with the relation of perception to social action and behavior. (6) A variety of research programs dealing with this area are now in operation. Studies are being conducted of the judgmental process in architectural evaluations; (18) of the perceptual features of neighborhoods and cities; (73, 74) and even of the impact of a region's visual characteristics on the community identification of residents. (75) So far, these studies have not demonstrated any link between visual properties and social pathology.

Measures of visual characteristics include, for example, classifications of street layout and facade and of landscaping and natural features; degree of vandalism, cleanliness, yard care, and deterioration; classifications of homogeneity or contrast of form, scale, architectural style, materials and color. One system of notation for the visual environment consists of path, node, edge, district, and landmark. (75)

(f) amenities: the social activities implied by the environment, ordinarily spoken of as the facilities which are programmed in the environment. Examples of amenities in a dwelling unit are: bathroom, kitchen, bedroom; in a housing project: community room, neighborhood store; in a region: shopping center.

There are some arguments against including the amenity concept among environmental properties. Unlike some of the properties mentioned earlier, its definition includes the behavioral as well as the physical level of reality, since to describe the amenity we must always identify a social or human activity in relation to a space. One seldom sees, designs, or thinks about a space or an environment without imagining its probable use, even though its actual use may differ from the expected use.

The close connection between the amenity concept and social activity has generated a good deal of interest in user requirement studies. In these studies, present or prospective users have been asked to indicate their degree of satisfaction with existing planning or housing arrangements, or to express their preferences among alternative proposals. (121) These studies have taken place mostly on the scale of housing, particularly low- and middle-income housing, and on the level of regional plans, especially with regard to new mass transportation systems. (51) Despite the growth of user requirement research, there have been very few studies of the effects of existing amenities on social behavior and social pathology. (119) Probably the major exception to this generalization are the studies of the social effects of slum rehousing, which have been conducted in the United States since the New Deal. (99)

Measures of amenity include the number and amount (floor area, space or number of facilities) of all service and support facilities.

These include recreation facilities and parks, shopping facilities, health care centers, and community centers. Specifically, measures identify number of tennis courts, square feet of shopping space, or number of hospital beds.

(g) *symbolic properties:* the social values, attitudes, statuses, and cultural norms which are represented or expressed by environments. Environments have been described as expressions of democratic or authoritarian order, of innovation and social change or continuity with the past, and of social equality or social hierarchy.

The symbolic meaning of the environment is a favorite theme of the design tradition, and the interpretation of the symbolism inherent in a building or an urban form is standard fare in the writings of architectural historians and critics. (*96*)

Discussions of the symbolic meaning of the environment have begun to crop up in the behavioral science literature. (*109*) Some sociologists use the fact that location in urban space varies in a patterned way with social class of residents as an index (and hence potentially a symbol) of income and occupational level in the American city. (*32*) Scholars interested in a social theory of city growth account for the failure of land-use expansion to follow a simple economic model in terms of the symbolic meanings which are associated with specific sites and neighborhoods. (*20, 38*) Social psychologists and psychoanalysts are now arguing that the response of the mentally ill to therapeutic settings can best be interpreted by understanding the attitudes and values which their hospital or home environments symbolize for them. (*40, 91*) The unconscious meaning of environmental symbols is said to apply equally at all scales. (*79, 98, 101*)

Measures which indicate symbolic properties include the number of church steeples, type and amount of street furniture, location and content of statues and monuments, the use of columns on buildings, and other architectural features, and the appearance of lawns and common areas.

(h) *architectonic properties:* the sensory or esthetic properties of an environment which arise from its unique qualities as a three-dimensional form, large enough to enclose the human organism. This property is independent of, and transcends, the visual and symbolic features of the physical environment.

The architectonic qualities occur when the physical form is evaluated independently, as a design product, for integrity and unity, for its structure, form, and for the spaces it creates. Sometimes a building is treated as a work of art or sculpture, and evaluation approaches esthetic criticism.

While these characteristics may be of most interest to designers, they also can elicit emotions in the users of buildings and spaces.

German estheticians of the last century called it *"Raumgefühl,"* and the Modern Movement in architecture claims that the self-conscious creation of this "sense of space" is its special contribution to the history of building. (*90*) However, so far, behavioral scientists have made little attempt to find ways to objectify this property or to study its social effects, with a few exceptions such as studying the effects of esthetic surroundings on well-being. (*80, 85*)

Architectonic properties derive from the structure of a building, method of construction, choice of materials, physical relation of spaces, and relationship to the environment. In addition, emotional responses are invoked by style, form, color, and other physical factors.

## 2. Behavioral Criteria

Ultimately, any evaluation of the built environment must be based on an accepted standard of what is good or bad for man, but no such generally accepted standard exists. However, the many scientific disciplines which have been concerned indirectly or explicitly with environmental effects have selected certain types of behavior for investigation. Although the study of these behaviors does not in itself resolve the debate about appropriate criteria, it does at least help us to understand both the possibilities and the problems involved in formulating an empirical approach to assessing environmental quality. In the following pages we first review the approach of each discipline to the question of the influence of the environment, and then proceed to develop a classification scheme aimed at providing a basis for the systematic evaluation of alternative built environments.

### a. *The Behavioral Focus of the Disciplines*

The *biological sciences* and their applied professions primarily focus upon the impact of man's environment upon biological processes, physical and mental health, and the pathology of disease. René Dubos, the microbiologist recently turned commentator upon the impact of environment, is mainly concerned with the long-term biological and genetic effects of man's adaptability to adverse environments. (*29*) Others in the field have been concerned with the incidence of mental illness in contrasting communities. (*33*) Still others place health factors high on the list of urban problems, including variables such as mental health and mental retardation. (*30*) More recently, attention has been turned to immediate environmental constraints, such as the delivery of medical health services within the community. (*24*) The measures utilized by these groups are usually objective and frequently comparative; they include mortality, incidence of disease, birth rate, life expectancy, and mental hospital admissions.

The research environment in these studies is usually large-scale at the "community" level, not the site plan or building scale. Few studies in the United States deal with sanitation and large-scale public health problems. Standards dealing with water, sewerage facilities, and sanitation are commonly accepted environmental controls in building and community development.

The *social sciences* deal with a broad range of human behavior—individual, group, social and institutional. Not all have been equally involved in consideration of environmental impact.

Sociologists probably have been the most active in the field, and their major concern has been with behavioral phenomena of groups and institutions. The setting in which social behavior and activities take place has always been of some concern within the discipline, if not always explicitly stated. Social pathology, including family disorganization, mental disorders, delinquency, and institutional disruptions, has been a traditional concern. (50) The social characteristics of people and their activities are increasingly being related to urban environments. (82) The measures which sociologists employ and can relate to the environment include communication and social interaction, class and value systems, family organization, life style, community organization and cohesion, mobility and social well-being. Research is undertaken at both the macro and micro scales; it covers subjective and objective evaluations, and includes comparative demographic characteristics and social indicators such as age, family structure, occupation, income, race, and ethnic backgrounds.

Anthropologists, too, with their concentration on cultural systems, have been involved with environmental considerations. The work of Edward Hall has been most popular with designers, as he introduces the concept of the experience of space as molded by culture. Environmental design must consider the sensory worlds of various cultures, since the perception and use of space are culturally determined. (54) For anthropologists, the behavior to be evaluated concerns human activity, life patterns, and the cultural traditions for carrying it out, including learning, defense, sexual behavior, child-rearing, eating, work patterns, authority, etc. Research in anthropology regards the environment as a territory adapted for carrying out an activity.

Psychology, more concerned with individual behavior, has considered the environment as a setting for individual behavior. (14, 56) Psychologists have studied attitudes, privacy, learning, visual perception, and the behavior of patients in mental hospitals. (93) Most of the work has been at the micro-environmental level, although some perception studies have dealt with large-scale environments. Some work has been experimental, usually involving the minor manipulation of seating or spatial arrangements. (103)

Political scientists and economists are less involved in environmental assessment at present. Implicit to both disciplines, however, are environmental constraints. Political boundaries are of major societal concern.

(31) Economists, in regional analyses do, of course, use physical bound-aries to define market areas. (66) Economic *measures* have also been used as criteria for evaluating environmental impact. More recently, some investigators with a legal bent have begun looking at environ-mental factors in anti-social behavior, such as crime, vandalism, and delinquency. (89)

As already indicated, measures used in assessing behavior generally fall into two categories: subjective and objective. Subjective measures have to do with attitudes, judgments, or feelings of the affected people or group. Objective measures include work productivity, health indica-tors, and degree of social interaction. The relation between subjective and objective responses is a field of research in itself. The development of gaming techniques is one attempt to bridge this problem, to aid in anticipating behavior.

Architects have internalized a basic knowledge of man's muscular-skeletal structure, certain assumptions about physical shelter, and the cultural traditions of their own societies. Books are available that pro-vide architectural standards, which relate to man's size and activities, including sizes and heights of doors, stairs, tables and traditional furnish-ings, as well as suggestions for room sizes, sports facilities, circulation spaces, etc. It is usually only when these considerations are absent from architecural work that they attract attention.

Because of a client orientation, architectural evaluation—when it goes beyond costs (client constraint) and evaluation of materials and struc-tures (a reflection of shelter)—may first consider maintenance and opera-tion of buildings. User evaluation, a more recent assessement criterion, is still largely oriented to circulation and access, and performance of functions. These factors reflect the design process which, in part, in-volves the structural assemblage of more or less traditional spaces for activities within a circulation system.

Because of his visual orientation and belief in "meaning" in archi-tecture, the architect's first interest may be visual perception and how people "read" buildings and spaces. He may, therefore, find ideas from psychology more readily applicable to his interests.

The planner, again a service- and client-oriented professional, is usually interested in larger scale environments, and more often, two dimensions. Because of a public-service orientation, evaluations of environments revolve around public costs and benefits—tax revenues, service costs, traffic generation, utility needs, community facilities. For a private client, usually a developer, the anticipated return must cover anticipated costs or the development will not take place. Measures that reflect the market place reaction to the built or buildable environment include land values, rents, and volume of sales. There is an implied health, social, and psychological concern in measures of density, land coverage, floor-area ratios, and land-use relationships, but these are not

160

yet used as standards. Zoning, long one of the planners' principal tools, was adopted, in part, out of consideration for the consequences to health, safety, and welfare of different land uses—for example, traffic, noise, smells, pollution and sanitation. Today zoning is more frequently used to regulate property values. When planners move from their more traditional concerns they tend to consider sociological factors, such as relocation, housing needs, community organization, and neighborhood identification, more than other aspects of social or biological sciences.

Engineers, the traditional designers of large-scale construction projects, concentrate on structural concerns but have looked at the impact of their work, sometimes more frequently than other designers. As pointed out in the previous sections of this report, they are eager to adopt measurement tools. Sometimes these are naive as far as human behavior is concerned. However, they tend to concentrate on the service and related benefits of the facilities they design, and are not usually concerned with psychological or sociological considerations. Measures they utilize to evaluate the impact of the environment they design include access time, user benefits, land-use generation, and energy or service provision.

b. *Dimension of a Behavioral Classification System*

In order to reduce the variation implied by the approach of the separate disciplines discussed above, we suggest that it would be useful to consider the following dimensions of behavior in studies of environmental quality. The classification is based on a distinction among three general categories of behavior and six scales of human activity or response at which this behavior occurs.

(1) *behavioral scale*

(a) the *individual*—individuals must be considered by age, principal occupation, economic and social groups, including race, religion, and ethnic background.

(b) the *family* or living unit—this interdependent unit is our basic economic group. There are significant variations often classified by household composition—the traditional family, the one-adult family, and the single person household, for example.

(c) the *performance* or (occupational) unit— this is basically an activity group, an office, factory, school (with subdivisions) or perhaps neighborhood, and is a relatively small group that can usually be physically located in one place.

(d) the social *institution*—larger than the previous group, this represents a professional or occupational group, an institution spread out in various locations, or any identifiable group within the population.

(e) the *community*—while difficult to define, it represents the agglomerated institutions and is the totality of these.

161

(f) the *larger political, economic, and national group*—which encompasses all the interdependent groups within a megalopolis or a nation.

(2) *behavioral categories*

There are three general behavioral categories which can include the various concerns of the disciplines and professions dealing with man's needs, attitudes, and activities. These are described below, together with suggestions of empirical measures which can be used to evaluate them.

(a) *survival and physical welfare*—the biological and physiological needs of man, affected by the environment, including his survival, security, comfort, safety, and general physical well-being. There are numerous measures of this; many are primarily health measures including disease rates, mortality, hospitalization, drug usage, alcoholism, and mental health. Other measures of safety and security can be derived from fire, crime, and arrest records; insurance rates; and security precautions such as burglar alarm systems and amount of street lighting.

(b) *satisfaction and attitude*—psychological set of users toward their environment. It is distinct from any abnormal psychological state covered under the previous category. This attitude can be measured directly by questioning users or inferred by determining the value people assign to factors in the environment. Inferential measures include the market value of properties, vacancy rates waiting lists for apartments, delinquent taxes, and turnover of properties. Other inferential measures of satisfaction have to do with how people treat the environment—whether they care for their property or vandalize it.

(c) *activity and performance*—covers the many varied social and functional activities of people within the built environment. There are many ways to measure behavior in this category. In general, time budgets and income budgets are good indicators of how people distribute their resources. Economic performance can be measured by productivity of workers, income, absenteeism, and unemployment. Recreation and leisure behavior can be measured by participation, attendance, and use of facilities. Educational activity is measured by school attendance, achievement, and enrollment. Commercial activity can be judged by sales volume per square foot. The performance of a transportation system for users is evaluated by travel times, traffic volumes, modal split, car usage, etc. Social activity can be measured by visits, friendships, and participation. In general, if choice is present in the built environment behavior should reflect preferences.

## 3. Research Design Strategies

Fundamental to a discussion of appropriate research designs for assessing environments is the distinction between strategies for studying environmental effects and strategies for studying environmental assessment. Studies of environmental effects examine the interrelations betwen the built environment and behavioral variables, with particular attention to the influence of the environment on behavior. Such stud· ies need not, and usually do not, raise questions about the adequacy of the environment as a setting for human activities or attempt to evaluate it by reference to established or hypothetical performance standards. It is just these issues, however, which are essential to inquiries in the area of environmental assessment. Without standards, either clearly stated or implied, the notions of assessment and evaluation are meaningless. In emphasizing this difference between studies of environmental effects and studies of environmental assessment, it is not our intention to call into question the close relationship between studies of the two types. On the contrary, given the present state of environmental studies in general, studies designed to evaluate the quality of the environment depend upon the development of deeper knowledge about the potential impact of the environment on behavior.

a. *Strategy One: Ex post facto* study of built environments ("natural experiments"). Here the researcher examines a specific built environment and evaluates it according to (not always) stated criteria. The built environment can range from the smallest to the largest scale.

Since, in this strategy, the built environment is already at hand, this is one of the more accessible methods. However, in such a method the researcher must isolate the effect of the environment from the effect of other factors, including the characteristics of the users, changes in user attitudes over time, and current management policies. Finally, the method can be used with any degree of rigor, ranging from the impressionistic "evaluations" of the architectural magazines to the multidisciplinary techniques of the Building Performance Research Unit. (*108*)

One technique used to isolate the relevant variables is to make a comparative study of two or more built environments. Wilner's study of the effects of the environment on health, for example, compared roughly matched groups, one of which moved to new housing while the other remained behind. (*120*) Mogey compared two roughly similar neighborhoods, one of which was new and the other old. (*86*)

b. *Strategy Two: Ex post facto* study of persons suffering pathological effects. Here the researcher begins with a specific group with pathological characteristics—disabled persons, the mentally ill, school underachievers—and attempts to determine the degree to which their problems can be linked to specific past environmental experiences. A control group, matched in terms of social and demographic characteristics, is usually necessary for this kind of study. It is a standard technique in studies of delinquency and criminal behavior, for example, the method was used by the Gluecks. (*42*) Loring's study of housing and social disorganization is also, in a sense, an example; he began with a group who had found their way into social welfare records and then matched them to control families. (72)

c. *Strategy Three:* Secondary analysis of already completed inquiries. The logic of this strategy is similar to that of the first two, except that here the researcher tries to use data already collected for other purposes. Some of Schmitt's studies of the relation between density and social pathology, for example, are based on re-analyses of already collected demographic data. (100) Although this method has the obvious disadvantage that it may not be possible to break down data collected for other purposes into categories that are meaningful for environmental assessment, it is nevertheless a relatively inexpensive method, and there must be many untapped sources of data—poll data, military records, National Health Survey data—which could yield much information.

d. *Strategy Four:* Large-scale, census-type studies, perhaps with a "piggy-back" component. Here the researcher would survey a large sample of the American population, asking questions both about environmental experiences and behavioral or attitudinal variables hypothetically related to these experiences. The strategy assumes that, in a large survey, enough respondents would turn up with similar environmental experiences to make it possible to correlate the environmental variables with the effect variables. Although, apparently there is no large-scale survey of this kind, the Midtown Manhattan Study, which used this technique for a small section of a city, might suggest some of the advantages and disadvantages of the method. (106)

e. *Strategy Five:* Experimental or intervention studies. Here the researcher takes advantage of demonstration programs; his research effort is incorporated as a fundamental component of plans to design a new environment. It is not necessary that the environment be specifically built as an experiment, although this has been done. A new hospital in Rochester, Minnesota, for example, included three different types of nursing stations, with the explicit intention of comparing them. (112) The Ministry of Housing and Local Government in Great Britain, on the other hand, does not build projects as experiments. Instead, it evaluates each project that it constructs and feeds the results of each evaluation into the program for the next similar scheme. (46, 47)

Environmental simulation is another type of experimental study. Here, hypothetical environments are constructed to see how people will react; the Environmental Research Foundation in Topeka, Kansas, has been using this approach. (43) It has obvious limitations in that only certain aspects of built environments can be simulated for less cost than building the actual environment.

## Part II Examples of Environmental Assessment

## A. Research on Residential Safety

Safety research suffers from the same difficulty as environmental assessment research in general; namely, a failure to relate hazards to specific features of the built environment. It also is similar to much environmental research in the sense that often it is easier to define a criterion for assessment negatively than positively, to measure accidents rather than health or well-being. However, safety research benefits from the fact that safety is indisputably a valued social goal, so that the issue of whether it is a suitable criterion for evaluating the environment is hardly debatable. Also, safety, although it may have to be defined negatively, is a relatively objective condition of the human organism or group and, therefore, is easier to measure.

### 1. Behavioral Criteria in Safety Research:

In the literature of safety research, safety is usually construed to mean avoidance of, or protection from, accidental injuries or death. This definition excludes any direct considerations of mental health, or of safety of property. There are no established comprehensive measurements of safety in residential areas, but there are extensive records of accidental injuries and deaths. However, there are three principal difficulties with using accidental injury and death data to measure safety in any given population or area. Many injuries are not recorded, or the records are not easily accessible. Severity of injury is a major factor; less serious accidents occur more often than do severe ones. Lastly, accidents resulting in serious injury or death are such relatively rare occurrences among any population that large samples are needed for statistical reliability.

The relative ease of measuring "safety" is reflected in the availability of data. The two best sources of data are the publications of the National Health Survey (Public Health Service) and the National Safety Council. The National Health Survey is a continuing, detailed survey of the population in which a national sample of about 40,000 households, or about 130,000 people, is interviewed each year. The National Health Survey had been conducted intermittently prior to 1956, but since that date it has been continuous.

The concepts by which injuries, accidents, and data related to them are classified in the National Health Survey are important to us. The classifications and concepts may not be ideal from the viewpoint of our inquiry, but they are generally suitable and the data are, by far, the most reliable and readily available. This also pertains to the data published by the National Safety Council.

An *injury* is defined to be "a condition of the type that is classified according to the nature of injury code numbers (N800–N999) in the

International Classification of Diseases." *(115)* Injured persons are classified in terms of the activity restrictions or medical attendance which result from an injury. An *activity-restricting injury* is one which causes at least one day of restricted activity. A *bed-disabling injury is* one which results in at least one day of bed disability (in hospital or at home). A *work-loss injury* or a *school-loss injury* is one which results in at least one day of work or school loss. A *medically-attended injury* is one for which a physician was consulted in person or by telephone, for treatment or advice. *(115)* These categories can be taken to be measures of the severity of accidental injuries.

In the National Health Survey, types of accidents are classified according to the following concepts:

"(A)   Accidents in which specific factors were involved, but which may or may not have caused the injury. Included in this group are moving motor vehicles, uncontrolled fire, explosion, firearms, and non-motor vehicles, such as train or bicycle.

"(B)   Accidents where injury was caused directly by an agent, such as machinery in operation, a knife, scissors, nail, animal or insect, foreign body in eye or other orifices, or a poisonous substance swallowed by the person involved.

"(C)   Accidents described in terms of the events leading to the occurence of the injury, such as falling, bumping into a person or object, being struck by a moving object, handling or stepping on sharp or rough objects, being caught in, pinched or crushed, coming in contact with hot object or flame, lifting, twisting, or stumbling.

" (D) Accidents resulting in injury that could not be classified in groups (A), (B), or (C)." *(116)*

Although we have emphasized that safety is a relatively accessible measurement, like all aspects of human behavior it also includes a subjective or cultural component. For example, the annual accidental death rate varies widely from country to country. In 1964 the highest death rate occurred in Chile and the lowest in the Philippines, according to data compiled by the World Health Organization. *(102)* The United States was eighth highest in the world. A sample of the national death rates is shown here:

| Country | Annual accidental death rate per 100,000 population for 1964 |
| --- | --- |
| Chile | 74.9 |
| France | 69.5 |
| Switzerland | 62.3 |
| West Germany | 60.6 |
| United States | 55.7 |
| Italy | 44.4 |
| England | 39.3 |
| Philippines | 12.1 |

The wide variations in these data may result from differing attitudes to safety or from different degrees of coverage in the data collection system. This wide variation in national accidental death rates also can be seen in national traffic death rates.

Two studies were encountered in which the measures for assessing the safety of the environment were the subjective responses of those interviewed. We found no studies in which subjective judgments of safety were compared with objective measures of safety for the same population.

Hall and Bennett undertook an empirical assessment of the recommended diameters of handrails in staircases. Different sizes of handrails were used in the experiment, and each subject was asked which diameter he found most pleasing to use and which he felt would have given the most security in the event of a fall. (55)

Miller and Cook did a user study of residential developments in Britain in which pedestrian and vehicular traffic had been separated. Those interviewed were asked about their awareness of danger from traffic hazards near their homes. Respondents perceived more danger in cases where major roads had to be crossed on the way to local shops and schools. (83)

A final characteristic of safety research that should be noted is that much of it is directed to testing operating standards of safety which have been developed on the basis of social convention.

Cestrone observes that his report, *Status of Safety Standards* is, to his knowledge, the first publication of an evaluation of the art of safety-standards setting in the United States. Cestrone describes two ways in which standards came into being. In the first, "substantial agreement is reached by concerned interests according to the judgment of a duly appointed authority." These are *consensus standards*. The other kind of standard is the *propietary standard,* which is developed for an industrial or professional organization or association by a membership committee. The two nationally recognized organizations producing consensus standards are the United States of America Standards Institutes (USASI) and the National Fire Protection Association (NFPA). Examples of organizations producing standards of the second kind are the American Society of Mechanical Engineers, the American Petroleum Institute, and the Underwriters' Laboratories. (21)

While there are no comprehensive safety standards for residential environments, many parts of these environments are the subjects of codes in which safety is a predominant consideration. The fire protection provisions of national, state, and local building codes are examples, as are codes for electrical wiring and appliances. All such codes are explicit or implicit expressions of safety standards. This can be seen in the statement of purpose of such codes. For example:

Section 102 of the Uniform Building Code states:

"The purpose of this Code is to provide minimum standards to safeguard life or limb, health, property, and the public welfare by regulating and controlling the design, construction, quality of materials, use and occupancy, location and maintenance of all buildings and structures within the city and certain equipment specifically regulated herein." (64)

Section 100.2 of the National Building Code states:

"The purpose of this code is to provide for safety, health and public welfare through structural strength and stability, means of egress, adequate light and ventilation and protection to life and property from fire and hazards incident to the design, construction, alteration, removal or demolition of buildings and structures." (2)

## 2. Environmental Properties in Safety Research

### a. Classification Schemes

Although there are a number of ways in which the physical environment is classified in safety research, in terms of the classification scheme we are proposing most of the work deals with the first four properties on our list: spatial organization, circulation systems, communications systems, and ambient properties.

In the National Health Survey the environment is recorded in two ways, in terms of both the place in which an accident occurred and the location of the residence of the person surveyed. Place of accident is classified as follows: (117)

"Home—The place of accident is considered as 'home' if the injury occurred either inside or outside the home but within the property boundaries of the home . . .

"Inside the house—'Inside the house' includes any room, attic, cellar, porch, or steps leading to an entrance of the house. However, inside the garage is not considered as inside the house.

"Outside the house—'Outside the house' includes the yard, driveway, garage, patio, gardens, or walks. On a farm, only the premises adjacent to the house are considered as part of the home . . .

"Street or highway—'Street or highway' means the entire area between property lines of which any part is open for the use of the public as a matter of right or custom . . .

"Farm—'Farm' as a place of accident refers to accidents occurring in farm buildings or on cultivated land, but does not include accidents occurring in the farm home or premises . . .

"Industrial place—'Industrial place' is the term applied to accidents occurring in an industrial place or premises. Included are such places as factories, railway yards, warehouses, workshops, logging camps, shipping piers, oil fields, shipyards, sand and gravel pits, canneries, and auto repair garages. Construction projects, such as houses, buildings, bridges, and new roads, are included in this category . . .

"School—'School' as a place of accident includes all accidents occurring in school buildings or on the premises. This classification includes elementary schools, high schools, colleges, and trade and business schools.

"*Place of recreation*—'Place of recreation' is used to describe accidents occurring in places organized for sports and recreation other than recreational areas located at a place already defined as 'home,' 'industrial place,' or 'school.' Bowling alley, amusement park, football stadium, and dance hall, are examples of 'place of recreation' . . .

"*Other*—Accidents which cannot be classified in any of the above groups or for which the place is unknown are classified as 'other.' Included in the classification are such places as restaurants, churches, business and professional offices, and open or wooded country."

In classifying the location of residence of a person, the National Health Survey follows the U. S. Census. Location of residence is described by:

1. Urban or rural residence
2. Size of place
3. Farm or nonfarm residence
4. Standard metropolitan statistical areas
5. Region of the United States

The precise definitions of these terms are given in *Health Survey Procedure*. (*117*)

The National Safety Council and other bodies involved in safety classify the environments in which accidents occur as follows: (*102*)

1. Motor-vehicle accidents
2. Public non-motor-vehicle accidents
3. Work accidents
4. Home accidents

Presumably this classification reflects the concerns of two important professional groups in safety: those in highway safety and those in industrial safety.

Within home safety alone a number of classifications of the environment can be found, each reflecting the characteristics of some safety phenomenon. As pointed out in the next section, in considering accidental falls on stairs, important environmental variables are the height of a stair riser or the diameter of a handrail. On the other hand, if we are considering the influence of the environment on injuries caused by fires, the critical questions are whether or not stairs exist in a house, whether the staircase is enclosed, and whether there are alternative means of egress from the upper floors. This is an example of the question of *scale* in classifying the environment. Many other similar examples could be noted. At the scale of organization of the dwelling unit, we could speak of high-rise or low-rise buildings, or of single-family, multi-family, or apartment buildings.

b. *The Influences of Environmental Parameters in Accidental Injuries and Deaths*

In this discussion, we shall examine environmental characteristics which have been related, or have been presumed to be related, to the occurrence of accidents in residential areas.

Stairs are one of the principal places where falls occur in the home. The Institute for Safer Living found that falls on stairs account for 13% of home accidents, and are more likely than other home accidents to result in serious injury or death. (63) Considerable attention has been given to safety considerations in the design of stairs. (22, 63, 67) The design recommendations deal with size, shape, uniformity of steps, adequate handrails, friction surfaces on treads, adequate lighting, the provision of landings at least at every half-floor level, the relationship of doors to the top and bottom of a flight of stairs, and the maintenance of good surfaces or coverings on the steps.

Flights of steps, or changes in level of less than three steps, have been found to be dangerous, especially for elderly people and those with poor eyesight. (22) Jones calls single steps a "very great hazard." (67) He suggests that if steps cannot be grouped into sufficient numbers, ramps would be better, and that handrails should be provided at any change in level for elderly people.

The environmental characteristic of most concern in falls on the same level is the frictional property of the ground surface. Indoors, attention is given to nonskid floor waxes, nonskid mats or textured surfaces in tubs and showers, and nonskid backing on small rugs. (88) Outdoors, in addition to nonskid surfaces on sidewalks and paths, keeping them free of ice and wet leaves is important. (10) There appears to be an increasing interest in energy-absorbing floor surfaces, to reduce injuries when falls do occur. Surfaces of this kind are already in widespread use in children's playgrounds.

There are three principal design considerations for safety against fires: preventing their occurrence, confining the spread of fires, and providing means of escape. Environmental factors which contribute to the prevention of fires are fire-resistant chimneys, lightning conductors, and proper maintenance of electrical equipment, furnaces, and fuel tanks. Once fires begin they can be contained, or their rate of travel can be retarded, through the use of fire-resistant building materials. Tight-fitting doors are recommended between the garage or basement and the other parts of a house.

Also recommended are insulated ceilings, walls, and floors near cookers, heaters, and furnaces. The open stairwell is considered a major hazard because most fires begin between midnight and 6 a.m. in living rooms, kitchens, or basements and extremely hot and lethal gases can rise through the stairwell and into bedrooms. Because of this, safety authorities advise that stairs should be enclosed and at either end have doors which are kept closed at night. For the same reason it is recommended that doors from landings into bedrooms should never have louvers or be other than solid, and should always be kept closed while people are asleep. Fire doors which close automatically in the case of fire have been suggested for isolating the different floors of a house.

Hot gases from fires in houses often cut off the normal means of egress: landings, stairs, and hallways. There should be a second exit for every room, especially bedrooms and basement recreation rooms which can be isolated by gases in the stairways. It is recommended that every room and habitable basement have at least one door to the outside, or one window low enough and large enough to be used as an emergency exit; it is also recommended that each upper floor room have a balcony, deck, or roof outside it which can be used as a refuge. (58) Otherwise fixed fire escapes or rope ladders are advised.

Seventy-four percent of all cases where people walk into, or fall through, glass doors or large areas of fixed glass occur at home. (92) When these doors or panels are of normal household glass they have little break-resistance, and major injuries can be caused by the jagged pieces. In all such instances, safety glass is now recommended. Wooden guard rails or large opaque door handles can be used as cues that glass panels exist.

The provision of safe storage areas and cabinets, which children cannot easily get to or open, for medicines, poisonous materials, or dangerous objects such as guns, is another safety consideration. (67)

The Small Homes Council of the University of Illinois has published designs and design criteria for model safe homes. (97)

Private swimming pools are the site of many accidental drownings. The principal recommendations for safety are the provision of a fence at least four feet high, of a gate with a latch mechanism which cannot be operated by children, and of a warning system against unauthorized or unsupervised use by children.

In the design fields, considerable attention has been given to the protection of pedestrians in residential areas from the dangers of traffic. An example of this is an extensive article entitled "Building Traffic Safety Into Residential Developments," published in *Urban Land*. (16) The most important principles which have been used in this area are:

1. The diversions of any traffic away from residential areas other than that which originates or has a destination there.

2. The segregation of vehicular traffic and pedestrian rights-of-way, and the provision of grade-separated crossings.

3. The careful control of traffic, and attention to safe street design principles within residential areas.

171

### 3. Current Research Projects Dealing with Residential Safety

Three federal research projects in environmental assessment, all dealing in part with residential safety, were found to be currently in progress. Two are sponsored by the Department of Housing and Urban Development and one by the Department of the Army. At present, no findings have been published for any of these undertakings.

The two HUD projects are part of Operation Breakthrough, the urban housing project. The first one is being conducted by Brown Engineering, Huntsville, Alabama, under an eighteen-month contract which began in 1969. Operation Breakthrough hoped to publish the results of this research by the middle of 1971. The research effort is limited to the residential structure and to specific locations within the dwellings. Generally, single-family buildings are being studied. There are three phases to the research contract. First, the major causes of home accidents, excluding fire, were investigated (kinds, numbers, severities of injuries, deaths, etc.) The second phase, which is to lead to recommendations for performance and prescriptive specifications for home safety, includes a study of the state of the art in the construction industry, an investigation of the equipment and design features of homes, and interviews with product manufacturers. In the third phase, which is getting under way presently, Brown Engineering will conduct an experimental study to test different aspects of safety. The results of these experiments will be incorporated in single-family and multi-family dwellings built by Operation Breakthrough.

Operation Breakthrough's second research project is being conducted jointly with the National Bureau of Standards. In this work, design criteria for Operation Breakthrough residential prototypes are being developed, using information drawn from a survey of existing practice. Safety is one of the factors being considered. (114)

The Department of the Army, through its Construction Engineering Research Laboratory, has begun a study of the quality of residential and working environments in military bases and in the surrounding areas. Safety is one consideration in this study, which aims broadly to find research methods that will enable designers to produce facilities which will be efficient and responsive to the individual's environmental requirements. The project is presently at the level of a review of the literature in environmental assessment.

### 4. Residential Safety Design Studies

Some examples of the research strategies discussed in Part I, C, 3 appear in residential safety studies. We did not find any studies exemplifying the first strategy where specific built environments are examined and evaluated against stated criteria. However, a common example of such a strategy used in practice is the inspection of buildings to see that they comply with local government codes.

Miller and Esmay's study of the nature and causes of stairways falls is an example of an *ex post facto* study of persons suffering pathological effects. *(84)* One hundred and one adults who had fallen on stairs were interviewed; both direct causes and contributing factors were sought. In each case the staircase was examined in detail, and correlations were sought between environmental factors and the incidence of falls.

Gowings also used this approach in *The Warren County Stair Design Survey.* *(45)* He further compared his findings about stairs with standards set forth in *Hazard-Free Houses For All,* by the Small Homes Council of the University of Illinois. *(62)*

To our knowledge, no large-scale, census-type studies of any aspect of residential safety, from an environmental assessment viewpoint, have been done. The National Health Survey offers a model for such studies in that it does record accidental injuries and the places in which they occur. An environmentally-oriented study of this kind would need much finer and more comprehensive data about the architectural environment.

Hall and Bennett undertook an experimental study of people's subjective reactions to handrail diameters. The continuous handrail in use on a flight of stairs was removed, and replaced by a handrail divided into four sections, each a different diameter. *(55)*

## B. The Example of Radburn

### 1. An Introduction to Radburn

The word "Radburn" represents to planners and designers a collection of concepts about neighborhood and community site planning. It includes the use of the super-block, cluster housing, separation of vehicular and pedestrian traffic, and common open space often linked to a walkway system. Many of these ideas are coming into vogue in the United States now, as the new zoning device of the planned unit development is gaining acceptance. These design ideas were introduced more than forty years ago with the planning of a new community in New Jersey, named Radburn.

The Radburn idea has long since transcended what was actually built at Radburn. But, like many ideas which gain currency, these concepts have never fully been studied. In fact, Radburn itself, for all the images it conjures up in architects' minds, has never been comprehensively evaluated. Because of the fame of the plan, and the impact it has had upon site planning, the community of Radburn would be an excellent candidate for environmental assessment.

In this section of the report, using the classification system developed in Part I,C, an approach to such an assessment is investigated. Many potential sources of data have been reviewed, and the result has provided some environmental measures which might be correlated with behavioral measures. Inevitably, in the discussion, some evaluation of Radburn is offered, and a number of research and theoretical questions raised.

The building of Radburn was undertaken in 1929 by a limited-dividend corporation in New York called the City Housing Corporation. The Corporation was comprised of men who wanted to demonstrate in the United States the benefits, practicality, and profitability of building better housing and communities than was the current practice. Any profit in excess of a limited return on investment was to be used for further development. After completing a successful apartment complex in New York City, the Corporation, with Henry Wright and Clarence Stein as planners, set out to build a new community to be patterned after the Garden Cities in England. (11)

Radburn was intended to be a community of 25,000 people, grouped in three neighborhoods of 7,500 to 10,000, each one-half mile in radius, centering on an elementary school and with its own shopping and community facilities. The Corporation acquired about two square miles of land in the Borough of Fair Lawn, New Jersey. Fair Lawn was a rural community, and Radburn, while having its own home owners' association, was to be part of the borough. The community is about 16 miles from the borough of Manhattan, adjacent to the Erie Railway. (11, 107)

The community was to be a complete departure from traditional speculative building. It was designed for families of moderate income, with the hope of meeting some of the problems confronting them. It was planned for the motor age, accepted the automobile, but provided for separate vehicular and pedestrian access. The two principal features of the Radburn plan were an innovative physical plan for the site, and an idea for community organizations with facilities allowing a wide variety of activities for the residents. To insure both, a protective legal compact, a Declaration of Restrictions was drawn up in 1929. (59)

Every owner of property at Radburn subscribes to the Declaration which sets forth the design controls, method of operation, government, and tax assessment to be used for the management and organization of Radburn. In fact, the Declaration, which imposes another level of government (of sorts) upon Radburn residents, has served as a model for home owners associations across the United States. The Radburn Association, run by a Board of Trustees, administers the Declaration. (94)

The major physical features of Radburn consisted of five design elements intended 1) to promote maximum use of land, light and air; 2) to provide safety from motor vehicles; and 3) to facilitate communication and friendship. (11) First, the housing was arranged in super-blocks, surrounded but not crossed by streets; houses in the super-block were serviced by culs-de-sac. Second, the circulation system was specialized,

174

with major roads, minor roads, service culs-de-sac, and pedestrian and bike paths. Third, primarily for safety, there was complete separation of pedestrian and automotive traffic, with pedestrian underpasses to enable crossing from one super-block to another. Fourth, the houses were turned around, with the kitchens facing the service court and the living rooms facing the front walks. Finally, within each super-block a park was built to serve as a spine to the development. (107)

The construction of Radburn was never completed. Two neighborhoods were begun, one on either side of Fair Lawn Avenue, and homes built on three super-blocks. The stock market crashed, the depression came, construction slowed and halted and, eventually, the City Housing Corporation went bankrupt. After 1934, when construction halted, a few homes were gradually added to Radburn. However, with the suburban sprawl following World War II, the remainder of Fair Lawn was developed in typical suburban patterns. Some of the houses that now comprise Radburn were not built in accordance with the plan. Radburn lost the opportunity to become a community. What remains is only a beginning of what was intended. Physically, it is divided by two blocks and a major thoroughfare. (13)

Today, the visitor to Radburn finds it difficult to locate, surrounded as it is by the more conventional site planning of the remainder of Fair Lawn. It is still controlled by the Declaration of Restrictions and managed by trustees and the Association. Physically, some elements of the site plan still exists. Chart A (pp. 178–181) gives some detailed description of Radburn following the classification used in Part I, C, 1. A summary description of the existing Radburn settlements is offered below.

Radburn consists of approximately 100 acres of land and 21 acres of park divided among three separate parks. There are about 550 attached and detached houses; there is also an apartment complex, Abbott Court, with 92 apartments. There are two swimming pools, one major playground, and an elementary school located within the inner-park system. Tennis courts, an archery field, a ball field, a church as well as the combination community center, library and gymnasium (Grange Hall) are located on nearby property. A small shopping center built with the original development, is adjacent to the housing.

The housing consists of a variety of types: detached housing, semi-detached duplex housing, and rows of townhouses with three or more structures built together. Some townhouses have two families (one over the other) and some are apartment units. Most of the houses have three bedrooms; some are two-bedroom houses. In all, including Abbott Court, there are about 750 households in Radburn; it has a population of about 2,400, perhaps one-tenth of what was intended.

175

## 2. Evaluating Radburn

Although a great deal has been written about Radburn, most of it is opinion. *(12, 15)* Two studies with some objectivity have been made, but neither has correlated any findings with specific physical features of the plan. One was completed in 1934, when about 340 families comprised Radburn. Basically a study of community participation, it found the population to be highly educated, generally well-employed, and with 97 per cent of the families participating in the community and its activities. *(59)* In the other study, Radburn was looked at together with nine other communities to determine the effects of a planned community upon the attitudes and activities of its residents. Here, the physical factors were not specifically considered, and the entire study was based on interviews with selected families. *(69)*

In undertaking any study of Radburn, two governmental organizations must be kept in mind: 1) the Borough of Fair Lawn and 2) the Radburn Association. Radburn is a part of Fair Lawn, now a suburban jurisdiction almost fully developed, with a population of about 40,000. It is located within Bergen County, contains about 3,500 acres, and has largely a dormitory population. It could provide a control group for any study of Radburn residents.

The Radburn Association is indispensable to the physical plan, for without it many of the planned facilities could not be maintained and operated. The Association maintains the parks, the common paths, the pools, and recreation fields. In the summer it sponsors a complete recreation program for the children. Throughout the year it operates the Grange, collects the assessments (ranging from $100 to $270 per household), and has the power to maintain unkept yards or houses and charge the negligent owners. In earlier days, before Fair Lawn had complete municipal services, the Association had its own sewerage disposal plant, collected garbage, operated street lighting, and policed the community. It once had a well-baby clinic, nursery and day-care center. *(11)* For partial evaluation, plan and photos, see *(123)* .

### a. *The Physical Variables*

The most innovative physical feature of Radburn is the site plan. The houses were conventional for their day, the novel features were their siting an small lots, with rear service courts for autos, and front pedestrian walks. Clarence Stein, one of the planners, states that the tight planning to economize on land and floor area has had its drawbacks. *(107)* The houses are relatively small, and there is some technical obsolescence. The kitchens are too small to confortably admit modern appliances. The garages no longer can serve the typical family car. The service courts are too narrow to easily allow large service and delivery trucks, and snowplows operate with great difficulty on culs-de-sac. Parking appears to be inadequate, and the closeness of the houses

176

reduces privacy. The parks and walkways have been maintained, but in contrast to pictures of the earlier days at Radburn, almost every house now has a fence or hedge around its small yard.

The remainder of Fair Lawn was subdivided and built without following the Radburn example. House lots were substantially larger; zoning did not permit the easy mixture of housing types. The super-block is not used.

The physical measures necessary for an assessment study of Radburn can be secured from plans and blue prints, public and private records, and observation. A great many possible measures are listed in Chart A. Sources of data about the Radburn houses and the site plan do exist. Plans filed with the Association can be found in the Grange and some have been published. (*107*) The building inspection departments of the municipal government have building plans on file, and subdivision plans are filed with zoning officials. However, these municipal functions did not exist at the time Radburn was built. Plan data will supply information on floor area, coverage, circulation, area of open space and other categories included under spatial organization, circulation systems, amenities, and architectonic properties.

Utility companies have records of hook-ups and usage that supply information about communication and ambient properties at the building scale. Public works departments, which operate and build sewerage systems, water systems, and roads, would be sources for data about ambient and circulation properties at the community level. Only observation and careful notation could quantify visual properties, symbolic properties, and some architectonic ones. However, our preliminary survey indicates that the Radburn maintenance crews are able to identify locations of vandalism, negligence, and littering.

b. *Behavioral Characteristics*

In many respects, perhaps because there has been more research conducted at this level, behavioral data sources seem better defined. Specific indices are listed in chart B and are discussed below.

With regard to the first behavioral classification, described in Part I,C, survival and physical welfare, a major design feature in Radburn was the separation of pedestrian and vehicular traffic. Stein and other planners have assumed that a significant reduction in such accidents followed from this design characteristic. However, the small size of Radburn's population (2,400) and the very low rate of occurrence of pedestrian accidents in general make it difficult to verify this assumption. At the national level, one pedestrial death could be expected among this size population every ten years. To improve the chances of statistical reliability long-term records are required, from Radburn's incorporation in 1929 if possible. In this instance, the police department in the Borough of Fair Lawn has kept records from the early 1930's to date on all reported pedestrian accidents. The data include

**Radburn: Description of the Built-Environment and Data Sources**

|  | SPATIAL ORGANIZA-TION | CIRCULA-TION SYSTEM | COMMUNI-CATION SYSTEMS | AMBIENT PROPERTIES |
|---|---|---|---|---|
| BUILDING: ..........<br><br>Housing | Small houses, primarily 3 bedrooms, two stories, lightly-planned kitchens<br>Source: building plans | Entrances—2 stairs absence of halls small garages small yards<br>Source: floor plans and plot plans | No television phones absence of picture windows fences<br>Source: survey | Small windows addition of air condi-tioning heating and power use screens humidifiers<br>Source: survey and utility company |
| SITE PLAN: ..........<br><br>Clusters and super-block | Small lots, houses close super-block park spine cluster housing several courts and walkways<br>Source: site plan | Narrow-culs-de-sac front side-walks separation of traffic pedestrian inner-blocks inadequate parking<br>Source: site plan | Many houses with fences, primarily chain-link absence of interior signs walkways | Shade trees summer houses minimum utility layout sound level<br>Source: observation |
| NEIGHBORHOOD:<br><br>Radburn Association | 550 separate lots 92 apart-ments 750 families, 2400 people 100 acres 21 acres park 3 super-blocks 2 divided neighbor-hoods | Underpass for pedestrians Radburn separated into two parts by strip of 2 blocks and Fair Lawn specialized roads | Absence of signs Bulletin boards Association paper | Utility lines difficult servicing on narrow roads original Radburn services<br>Source: public works |

Radburn: Description of the Built-Environment and Data Sources

| VISUAL PROPERTIES | AMENITIES | SYMBOLIC PROPERTIES | ARCHECTONIC PROPERTIES |
|---|---|---|---|
| High level of maintenance well cared for yards, planting lack of vandalism no deterioration on 40-year-old houses | Appliances conversion of garages, basements architectural changes porches | Split-rail fences plants and flowering shrubs lawn furnitures chain-link fences lawn care | Conventional design of houses pseudo-Tudor and New England Brick, white clapboard shingles |
| Park maintenance walk and paving condition landscaping Source: observation | Sandboxes playgrounds tot lots, sandboxes 3 parks summerhouses benches | Private internal walkways | Design'recognition of super-block and Radburn Idea |
| Writing on underpass Radburn facilities maintenance landscaping Source: observation | 2 pools tennis and archery courts baseball field Grange Hall shopping center church | Church in Radburn | Reputation of Radburn widely published |

(Continued next page)

Radburn: Description of the Built-Environment and Data Sources

|  | SPATIAL ORGANIZA-TION | CIRCULA-TION SYSTEM | COMMUNI-CATION SYSTEMS | AMBIENT PROPERTIES |
|---|---|---|---|---|
| LOCAL COMMUNITY: ........ <br><br> Fair Lawn, New Jersey | 3500 acres 40,000 people largely dormitory suburb fully developed Source: land use map | Typical suburban street plan access via express-ways served by Erie com-mutor railroad suburban bus system | Street signs traffic lights commercial signs | Public utilities public service corporation pollution |

REGION: ...............The general region has little relevance to Fair Lawn ex-
New York       cept as the transportation and employment opportunities
               allow it to function as a subsidiary unit of the Metro-
               politan area

MACRO-REGION: ..Data about the macro-region are largely irrelevant to an
N.E.           evaluation of Radburn
Seaboard

date and time of accident, location, weather, number of pedestrians injured, home address, sex, and injury of victims. From these sources, accident data within Radburn or to Radburn residents can be gathered.

With regard to other aspects of health and accident measurement, data are not so readily available, and require the collection of information through a special survey. Hospital admission and emergency accident records do seem to be collected by the regional hospitals which serve the Radburn population. However, the hospitals regard these records as confidential information, and apparently are unwilling to breach this confidence for studies of the kind that interest the researcher on environmental assessment. The New Jersey State Health Department does not keep records by small areas; this is standard practice throughout the United States. In general, mortality and disease statistics are not tabulated in terms of areas as small as Radburn. Furthermore, even when these data are available by municipal units and other political jurisdictions or health reporting districts, they usually fail to record the specific environmental conditions under which the accident took place.

Other possible records about physical welfare have to do with fire

**Radburn: Description of the Built-Environment and Data Sources**

| VISUAL PROPERTIES | AMENITIES | SYMBOLIC PROPERTIES | ARCHECTONIC PROPERTIES |
|---|---|---|---|
| Appearance of upper-middle-class suburban community limited deterioration Source: observation | Community facilities shopping recreation one swimming pool | Suburban neighborhoods | General, undistinguished conventional Post War II |

hazards and the need for policing. The number of fires and the number of crimes and arrests are potential measures of the safety of an area, defining safety not in terms of accidental injury but rather in terms of property protection, freedom from vandalism and personal attack. Other possible indicants are fire insurance and home property insurance rates. Such data are more easily obtainable than much of the information relating to health and accidents, and presumably could be used as a basis for environmental assessment.

With regard to satisfaction and attitude, the use of survey research to investigate subjective responses of individuals and families, such as was done in the University of Michigan study, (69) is a common method but requires the special collection of data. More objective measures of satisfaction can be secured through investigation of the local real estate market. The resale prices of homes, the waiting lists for apartments, the vacancy and turnover rates of housing units, and the length of residence of households can all be used as measures of satisfaction and attitude toward Radburn. However, since such measures are also dependent on the general state of supply and demand in the housing market, they must be interpreted with care.

**Radburn: Data and Measurements of Behavioral Criteria**

|  | Survival and physical welfare | Satisfaction and attitude | Activity and performance |
|---|---|---|---|
| Individuals ............. by age groups | Safety and accident records crime records health and mortality | Subjective responses | Time budgets school records employment records juvenile records |
| Family ..................... by type | Medical expenditures absentee records health statistics | Subjective responses turnover, length of residence | Income budgets family cohesion divorce rates |
| Performance unit .... housing types, neighborhoods | Fire and insurance rates fire occurrence break and entry cases | Low vacancy rates market demand assessment records delinquent taxes | Maintenance costs operating costs friendship patterns |
| Institution ............... Radburn Association | Could have been eliminated in 1960 Association rules Declaration changes | Length of existence long-term residents architectural changes vandalism minutes of meetings | Participation in activities census data voting statistics extent of activities social cohesion |
| Community .............. Fair Lawn | Safety records, accidents police and fire records | Resentment of Radburn | Public services community activities |
| National group ........Relevant for comparison with national or regional norms upper-middle class | | | |

The manager of Abbott Court reports there is no vacancy and little turnover in his apartments; however, he also reports that his are the lowest rents in Fair Lawn, which has a shortage of apartments. The manager of the Radburn Association said that about 60 of the original Radburn inhabitants were still in the community. Although 28 property transfers occurred last year, this represented only 8 new families; the rest were intra-Radburn switches. Reported sales prices are high, sometimes $60,000 to $75,000 for a larger single-family detached house facing "B" Park. According to the Borough assessor, there is no way to make comparisons on the sales of houses in Radburn with those in Fair Lawn, for they are smaller units with smaller lots than houses in Fair Lawn. In general, demand for property in Radburn is reported to be strong.

The assessor has a file on every property in Fair Lawn that indicates age of structure, deed transfers, sales, assessment over time and other information relative to sustained value. A comparison of Radburn properties with a selected control group in other sections of Fair Lawn built in the same era would permit analysis of turnover, length of residence, resale price, and assessment changes over time.

The Association has some records that are useful. There are Minutes of Association meetings which would give a report of the concerns of the community over time. There are also records of architectural changes to the properties, since these had to be approved by the Association. Unfortunately, there are no historical records of membership in the Association.

With regard to the investigation of the behavioral area of performance and activity, the Association activities and the summer recreation program become very relevant. Whether the Radburn residents participate in more activities or sports than others of similar characteristics is unknown. The budget for the Radburn Association is roughly similar to the Recreation budget for the Borough of Fair Lawn. The Borough claims that one out of every two residents participates in its recreation program. How this might compare with the activity of Radburn residents has not been studied although obviously it could be. In assessing the quality of Radburn it would be of particular interest to secure time budgets and income budgets to see if the benefits of Radburn are discernible in how people spend their time or money, compared to a control population. These data are not available, and would have to generated.

Other differences in performance and activity levels, for the most part, would have to be studied through the collection of original data. Topics that might be meaningful in assessing Radburn include friendships and social contacts related to the physical design of the community and transportation patterns and methods of movement. There is some evidence that residents of planned communities use automobiles less often. (69) Behavioral data that might be available on a small area basis which would identify Radburn include census data, voting data, and school records. Juvenile records, which might indicate the behavior of youths, are usually confidential but might be secured. Other data which would be useful are difficult to assemble: employment records, divorce records, and other indicators of performance are not assembled by residence of the indivdual.

# Part III Conclusions, Appendix, and Bibliography

## A. Conclusions

There has been a great surge of interest recently in this country and throughout the world in the problem of environmental quality. This new concern is expressed in the statement of a leading American ecologist that our physical environment existed before man was created and the challenge is how to enable man to adapt to this environment and, at the same time, achieve the human goals which have been generated through five millennia of civilization. The search for standards and criteria in terms of which to evaluate the quality of the environment is the principal response of the scientific community to this new concern.

The research inquiry reported in this document was undertaken in an effort to pinpoint some of the key issues which arise in one area of environmental quality research, namely, the assessment of the quality of the built environment in terms of criteria related to the behavioral and social dimensions of human activity. Although presumably among the most important set of criteria according to which the built environment should be assessed, behavioral dimensions have been less researched than dimensions dealing with economic cost, materials technology, and building engineering. We knew this before we undertook our project and, for this reason, we put our emphasis on understanding the institutional, conceptual, and methodological obstacles to efficient and competent assessment studies rather than on trying to conduct specific empirical studies as such. However, we also explored the feasibility of many of the ideas which emerged by considering them in the context of a specific residential environment, the planned settlement of Radburn, New Jersey.

The conclusions that have emerged from our inquiry can be stated as follows:

1. Environmental assessment research is a form of applied social science. As an applied social science it depends upon the development of fundamental knowledge about the way in which the built environment interacts with other environmental variables to influence behavioral and social organization.

2. There is no logical reason why this fundamental knowledge cannot be developed. The kinds of conceptual and methodological problems that arise are similar to those which the social and biological science disciplines have dealt with successfully in the past.

3. It will require a good deal of institutional experimentation to discover the most efficient system for organizing the responsibility for environmental assessment. Several different design professions have an interest in the area and one group is obviously best suited to take in this responsibility.

4. Although assessment research may properly be located within a professional setting because of its nature as an applied discipline or social technology, the development of the knowledge base for assessment will depend upon cooperation among several scientific disciplines. We have tried to indicate the potential for this development by describing what is already understood about the effects of the built environment due to efforts of various social and biological science disciplines.

5. An important requirement for the development of basic knowledge in the field, and also for the conduct of assessment studies, is the formulation of a set of concepts for describing the characteristics of built environments objectively. We have set forth an example of such a scheme and have indicated how it might be applied to the description of a residential environment.

6. A second important requirement for the advancement of assessment research is to establish a list of behavioral criteria which, at the same time, relates to critical elements of human response and offer a fair chance of being translated into empirical measures. We have offered the rudiments of such a list, and by considering these criteria in the context of Radburn have tried to indicate the kinds of data sources which either are available or must be assembled for measuring them.

7. A third requirement is to decide on research designs which provide opportunities either for studying behavioral effects of the environment or for assessing environmental quality. A number of alternative designs or strategies have been described, some of which point to the need for original studies; others emphasize the value of utilizing data collected previously for purposes other than environmental assessment.

8. Epidemiological research on residential safety serves as a model to support our conviction that the established tradition of scientific research is appropriate for handling the problems that arise in the study of environmental effects and in the conduct of assessment research. At the same time, the more advanced state of research in this area also suggests many problems that are likely to be encountered as environmental research moves beyond an interest in medical and biological variables. Two of these problems which are particularly onerous are (1) the need to find ways of overcoming the incompleteness of statistical data already being collected by public agencies that potentially could be useful for assessment research, and (2) the need to begin tabulating official records in terms of small geographical and spatial units.

9. Our review of the literature on residential safety, as well as our preliminary forays in applying our conceptual and methodological model to Radburn, suggest that progress in the area of environmental research will depend very heavily on the capacity of the scientific community to launch several large-scale empirical studies for the purpose of collecting original data on built environments. We cannot rely on

existing data resources, and despite their already-demonstrated concern and achievement, we will have to find new ways of organizing the intellectual and institutional resources of the design professions and the social and biological science disciplines.

## B. Appendix

### 1. *Periodicals*

A growing number of journals are partially or primarily concerned with the relationship of man and his built environment. We have not included single special issues of other journals.

*DMG News letter,* publication of the Design Methods Group established in 1966. Compilation of news, abstracts and reviews of interest to architects, planner and regional scientists concerned with scientific research in design methodology. Sponsored by the College of Environmental Design, University of California, Berkeley, and the School of Architecture, Washington University, St. Louis. Ten issues yearly, Sage Publications, Inc., Beverly Hills, California.

*Design and Environment,* commercial journal, for translating findings of environmental sciences for use of designers. Designed for interprofessional use with articles about studies, federal funding, on-going research and seminars. For architects, engineers, planners, designers and industry concerned with this area. Begun 1970, quarterly, RC Publications, Inc., New York City.

*Environment and Behavior,* scholarly interdisciplinary journal, concerned with study, design and control of the environment and its interaction with human behavioral system. Reports rigorous experimental and theoretical work relating physical environment to human behavior at all levels. For social scientists and designers. Begun 1969, quarterly, Sage Publications, Inc., Beverly Hills, California.

*Environment and Planning,* British journal, an international journal to accelerate advances in environmental science, particularly locational, transportation and structural aspects of human activities in cities and regions. Begun 1969, quarterly, Pion Limited, London, England.

*Journal of Environmental Systems,* professional journal for reporting papers by those concerned with analysis, design and management of environment. Large-scale environmental systems considered. Primarily concerned with problems of engineering, systems analysis, operation research, computer and information systems, management economics, pollution control. New publication, quarterly, Baywood Publishing Company, Wantagh, New York.

*Man-Environment Systems,* academic journal reporting, in loose-leaf access form, on-going research, news, and abstracts of reports

186

concerned with man and his social and physical environment. Concerned with interface between research in behavioral and social science and design and management of physical environment. Merged from *Man and his Environment* and *Architectural Psychology,* as a communication forum. Begun 1969, bi-monthly, Pennsylvania State University, University Park, Pennsylvania.

*Milieu,* mimeographed newsletter of Environmental Research Foundation, reporting research theory and findings of interest to design and behavioral disciplines. Begun 1965, three issues yearly, Environmental Research Foundation, Topeka, Kansas.

## 2. *Established Research Centers*

Below are listed the more established applied research centers, primarily affiliated with architectural and design programs which have established some reputation in the field of man-environment relations.

a. U.S. Universities

University of California, Berkeley, College of Environmental Design

The Center for Planning and Development Research, part of the Institute for Urban and Regional Development which is the research arm of the College, has since 1962, conducted studies related to city and regional planning, social and technical processes. In part, it attempts to develop new techniques for urban problems. Several recent studies have been concerned with the social and attitudinal implications of residential developments.

Under a grant from the National Science Foundation, a research training unit will be established within the Department of Architecture to develop methods and teach architectural students how to conduct research on behavioral responses to architecture.

Carnegie-Mellon University, Institute of Physical Planning

Sponsored by the School of Urban and Public Affairs and the Department of Architecture. To conduct research and graduate education on effects of the physical environment on people, land use, housing, and crime.

City University of New York, Environmental Psychology Program

A research and graduate program concerned with psychology and environmental impact. Many studies have involved patients in psychiatric hospitals and perception of environments, both closely related to traditional psychological subject areas, but concentrating on environmental factors.

Cornell University, Division of Urban Studies, Center for Urban

Development Research

An interdisciplinary research center, formerly the Center for Housing and Environmental Studies, which has conducted architectural, planning and behavioral research relating to urban life.

University of Michigan, College of Architecture and Design, Architectural Research Laboratory

Has conducted building evaluations (largely materials and structures) and currently is developing prototype designs for educational facilities, judicial facilities, and criteria for these facilities, related to behavioral and community needs.

New York University, Institute of Planning and Housing

Research institute closely allied to legal and public administration aspects of urban environment. Work involves designing residential environments to reduce anti-social behavior; law enforcement; public housing project protection; concern with vandalism; and development of housing codes.

University of Oregon, School of Architecture and Allied Arts, Center for Environmental Research

Research center doing field projection design and setting for behavior as well as use of buildings through time.

Pennsylvania State University, College of Human Development, Division of Man-Environment Relations

One of stronger programs developing around environmental behavior studies, research and design. Directly related to design professions of architecture and planning and bringing social and behavioral considerations to the professionals' attention. Founded in 1968.

University of Southern California, Graduate Program of Urban and Regional Planning

A major research effort funded by the U. S. Public Health Service is underway here to develop criteria and concepts for the residential neighborhood. Research by planners, social scientists and medical personnel will assess preferences and the social and psychological well-being within residential environments. Designed to develop a replacement for *Planning the Neighborhood,* 1948 guide prepared by the American Public Health Association's Committee on the Hygiene of Housing.

University of Utah, Department of Architectural Psychology

Collaboration between departments of architecture and psychology to develop programs for graduate architectural students.

University of Wisconsin, Environmental Design Center
Doing interdisciplinary research evaluating information from behavioral and natural sciences which can be related to human behavior and environmental variables and applied with design disciplines. Areas included are: vision, body mechanics, and form perception.

b. British Universities

University of Cambridge, School of Architecture, Land Use and Built Form Studies
Research to determine interrelationships between building and land use, including traffic networks. Studies have included environmental evaluation of buildings and spatial distribution of built form.
University of Strathclyde, School of Architecture, Building Performance Research Unit
Unit developing techniques by which designers can appraise the quality of their work and designs. Measures of performance include architectural, operational, psychological, physical, and economic consequences of space decisions. Building appraisal includes user subjective and objective responses.

c. Other Groups

Environmental Research Foundation, Topeka, Kansas
Established as nonprofit center in 1965 to conduct research in area of man's behavior and architectural environment. Promotes communication and coordination between design professions and social and medical sciences. Work has included mental health evaluations in psychiatric facilities, housing environment and behavior, and human movement and architecture.
Ministry of Technology, Building Research Station, United Kingdom
Since 1921, Station has conducted a number of studies on properties of buildings and their structures. Began performance studies of buildings in 1956; building as a functioning entity. Primarily concerned with materials, maintenance and structure. Minimum user evaluation.
National Bureau of Standards, Building Research Division, United States
Federal agency for testing materials and structures. Playing a major role in developing criteria for assessing Operation Breakthrough prototypes. Has not, as yet, gotten into user experiments, or social evaluation of buildings.

# Bibliography

1. American Institute of Architects. THE ARCHITECT'S HANDBOOK FOR PROFESSIONAL PRACTICE. Washington: The Institute, 1964.
2. American Insurance Association. NATIONAL BUILDING CODE. New York: The Association, 1967.
3. American National Standards Institute. AMERICAN NATIONAL STANDARDS INSTITUTE CATALOG. New York: The Institute, 1971.
4. American Public Health Association, Committee on the Hygiene of Housing. PLANNING THE NEIGHBORHOOD. Chicago: Public Administration Service, 1960.
5. American Society for Testing and Materials. ASTM STANDARDS IN BUILDING CODES: SPECIFICATIONS, METHODS OF TEST, DEFINITIONS. Philadelphia: The Society, 1965.
6. Appleyard, Donald, Kevin Lynch and John R. Myer. THE VIEW FROM THE ROAD. Cambridge: M.I.T. Press, 1964.
7. *The Architects' Journal.* London: The Architectural Press, Ltd.
8. Ardrey, Robert. THE TERRITORIAL IMPERATIVE: A PERSONAL INQUIRY INTO THE ANIMAL ORIGINS OF PROPERTY AND NATIONS. New York: Atheneum, 1966.
9. Arnheim, Rudolf. ART AND VISUAL PERCEPTION: A PSYCHOLOGY OF THE CREATIVE EYE. Berkeley: University of California Press, 1954.
10. Associaiton of Casualty and Surety Companies. AND WE ALL FALL DOWN. New York: The Association, 1964. (Pamphlet).
11. Augur, Tracy B. "Radburn: The Challenge of a New Town," *Michigan Municipal Review,* February 1931, pp. 19–22; March 1931, pp. 39–41.
12. Bailey, Anthony, "Fair Lawn, New Jersey Profile: Through the Great City," *New Yorker,* Vol. 43, July 29, 1967, pp. 50+.
13. ——, "Radburn Revisited," *New York Herald Tribune,* September 27, 1964, pp. 9–12.
14. Barker, Roger G. ECOLOGICAL PSYCHOLOGY. Stanford: Stanford University Press, 1968.
15. "Brave New Towns that Aged Awkwardly, Radburn, New Jersey, and Greenbelt, Maryland," *Business Week,* January 9, 1971, pp. 22+.
16. "Building Traffic Safety into Residential Developments: A New Edition," *Urban Land,* Vol. 20:7, July–August 1961, pp. 1–14.
17. California, University of, University Residential Building System. *CONTRACT DOCUMENTS AND PERFORMANCE SPECIFICATIONS.* URBS publication 1. Berkeley: University of California, 1967.
18. Canter, David. "An Intergroup Comparison of Connotative Dimensions in Architecture," *Environment and Behavior,* Vol. 1:1, June 1969, pp. 37–48.
19. Caplow, Theodore, Sheldon Stryker and Samuel E. Wallace. THE URBAN AMBIENCE: A STUDY OF SAN JUAN, PUERTO RICO. Totawa Totowa, N.J.: Bedminster Press, 1964.
20. Caplow, Theodore. "Urban Structure in France," *American Sociological Review,* Vol. 17, October 1952, pp. 544–549. Reprinted in George A. Theodorson, editor, STUDIES IN HUMAN ECOLOGY. Evanston: Row, Peterson and Company, 1961, pp. 384–390.
21. Cestrone, Patrick F. STATUS OF SAFETY STANDARDS. Washington: Bureau of Safety Standards, U.S. Department of Labor, 1968.
22. Clifton, Carol. "Stairs Can Be Your Downfall," *Family Safety,* Fall 1970, pp. 4–6.
23. Coleman, James Samuel. COMMUNITY CONFLICT. Glencoe: Free Press, 1957.
24. Comprehensive health planning is becoming a part of regional planning activities.

25. Dahir, James. THE NEIGHBORHOOD UNIT PLAN. New York: Russell Sage Foundation, 1947.
26. Deasy and Bolling, Architects A.I.A. ACTION, OBJECTIVES AND CONCERNS. HUMAN PARAMETERS FOR ARCHITECTURAL DESIGN. A PLANNING STUDY. Los Angeles: California State College.
27. Deutsch, Morton and Mary E. Collins. INTERRACIAL HOUSING: A PSYCHO-LOGICAL EVALUATION OF A SOCIAL EXPERIMENT. Minneapolis: University of Minnesota Press, 1951.
28. Donaldson, Scott. SUBURBAN MYTH. New York: Columbia University Press, 1969.
29. Dubos, René. MAN ADAPTING. New Haven: Yale University Press, 1965.
30. Duhl, Leonard J., editor. THE URBAN CONDITION: PEOPLE AND POLICY IN THE METROPOLIS. New York: Basic Books, Inc., 1963.
31. Duncan, Otis Dudley, W. Richard Scott, Stanley Lieberson, Beverly Duncan and Hal H. Winsborough. METROPOLIS AND REGION. Published for Resources for the Future. Baltimore: Johns Hopkins Press, 1960.
32. Duncan, Otis Dudley and Beverly Duncan. "Residential Distribution and Occu-pational Segregation," American Journal of Sociology, Vol. 60, March 1955, pp. 493–503. Reprinted in Paul Hatt and Albert Reiss, editors, CITIES AND SOCIETY. Glencoe: The Free Press, 1957, pp. 283–296.
33. Dunham, H. Warren. COMMUNITY AND SCHIZOPHRENIA. Detroit: Wayne State University Press, 1965.
34. Educational Facilities Laboratories. SCSD: THE PROJECT AND THE SCHOOLS. New York: The Laboratories, 1967.
35. Elkins, Stanley and Erik McKitrick, "A Meaning for Turner's Frontier." Part I. Political Science Quarterly, 69, September 1954, pp. 321–353. Part II. Political Science Quarterly, 69, December 1954, pp. 565–602.
36. Faris, Robert E. L. and H. Warren Dunham. MENTAL DISORDERS IN URBAN AREAS. Chicago: University of Chicago Press, 1939.
37. Festinger, Leon, Stanley Schachter and Kurt Back. SOCIAL PRESSURES IN INFORMAL GROUPS: A STUDY OF HUMAN FACTOR IN HOUSING. New York: Harper & Bros., 1950.
38. Firey, Walter. "Sentiment and Symbolism as Ecological Variables," American Sociological Review, Vol. 10, April 1945, pp. 140–148.
39. Forde, Caryll C. HABITAT, ECONOMY AND SOCIETY. New York: E. P. Dutton, 1963.
40. Garfinkle, Harold. STUDIES IN ETHNOMETHODOLOGY. Englewood Cliffs: Prentice-Hall, 1967.
41. Geddes, Robert and Bernard P. Spring. A STUDY OF EDUCATION FOR ENVIRONMENTAL DESIGN. Sponsored by the American Institute of Architects. Princeton: Princeton University, 1967.
42. Glueck, Sheldon and Eleanor T. Glueck. FIVE HUNDRED CRIMINAL CAREERS. New York: A. A. Knopf, 1930.
43. Good, Lawrence R., Saul M. Siegel and Alfred Paul Bay, editors. THERAPY BY DESIGN: IMPLICATIONS OF ARCHITECTURE FOR HUMAN BE-HAVIOR. Springfield, Illinois: Thomas, 1965.
44. Goodman, William I. and Eric Freund, editors. PRINCIPLES AND PRACTICE OF URBAN PLANNING. Published for the Institute for Training in Munici-pal Administration. Washington: International City Managers' Association, 1968.
45. Gowings, D. THE WARREN COUNTY STAIR DESIGN SURVEY, PART 2. Harrisburg: Division of Environmental Safety, Pennsylvania Department of Health, [Fall 1962?].

46. Great Britain, Ministry of Housing and Local Government. GROUPED FLAT-LETS FOR OLD PEOPLE: A SOCIOLOGICAL STUDY. London: Her Majesty's Stationery Office, 1962.

47. Great Britain, Ministry of Housing and Local Government. SOME ASPECTS OF DESIGNING FOR OLD PEOPLE. London: Her Majesty's Stationery Office, 1968.

48. Gutman, Robert. "Library Architecture and People," *In* Ernest de Prospo editor, *The Library Building Consultant.* New Brunswick: Rutgers University Press, 1969.

49. ———. "The Questions Architects Ask," *Transactions of the Bartlett Society,* Vol. 4, 1965–66, pp. 47–82.

50. ———. THE SOCIAL EFFECTS OF THE URBAN ENVIRONMENT. A mimeographed report. n.d.

51. ———. "Urban Transporters as Human Environments," in *Journal of the Franklin Institute,* special issue: *New Concepts in Urban Transportation Systems,* Vol. 286:5, November 1968, pp. 533–539.

52. Haig, Robert M. and Roswell C. McCrea. MAJOR ECONOMIC FACTORS IN METROPOLITAN GROWTH AND ARRANGEMENT. Vol. 1 of REGIONAL SURVEY OF NEW YORK AND ITS ENVIRONS. New York: Committee on Regional Plan of New York and Its Environs, 1927.

53. Hall, Edward T. THE HIDDEN DIMENSION. New York: Doubleday, 1966.

54. ———. THE SILENT LANGUAGE. Garden City: Doubleday, 1959.

55. Hall, Norman B., Jr. and Edward M. Bennett. "Empirical Assessment of Handrail Diameters," *Journal of Applied Psychology,* Vol. 40:6, 1956, pp. 381–382.

56. Haythorn, William W. A "NEEDS" BY "SOURCES OF SATISFACTION" ANALYSIS OF ENVIRONMENTAL HABITABILITY. Tallahassee: Florida State University, May 1970. Paper prepared for the First National Symposium on Habitability.

57. Hediger, H. WILD ANIMALS IN CAPTIVITY. New York: Dover, 1964.

58. "House Hunting for Safety," *Home Safety Program Guide,* Vol. 12, pp. 1–8.

59. Hudson, Robert B. RADBURN: A PLAN FOR LIVING. A study made for the American Association for Adult Education. New York: J. J. Little and Ives Company, 1934.

60. Hunt, William Dudley, Jr., editor. COMPREHENSIVE ARCHITECTURAL SERVICES: GENERAL PRINCIPLES AND PRACTICE. Published for the American Institute of Architects. New York: McGraw-Hill, 1965.

61. Hunter, Floyd. COMMUNITY POWER STRUCTURE. Chapel Hill: University of North Carolina Press, 1953.

62. Illinois, University of, Small Homes Council, Building Research Council. HAZARD-FREE HOUSES FOR ALL. Champaign: The Council.

63. Institute for Safer Living. HOW NOT TO GET THE BREAK OF YOUR LIFE. Wakefield, Mass.: The Institute, 1967. (Pamphlet).

64. International Conference of Building Officials. UNIFORM BUILDING CODE. Pasadena: The Conference, 1967.

65. International Council for Building Research, Studies and Documentation. DIRECTORY OF BUILDING RESEARCH AND DEVELOPMENT ORGANIZATIONS. Rotterdam: C.I.B. Bouwcentrum, 1963.

66. Isard, Walter. METHODS OF REGIONAL ANALYSIS: AN INTRODUCTION TO REGIONAL SCIENCE. Cambridge: Technology Press of Massachusetts Institute of Technology; New York: John Wiley and Sons, Inc., 1960.

67. Jones, Rudard A. "The Safer Home—Will It Come to Be?," *National Safety Council Transactions,* 1969.

68. Keller, Suzanne Infeld. THE URBAN NEIGHBORHOOD: A SOCIOLOGICAL PERSPECTIVE. New York: Random House, 1968.

69. Lansing, John B., Robert W. Marans, and Robert B. Zehner. PLANNED RESIDENTIAL ENVIRONMENTS. Ann Arbor: Survey Research Center, Institute for Social Research, University of Michigan, 1970.

70. Litwak, Eugene. "Reference Groups, Theory, Bureaucratic Career and Group Cohesion," *Sociometry*, Vol. 23, March 1960, pp. 72–84.

71. ———. "Voluntary Associations and Neighborhood Cohesion," *American Sociological Review*, Vol. 26, April 1961, pp. 258–271.

72. Loring, William C. "Housing Characteristics and Social Disorganization," *Social Problems*, Vol. 3:3, 1956, pp. 160–168. See note 189 on p. 119 above.

73. Lowenthal, David, editor. ENVIRONMENTAL PERCEPTION AND BEHAVIOR. Chicago: University of Chicago, Paper in Geography, 1967.

74. Lukashok, Alvin and Kevin Lynch. "Some Childhood Memories of the City," *Journal of the American Institute of Planners*, Vol. 22, Summer 1956, pp. 142–152.

75. Lynch, Kevin. THE IMAGE OF THE CITY. Cambridge: M.I.T. Press, 1960.

76. ———. SITE PLANNING. Cambridge: M.I.T. Press, 1962.

77. Lyndheim, Roslyn. UNCOUPLING AND REGROUPING THE HOSPITAL SYSTEM. Berkeley: Institute of Urban and Regional Development, University of California, 1967.

78. McCue, Gerald M., William R. Ewald, Jr., and the Midwest Research Institute. CREATING THE HUMAN ENVIRONMENT. A report of the American Institute of Architects. Urbana: University of Illinois Press, 1970.

79. Marcuse, Herbert. EROS AND CIVILIZATION: A PHILOSOPHICAL INQUIRY INTO FREUD. Boston: Beacon Press, 1955.

80. Maslow, A. H. and N. L. Mintz. "Effects of Aesthetic Surroundings," *Journal of Psychology*, No. 41, 1956, pp. 247–254.

81. Meier, Richard. A COMMUNICATIONS THEORY OF URBAN GROWTH. Cambridge: M.I.T. Press, 1962.

82. Michelson, William H. MAN AND HIS URBAN ENVIRONMENT: A SOCIOLOGICAL APPROACH. Reading: Addison-Wesley, 1970.

83. Miller, A. and J. A. Cook, "Radburn Estates Revisited: Report of a User Study," *Architects' Journal*, 1 November 1967, pp. 1075–1082.

84. Miller, J. A. and M. L. Esmay. "Nature and Causes of Stairway Falls," *Transactions of the American Society of Agricultural Engineers*, Vol. 4:1, 1961, pp. 112–114.

85. Mintz, N. L. "Effects of Aesthetic Surroundings," *Journal of Psychology*, No. 41, 1956, pp. 459–466.

86. Mogey, John M., FAMILY AND NEIGHBORHOOD: TWO STUDIES IN OXFORD. London: Oxford University Press, 1956.

87. Moore, Gary T., editor. EMERGING METHODS IN ENVIRONMENTAL DESIGN AND PLANNING: PROCEEDINGS OF THE DESIGN METHODS GROUP FIRST INTERNATIONAL CONFERENCE, 1968. Cambridge: M.I.T. Press, 1971.

88. National Safety Council. THE HAZARD HUNTER. Chicago: The Council, 1968 (?). (Pamphlet).

89. Newman, Oscar and George Rand. CRIME AND HOUSING. Study being undertaken at New York University.

90. Norberg-Schulz, Christian. INTENTIONS IN ARCHITECTURE. Cambridge: M.I.T. Press, 1966.

91. Osmond, Humphrey, "Some Psychiatric Aspects of Design," in Laurence B. Holland, editor, WHO DESIGNS AMERICA? American Civilization Conference, Princeton University. Garden City: Anchor Books, Doubleday, 1966. pp. 281–318.

193

92. "People Who Live in Glass Houses," *Home Safety Program Guide*, Vol. 11, pp. 1–8.
93. Proshansky, Harold M., William H. Ittelson and Leanne G. Rivlin, editors. ENVIRONMENTAL PSYCHOLOGY: MAN AND HIS PHYSICAL SETTING. New York: Holt, Rinehart and Winston, 1970.
94. Radburn Management Corporation. RADBURN: PROTECTIVE RESTRICTIONS AND COMMUNITY ADMINISTRATION. Fair Lawn: The Corporation, n.d.
95. Regional Plan Association. SPREAD CITY: PROJECTIONS OF DEVELOPMENT TRENDS AND THE ISSUES THEY POSE. THE TRI-STATE NEW YORK METROPOLITAN REGION, 1960–1985. New York: Regional Plan Association, 1962.
96. Rowe, Colin. "The Mathematics of the Ideal Villa," *Architectural Review*, March 1947, pp. 101–104.
97. "Safety's Role in Urban Renewal," *Home Safety Program Guide*, Summer 1961, pp. 1–7.
98. Schilder, Paul. THE IMAGE AND APPEARANCE OF THE HUMAN BODY. London: Kegan Paul, French and Trubner and Company, 1935.
99. Schmitt, Robert C. "Density, Health and Social Disorganization," *Journal of the American Institute of Planners*, Vol. 32:1, January 1966, pp. 38–40.
100. Schorr, Alvin Louis. SLUMS AND SOCIAL INSECURITY. London: Nelson, 1964.
101. Searles, Harold F. THE NON-HUMAN ENVIRONMENT IN NORMAL DEVELOPMENT AND IN SCHIZOPHRENIA. New York: International Universities Press, 1960.
102. Seaton, Don Cash, Herbert J. Stack and Bernard I. Loft. ADMINISTRATION AND SUPERVISION OF SAFETY EDUCATION. New York: Macmillan Company, 1969.
103. Sommer, Robert. PERSONAL SPACE: THE BEHAVIORAL BASIS OF DESIGN. Englewood Cliffs: Prentice-Hall, 1969.
104. ———. "Studies in Personal Space," in *Sociometry*, Vol. XXII:3, September 1959, pp 247–260.
105. Sonnenfield, J. "Variable Values in Space and Landscape: An Inquiry into the Nature of Environmental Necessity," *Journal of Social Issues*, Vol. XXII:4, 1966, pp. 71–82.
106. Srole, Leo. MENTAL HEALTH IN THE METROPOLIS: THE MIDTOWN MANHATTAN STUDY. Thomas A. C. Rennie series in Sociological Psychiatry. New York: Blakiston Division, McGraw-Hill, 1962.
107. Stein, Clarence S. TOWARD NEW TOWNS FOR AMERICA. New York: Reinhold Publishing Corporation, 1957.
108. Strathclyde, University of, Building Performance Research Unit. "Building Appraisal: St. Michael's Academy, Kilwinning," *Architects' Journal*, January 7, 1970, pp. 9–50.
109. Strauss, Anselm. THE AMERICAN CITY: A SOURCEBOOK OF URBAN IMAGERY. Chicago: Aldine Publishing Company, 1968.
110. "Study Points National Science Foundation at Social Needs," *Engineering News-Record*, Vol. 186:7, February 18, 1971, p. 7.
111. Thiel, Phillip. "A Sequence-Experience Notation for Architectural and Urban Space," *Town Planning Review*, Vol. 32:1, April 1961, pp. 33–52.
112. Trites, David K., Frank D. Galbraith, Jr., Madelyne Sturdavant and John F. Leckwart. "Influence of Nursing-Unit Design on the Activities and Subjective Feelings of Nursing Personnel," *Environment and Behavior*, Vol. 2:3, December 1970, pp. 303–334.

113. U.S. Department of Commerce, Bureau of Public Roads. HIGHWAYS AND ECONOMIC AND SOCIAL CHANGE. Washington: Government Printing Office, 1964.
114. U.S. Department of Housing and Urban Development. GUIDE CRITERIA FOR THE EVALUATION OF: OPERATION BREAKTHROUGH. 5 volumes, interim draft. Washington: The Department, 1971.
115. U.S. Public Health Service. HEALTH STATISTICS: PERSONS INJURED BY DETAILED TYPE AND CLASS OF ACCIDENT. Series B-No. 37. Washington: U.S. Department of Health, Education, and Welfare, 1962.
116. ———. HEALTH STATISTICS: PERSONS INJURED IN THE HOME AND ASSOCIATED DISABILITY. Series B-No. 39. Washington: U.S. Department of Health, Education, and Walfare, 1963.
117. ———. HEALTH SURVEY PROCEDURE. Series 7, No. 2. Washington: U.S. Department of Health, Education, and Welfare, 1964.
118. Wacks, Martin. BASIC APPROACHES TO THE MEASUREMENT OF COMMUNITY VALUES. Occasional Series Paper No. 8. Urbana: Center for Urban Studies, University of Illinois, 1970.
Prepared for presentation to the 49th annual meeting of the Highway Research Board.
119. Wallace, Anthony F. C. HOUSING AND SOCIAL STRUCTURE. Philadelphia: Philadelphia Housing Association, 1952.
120. Wilner, Daniel M., R. P. Walkey, T. Pinkerton, and M. Tayback. THE HOUSING ENVIRONMENT AND FAMILY LIFE. Baltimore: Johns Hopkins Preses, 1962.
121. Wilson, Robert L. "Livability of the City: Attitudes and Urban Development," In F. Stuart Chapin, Jr. and Shirley Weiss, editors, URBAN GROWTH DYNAMICS. New York: John Wiley and Sons, 1962, chapter 11.
122. Wohlwill, Joachim F. "The Physical Environment: A Problem for a Psychology of Stimulation," Journal of Social Issues, Vol. XXII:4, 1966, pp. 29–38.
123. Hanke, B., J. Krasnowiecki, and W. C. Loring. THE HOMES ASSOCIATION HANDBOOK, ULI TECHNICAL BULLETIN No. 50. Washington: Urban Land Institute, 1964 & revised printing 1970, pp. 73–76, 145, 153, 155, 161, 165, 175, 177, 179, 243, 277–279, 282, & 412.

# Chapter VII

## Measurement of the Effects of the Environment Upon the Health and Behavior of People

LAWRENCE E. HINKLE, JR.

### Introduction

It is widely recognized that there is a need for better means of measuring what is often called the "quality" of the environment. (1) The word "quality," as it is used in this context, has an evaluative sense—it implies that there is a relative "value," "goodness," or "appropriateness" of the environment, which can be measured in terms of its relation to something else. Under various circumstances this "something else" may be the health and survival of the natural systems that are part of the environment, the integrity of the natural physical features of the environment, the beauty of the landscape, or the appropriateness of the man-made parts of the environment to the activities for which they are used. However, most of the time this "something else" is the "quality of human life" in the environment. The need that is most often remarked upon is a need for a way of evaluting how the "quality of human life" is affected by the environment, or by a part of the environment.

It should be emphasized that the various methods that might be proposed for measuring the quality of the environment will not necessarily yield parallel answers. What is most beneficial for the natural systems in the environment may not be conducive to its physical inintegrity or to its natural beauty, and what produces the finest quality of life for people in the environment may not be conducive to the preservation of its physical integrity or to the survival of some of the natural systems in it. It is quite clear that under many circumstances there is a conflict between the needs of men and the needs of the natural environment. (2, 3)

This paper is man-oriented. It is directed at the problem of measuring the effect of the environment upon the health and behavior of people as individuals or as populations of individuals. It is not primarily concerned with the effects of people upon the environment, nor is it concerned with the effect of the environment upon human social groups as such. It is directed at the question of how to make measurements upon individuals which may reflect the effect of the environment upon their health and behavior. It is concerned with the matter of how people are affected by their interaction with the environment in which they live.

The comments in this article are intended to be general, and to suggest a method that might be adaptable for general use. However, I have added, separately as a section of notes, comments based upon the experience of the Division of Human Ecology at Cornell University Medical College, during the period since 1954, and some indications of the methods that we have used at various points.

## Part I Discussion

### A. Theoretical Considerations

#### 1. Definition of "Man" and "Environment"

This paper is written from the biological point of view that is shared by the natural sciences. This point of view does not appear to be in fundamental conflict with that of the social and behavioral sciences. In the interest of specificity, we shall begin by defining "man" and "environment" in the technical language that is used in the biological sciences, because such a definition is important to the logical structure of the argument that follows.

The definitions of "man" and "environment" that are used here are based upon the biological concept that the higher forms of life exist as discrete and more or less independent organisms, and that each organism is surrounded by an "environment." The maintenance of the life of the organism is dependent upon a constant interaction between the organism and its environment. In technical terms, the living organism is regarded as a finite, highly organized, biological system, which maintains itself in a "dynamic steady state" over a limited period of time by the consumption of free energy and by the constant interchange of matter, energy, and information with the environment. (4) The "dynamic steady state" is an equilibrium of constantly interacting and inherently unstable biochemical systems which is maintained by an input of free energy and information. (5)*

The "environment" of an organism, in the broadest sense, is defined as all of the universe that is outside of its boundaries; more specifically it is considered to be made of those parts of the universal system with which the organism interacts.

In this paper a "man" is considered to be a living organism in the sense in which we have just defined this term, and his "environment"

---

* See Note 1, on Page 222.

is considered to have the same general characteristics as the environment of other living organisms as these have just been described.

## 2. Interfaces Between Men and the Environment

The boundaries of the living organism that is "man" are considered to be his skin, the lining epithelium of his respiratory tract, the lining epithelium of his gastrointestinal tract and the lining epithelium of his kidney and urinary tract. These, and his "organs of special sense" are the primary interfaces between him and his environment. The "organs of special sense" are the eyes, the ears, the olfactory organs, the taste organs, and the special organs within the skin and inside the body which provide for the senses of touch, pain, temperature, pressure position in space, and acceleration.

It is important to note that, by this definition, the clothing on a man's back, the air in his lungs, the food in his gastrointestinal tract, and the urine in his bladder are parts of the environment. All of these are outside of the boundaries of the organism. The gastrointestinal tract, the respiratory tract, and the genito-urinary tract are looked upon as special biological arrangements facilitating interchanges with the environment. The contents of the lung and and of the gastrointestinal tract are parts of the environment which have been ingested and brought into intimate contact with the organism in order to effect these interchanges. The contents of the urinary tract are waste products from the organism which are being excreted back into the environment. Thus men, like other living organisms, are in constant and intimate contact with their environment, and ingest or enclose a part of it in order to facilitate their interchanges with it.

## 3. The Nature of Man-Environment Interchanges

The maintenance of human life is dependent upon a constant interchange of water and heat across the skin; of water, carbon dioxide, and oxygen across the epithelium of the lung; of food, minerals, and water across the epithelium of the gastrointestinal tract; of water, salts, and organic substances across the epithelium of the kidneys.

All of these processes are associated with an interchange of information—as well as an interchange of energy.* This interchange of information is essential to the maintenance of human life. However, the information processing that goes on within these organs may be looked upon as largely incidental to the transfer of energy, gases, fluids, minerals, and organic substances that are the primary activities of these interfaces between the organism and its environment.

The organs of special sense represent the interface between the man and his environment that is primarily concerned with the acquisition of information, as such, from the environment. These organs are closely

---

* See Note 2, on Page 222.

coupled with the central nervous system, and through this, to the neuro-endocrine effector systems. This arrangement makes it possible for the human organism to use the information acquired from the sense organs to draw inferences about those aspects of the environment which do not impinge upon it directly, but are distant from it in time and place, and also makes it possible for the organism to organize adaptive responses to the environment which involve the entire human system.

## 4. Types of Interchange with the Environment

The gross energy interchanges between a man and his environment amount to approximately 2,500 to 4,000 kilogram calories per day. These are carried out primarily through interchanges of food and water through the gastrointestinal tract; of water, gas, and heat through the lungs; of water, minerals, and organic substances through the kidneys; and of heat and water through the skin. There is also some exchange of energy as kinetic energy from the muscular activity of the man, and some interchanges of radiant energy through the skin. Altogether, the gross energy interchanges between a man and his environment are numerically rather few, and of small variety, but any interference with them can present a serious and immediate threat to life.

By far the largest number and variety of interactions between men and their environment are based upon interchanges of information. It has been mentioned that such procedures as the digestion of food, the immune responses to chemical and microbial agents, and the elaboration of defense mechanisms against these, involve information processing of a rather high order, much of which is carried out at a cellular level outside of the nervous system. Quite over and above these is the large proportion of the adaptive reactions of men to their environment which are carried out through the mediation of the sense organs and the central nervous system. A large part of these adaptations are to aspects of the environment which do not impinge upon the man directly, but are at distance from him in time and place.

## 5. Important Features of the Environment

Informational interchanges with all aspects of the environment, whether these represent food, bacteria, people, or distant events, involve reactions to information acquired by the organism. The reaction of the organism is based upon the biological meaning of this information to the organism, and is based upon its own evaluation of the information. The "biological meaning" is in part "programmed" into the organism, but it may be seriously modified by the past experiences of the organism. That is to say, biological reactions to the environment, at all levels, are not only inherited (genetically programmed) but also learned.

In effect, a man reacts to most of his environment, not in terms of gross quantitative interchanges of energy with it, but in terms of the information he acquires from it. His reaction to this information is based upon the "meaning" (in the biological sense) of the information to him. This meaning may be, in many respects, highly special to a particular person, and to the environmental situation in which he exists at a given time. Concepts such as "stress," which are useful in describing gross, quantitative energy interchanges, are not helpful in describing the interactions between man and his environment which are based upon informational interchanges.

In general, the aspects of the environment which are most important to a man are those which impinge upon him directly, those which immediately surround him, and those which are most meaningful to him. Food, water, air, and clothing are extremely important features of the human environment, as are the chemical and microbial agents which impinge upon the skin, the lungs, and the gut. Since men live and work in buildings and cities of their own creation, and since they spend much of their time utilizing complex tools and other artifacts of human society, these are extremely important parts of the environment. Also, since men are social animals who always exist as members of social groups in which there are complex social roles and elaborate rules governing interpersonal relationships, other people are among the most meaningful features of the human environment; and since social groups are among the most meaningful features of the human environment, these are also among its most important features.

Learned behavior, which is directed toward maintaining a man's relationship with other people around him, and toward maintaining his position in the social group, accounts for a major portion of a man's reactions to his environment.

In the biological sense, there is only one environment. Other people and the artifacts of human society are among the most important parts of it. Despite the fact that the ultimate welfare of man depends upon the integrity of other parts of the natural system, the forests, the oceans, and the open fields are relatively unimportant features of the human enviroment in terms of their immediate influence upon human health and behavior.

## 6. Changing Features of the Human Environment Throughout Life

Men, like other metazoan organisms, have a limited span of life. The human life span is of the order of 75 years. Although some believe that this life span might be extended significantly if the chronic and degenerative disorders of old age should be overcome, the prevailing opinion is that it is more or less programmed into the organism at birth. The limitations of the human life are created partly by the limited number of cell divisions that can take place in such self-reproducing tissues as the bone marrow, and partly by the limitations on the life of the cells of the central nervous system, which cannot reproduce themselves, and drop out gradually, over a period of years, until their number is reduced to the point at which the brain loses so much of its functional capacity that it can no longer sustain independent human life.

During the course of his life span, a human follows an orderly progression of growth and development to maturity and, finally, to death. At any stage of his development, there is a limited range of forms and functions of his organs which are compatible with the full maintenance of all human activity.

During the approximately "three score years and ten" that are allotted to it, the human organism maintains its life processes precariously by constant adaptation to an environment that is always hostile in the sense that the external environment is always different from the internal milieu which surrounds the cells and which must be maintained in a state of relative constancy if the organism is to survive.

The life span of a human begins, in effect, when an ovum is fertilized by a sperm. During the first nine months of its life, the environment of the human organism is represented by the amniotic fluid and by the interface between the placenta and the circulation of its mother. The characteristics of this environment are clearly dependent upon the health and behavior of the mother.

When the human infant leaves the uterus, it is exposed to an environment in which it must maintain its body temperature, and with which it must carry out its own interchanges of gases, food, and water. It must now cope with the pathogenic microorganisms and potentially damaging materials that it may encounter. It is still quite immature, and must depend upon the assistance of another human being in order to survive. Biologically, the mother is cast in the role of protector and nurturer of the newborn infant, but social group practices may cause this role to devolve upon others, in whole or in part.

The person, or persons, who are in the role of caring for and protecting the developing infant are among the most important features of the environment that a human encounters during his lifetime. In the first few years of its life, these people provide the infant with most of its nutrition, as well as its protection from injury, pathogens, and exposure to extremes of temperature. Moreover, these people, who are in the most intimate contact with the infant, begin to provide it with that store of acquired information which is its "cultural inheritance." They enable the infant to learn how to speak, and how to use clothing, household articles, and other artifacts which men depend upon for most of their adaptive behavior. They also enable the infant to learn its place in the social group, its status in relation to the people around it, and the rules of behavior in relation to other people and to society. They impart this information to the infant not so much by their explicit acts, as by the implications of their behavior toward the world around them and toward the child.

The environment of a child, from the first few years of life until it becomes an adult, changes in gradual stages, but it is never entirely different from the environment into which the child was born. As a human grows, he continues to require protection from the significant fluctuations in the physical features of his natural environment; he continues to require adequate nourishment, protection from trauma, noxious agents, and pathogens; and he continues to develop the learned behavior and the ability to handle cultural artifacts upon which much of his adaptive capacity depends. Although he is less directly dependent upon others around him for immediate assistance, he is now, and remains throughout his life, dependent upon other people, and upon the entire society for almost all of the goods and services that he utilizes. The "division of labor" or, in other words, the division of social roles, is so great in any human society that no man makes or provides even a small proportion of the goods and services that are necessary to the maintenance of his life.

As he grows older, the social roles of a developing human change and become more complex, and his relationships with other people change, but he remains dependent upon the people immediately around him, and those most closely related to him, for the satisfaction of many of his most important needs. During this period of his life, also, he is likely to be exposed to formal education or training, which gives him the opportunity to acquire parts of the cultural heritage which cannot be learned by simple association with others. The nature, quality, and duration of his education largely determine the ultimate extent to which a man develops his basic intellectual capacities, and may determine to a large extent the nature of his ultimate social role.

The period of mature life is one in which most people in modern society continue to carry through a changing progression of relationships with others around them. In the latter part of adult life, as the gradual degeneration of old age begins, the cumulative effects of exposure to environmental conditions and noxious agents may cause breakdowns in organ function which ultimately lead to death. During this stage of life, it is difficult to tell how much of the deterioration of the human organism is due to inevitable biologic senescence, and how much is the result of exposure to adverse environmental conditions. Also, during this period of life, a person experiences removal from many active social roles which have sustained him in the past. He must endure the disruption of important interpersonal relationships because of death and illness, and he must adapt himself to resuming the role of dependency. All of these adaptations must be made by the aging at a time when adaptive capacities are becoming progressively more feeble.

## B. The Effects of the Environment upon People

### 1. The Theoretical "Ideal Environment"

If one were to set up a theoretical "ideal" environment for a man, it appears that this environment would have the following characteristics:

a. It would be an environment in which the man would live out his full span of life.

b. It would be an environment in which his life would be free from any period of illness or disability caused by interaction with the environment, and in which he would develop none of the impairments which are the results of illness.

c. (1) It would be an environment in which his physical growth and development would be unimpaired.

(2) It would be an environment in which he would be able to acquire all the cultural information, including all of the skills and all of the formal education, that his innate biological equipment make possible for him to assimilate.

(3) It would be an environment in which he could acquire the ability to enter into and undertake any role in the society which might be desirable for him and for the social group.

(4) It would be an environment in which he could acquire the ability to relate to other people around him to the social group in a manner such that he would be able to satisfy his biological and psychological needs within the framework of a behavior acceptable to the group and to the people around him.

One might epitomize these four points under 'c' by saying that an ideal environment for a man would be one in which he would be able to realize his full biological potential.

d. It would be an environment that would not, in itself, hinder the man in the performance of any activities essential to the satisfaction of his roles in his society, or require him to undertake any activities to deal with the environment which he would not have to undertake if adverse characteristics of the environment were not present.

e. Finally, it would be an environment in which it would be possible for him to obtain pleasure and satisfaction.

Such an ideal environment undoubtedly has not been enjoyed by any man, and probably it never will. The reason for putting it forth as a concept is that such a concept can be used as a basis for estimating to what extent any given environment may be less than optimal for any given person, and for comparing environments in terms of their effect upon individuals or groups of individuals. The concept of an "ideal environment" can also provide a basis for estimating the effect upon people of features of the environment or of changes in the en-

204

vironment, in terms of whether or not, or how much, these cause the environment to move toward or away from a theoretical optimum for the people in it.

## 2. Effects upon Health and Behavior Created by Interactions with the Environment

Since the environment is, in general, "hostile" in the sense that it is different in many ways from the characteristics of the internal milieu which must be maintained by the human organism if life is to continue, any change in the relation of a man to his environment is likely to require an adaptation on his part. This means that a likely result of any interaction with the environment will be an adverse effect on the man—it will require him to make a new adaptive effort. In spite of this, there may be a significant proportion of environmental interactions which have the ultimate effect of lessening the adaptive demands upon the human organism, because the new man-environment relationship may be less demanding for the man.* Thus, the result of an interaction between a man and his environment, or a change in the environment, may move it in the direction of an "ideal" environment for the man, as we have described in the previous section, or move it away from this "ideal."

In spite of the diversity of environmental situations and the many specific effects that interactions with these can create upon the health and behavior of people, it appears that all of these effects can be grouped into a relatively small number of categories:

### a. Lethal Effects

Interactions with the environment can increase the likelihood of the death of a person before he attains his expected span of life, or they can lessen the likelihood that he will die before he attains his expected span of life.

There are a number of mechanisms that are commonly involved in life-threatening interactions with the environment. These include effects upon the essential supplies of food, air, or water; interference with heat exchange; poisoning or intoxication with chemical agents; traumatic damage to the organism caused by physical energy; and the effects of invasion of microbial agents; but they also include changes in the relation of a man to his social group, or to the others around him, which cause him to behave in a manner—sometimes overt and straight-forward but sometimes complex and inapparent—which shortens his life.

The interactions between people and the environment that threaten life often take place insidiously over long periods of time. They may lead to the development of "chronic disease processes" which create no

---

* See Note 3, Page 222.

apparent impairment of the activities of the human organism for many years, but ultimately cause death. Classic examples of this are athero-sclerosis and arterial hypertension which are so common in modern societies.

b. *Disabling Effects*

Interaction between a person and his environment may lead to an impairment of the function of one or more of his organ systems, which may or may not be reversible. This impairment of the function of organs, in turn, may lead to some impairment of the bodily functions of the man, as a whole, or to some disturbances of his mood, thought, or behavior. The disability of the person, as a whole, may be temporary and wholly reversible, or prolonged and not wholly reversible. It may or may not lead to some shortening of his life span. Often it does not do so.

Typically, environmentally induced disorders of bodily function and disturbances of mood, thought, and behavior are thought of as "ill-nesses" or "injuries" except when they are of the most transient or superficial nature. The term "illness" is usually reserved for active processes, even though these may be long term and chronic. When the active process which is the "illness" has ended, the person may be permanently damaged. The residential damage is usually referred to as an "impairment." Typical "impairments" are the paralysis of an ex-tremity which follows poliomyelitis, the deafness which may follow otitis media, or the loss of teeth, which may result from dental caries.

Illnesses, injuries, and impairments usually carry with them a threat to life in the sense that those who exhibit illnesses, as a group, have a greater likelihood of not living out their expected span of life, than those who do not. However, the threat to life that is associated with an illness is not necessarily parallel to the degree of impairment that is created by this illness. Many illnesses that are quite prostrating for short periods of time may be associated with little or no threat to life.* Similarly, the impairments that may result from illnesses or injuries may not seriously affect longevity. People who are totally deaf or blind, for instance, or those who have lost the use of their extremities may be seriously disabled, but they may, neverthless, live out a full span of life.

Because the "'seriousness" of an illness (the extent to which it threatens life) is not necessarily parallel to its "severity" (the extent to which it disables the person), it is useful to have separate methods for measuring threat to life created by an illness, and for measuring the disability it produces so that one can have an independent indication of the extent to which an aspect of the environment threatens life, and the extent to which it leads to temporary or permanent disability.

* See Note 4, Page 222.
* See Note 5, Page 223.

Interactions with the environment may decrease disability as well as increase it. It is the goal of medical treatment to decrease disability and impairment as well as to increase longevity. Changes in people's activities, changes in their exposure to environmental agents, and changes in their interpersonal relations may also be associated with a decrease in the frequency or severity of various kinds of disability and in the frequence of the impairments that follow illness.

Periods of illness, like fatalities, may be produced by a variety of forms of interaction with the environment.*

c. *Effects Upon Growth and Development*

Interactions with the environment may have effects on human development, even when they do not lead to the creation or prevention of those defects which might be called "impairments."

The exposure of pregnant women to environmental agents such as German measles virus or thalidomide may create serious "congenital" defects in their unborn children. Even when the health and behavior of mothers produce no definite "defects" in their children, these might, nevertheless, be responsible for a wide range of variation in such important biological characteristics of the newborn as the duration of their gestation and their maturity at birth, their birth weight, and their ability to resist infectious agents. (7)

Similarly, it is well known that the exposure of newborn infants to infections, inadequate nutrition, injuries, rejection, and neglect can cause serious and irreparable damage to them. Among growing children, differences in food intake, in activity, in the sanitation of the surroundings, and in the frequency of minor illnesses, can be associated with subsequent differences in the amount of deafness, dental caries, atherosclerosis, and obesity that they experience in adult life. Over and above this, variations in such environmental factors may also be associated with variations in rates of growth of children, in their ultimate stature, in the onset of their maturity, and in their advancement in school.

The availability of medical care for such stigmata as malocclusion, strabismus, or serious acne may have an effect not only on a child's physical well-being, but also on its self image, and its role in society. The attitudes and behavior of other people around the child and the interaction of the parents with each other can be determining factors in the ultimate ability of a child to handle interpersonal relations, and the ability to deal with its own needs and drives within an acceptable social framework. The speech, the dress, and the level of education of the parents, the place they live in, and the way other people treat them become an important part of the cultural inheritance of a child. The appearance of a child's clothing, the work that his father does, and the

---

* See Note 6, Page 224.

quality of the school he attends may have little or no effect upon his longevity or disability, but they may be extremely important determinants of his ultimate role in society and the extent to which he realizes his full biological potential.

d. *Constraints upon Behavior*

The environment places important constraints upon human behavior; and changes in the environment may alleviate these or make them more severe.

Over and above the effects of the environment on the length of life, on the occurrence of disability and impairments, and on the growth and development of people, it may also place limits upon the ability of a people to carry out actions which are desirable or necessary for them, in the biological sense, including some of those activities which are desirable or necessary for them if they are to fulfill their social roles. Conversely, the character of the environment in which they live may make it necessary for them to undertake activities in which they would not other wise engage, and these activities may make important biological and social demands upon them.*

The constraints upon human activities that may be created by environmental conditions, and the otherwise unnecessary activities that are engendered by the effort of people to deal with environmental conditions are not, strictly speaking, "health effects." While it is quite clear that an interrupted night's sleep, the fatigue of a long journey, the inability to have a bowel movement when the desire is upon one, the unavailability of hot water, the draft from a broken window, or the lack of privacy in a bedroom, are all relevant to human health, the effect of these upon the health of people may be hard to detect.

Over the long run, by carefully controlled studies, it would probably be possible to demonstrate effects that conditions such as these have on the health of otherwise vigorous people; but, at the present time, it is much easier to demonstrate that these conditions have an effect upon people whose adaptation is precarious—upon the aged, the ill, and the newborn, for example.

In general, it may be said that environmental conditions which place constraints upon human behavior may have a markedly adverse effect on the health of some people, but that they have little demonstrable effect on the health of most people. Most healthy, vigorous people, might live at the end of a runway, or in a drafty house for a long period of time without demonstrable effect upon their morbidity, mortality, growth, or development. Under most circumstances the discomfort that arises from a noisy environment or a drafty room, cannot, strictly speaking, be regarded as an illness. Yet this does not mean that phenomena such as noise and drafts may not have seriously adverse effects

---

* See Note 7, Page 224.

upon the "quality of life." Conditions such as these lay important constraints upon those who are exposed to them. They impair the freedom of action of the people who have to deal with them, and they make it very difficult, if not impossible, for these people to perform effectively in many kinds of social roles, and to carry out many kinds of activities that are necessary or desirable for them and that may be extremely important to them.

In general, experience suggests that the differences in the artifacts of human society—limitations in the design, arrangement, construction, or state of repair of machines, buildings, roadways, parks, neighborhoods, cities, and the like—are more likely to place constraints upon the activities of people who live in them or use them, than they are to produce immediate "health effects."

Many of the major constraints on human behavior that are created by the environment, are created not so much by its physical features as by the requirements of social groups. Even when the physical characteristics of the environment are optimal, the satisfaction of the fundamental biological needs, and the personal desires of people, (such as the need for sleep, food, and rest, the desire for comfort, the expression of aggression, or the gratification of sexual drives) are severely constrained by socially determined rules for human behavior, and by the requirements of social roles. The society does not expect a mother to neglect her crying child in order to get a good night's sleep, a workman to neglect his job simply because he feels tired, or a combat soldier to exhibit a greater concern for his own health and well-being than for his role. Even when the physical characteristics of clothing, housing, means of transportation, or places of work, in themselves, place limitations upon human behavior, it appears that these limitations are likely to be based upon social determinants or markedly influenced by them.*

e. *Effects of Pleasure and Satisfaction*

Interactions with the environment may affect the pleasure and satisfaction of people.

Even in the absence of any important constraints upon their behavior, people may derive more or less satisfaction and pleasure from their environment because of its beauty, familiarity, values, or social implications, or because of other qualities which they perceive in it. Pleasure and satisfaction are part of the experience of the individual, and they cannot be separated from this. They are in many ways unique to each person, even though it is true that many features of the environment which are perceived as a source of satisfaction to one member of a group, may be a source of satisfaction to many others also. Although pleasure and satisfaction are often denigrated as values, the

_____
* See Note 8, Page 225.

209

pleasure and satisfaction that people obtain from their environment is not a trivial feature of it. Often people will sacrifice other aspects of their environment in order to create an environment which gives them pleasure and satisfaction.

### 3. The Hierarchy of Environmental Effects upon Humans

The five categories of environmental interactions and their effects upon humans, which we have just discussed, have been listed in the general order of the "seriousness" of the consequences that these interactions may have for the individuals who experience them. Environments, or portions of environments, which may have lethal effects upon people have been assumed to have consequences which are "more serious" than those which are likely to cause only disability among people. Similarly, features of the environment which cause some permanent disability among people have been assumed to have more serious consequences than features which cause only transient periods of disability. Features of the environment which prevent people from obtaining an optimal development have been regarded as "more serious" for the individuals exposed to them than those which cause transient periods of disability provided these latter do not create any clear-cut impairment. Aspects of the environment which prevent people from attaining an optimal development have also been regarded as having "more serious consequences" than those which merely place constraints upon people's behavior. Finally, those which place constraints upon human behavior have been assumed to have more serious consequences than those which merely prevent people from attaining pleasure or satisfaction.*

### C.   The Measurement of the Effects of the Environment upon People

The scheme for measuring the effects of the environment upon the health and behavior of people, which is here proposed, is based upon an attempt to measure independently:

(a) the extent to which an environment shortens the life of those who are exposed to it,

(b) the extent to which an environment creates disability or impairments among those who are exposed to it,

(c) the extent to which those who are exposed to an environment do not realize their full biological potential for growth and development,

(d) the extent to which the environment places constraints upon the ability of those who are exposed to it to engage in activities that they find necessary or desirable, and

(e) the extent to which an environment fails to provide pleasure and satisfaction for those who are exposed to it.

---

* See Note 9, Page 225.

This apparently negative approach is based upon the evidence that all environments are less than ideal, and that the adverse features of an environment are the more readily observed and counted.

## 1. Lethal Effects

a. The lethal effects of environments are more readily measured than any others, probably because death is, in the words of the epidemiologist, a "clear-cut end point" with such serious social implications that it is almost always taken note of, recorded, and accounted for. "Death rates" among human populations by age, sex, race, area of residence, and many other demographic characteristics, are commonly calculated and published. With more or less accuracy, depending upon the accuracy and completeness of the diagnostic data, they may be calculated for various environmental agents which are "causes of death." Death rates for automobile accidents, tuberculosis, or malaria, are rather easy to obtain, and those attributable to cigarette smoking or lead poisoning can be estimated with some accuracy.

b. Death rates for human populations living under a given set of environmental conditions over a period of time may be determined from the prospective observation of these populations, or, less accurately, from past records. When there is a question of an exposure to a particular feature of an environment which has a suspected lethal effect, the determination becomes more difficult, because it is then necessary to determine the extent of the exposure which may vary from individual to individual, and to estimate how much of any mortality that is observed in a population may be due to the environmental factor under consideration, and how much may be attributable to other factors that cause mortality.

When the exposure to a supposed lethal factor and the death attributable to it occur in rather quick succession, and when the lethal factor produces a fatal lesion with distinctive characteristics (for example in the case of an automobile accident) death rates attributable to the environmental factor may be relatively easy to compute. However, when there is a long or variable time between the exposure to the supposed lethal factor and the death, and when the factor produces no characteristic lesion, but appears to combine with a number of other factors to produce any one of a number of fatal lesions that may also have other causes (as in the case of cigarette smoking), then death rates attributable to the environmental factor may be more difficult to compute. The use of carefully chosen comparison populations and techniques such as partial correlation may be helpful in this regard.

c. A problem arises when one undertakes the study of lethal effects in small populations, or when one wishes to obtain a quick estimate of lethal effects in a large population. In modern societies such as our own, death rates for all causes are quite low except among the new-born and the very old. Even when environmental factors such as cigarette smoking have a highly lethal effect, the action of this effect may be long delayed and the number of deaths apparently attributable to this factor that occur per unit of time in the population available for study may be quite small. Retrospective data may be absent or inadequate and a prospective study might be prohibitively time consuming. Under these circumstances some investigators have attempted to use cross sectional surveys of population at a given point in time in order to estimate the past and present risk of premature death in this population.

Such a procedure is based upon relatively unproven methods, and the results are subject to more uncertainty than those that are obtained with more standard methods. However, one can obtain some estimate of the risk of premature death in a population provided one has information about the deaths that have occurred in the population in the past and about those people who have entered the population and who have left it during the period of study, and provided one can examine a probability sample of the population. It is based on the probability of death which has, in the past, been associated with various kinds of illness, and upon the amount of illness that is exhibited by or experienced by, the people in the sample.*

## 2. The Measurement of Disabling Effects of the Environment

There are established methods for measuring the amount of disability that is present in a population over a period of time. These methods have grown out of the experience of employers, school authorities, military authorities, and others who must be concerned with such matters as absence from work and the number of effective members of a population who are on hand at any one time. Other methods for measuring disability have arisen from the needs of those who are concerned with the requirements for medical care, and the number of hospital beds and physicians which must be available.

In general, the theoretical framework for the measurement of disability is similar to that which is used by the National Health Survey. (8) Since most disability is temporary, the period of disability experienced by a person may be defined as an "episode," and the duration of the episode may be measured in days.† The "severity" of an episode of disability is measured in terms of the extent to which a person is unable to carry out his primary social role, and to maintain his normal bodily functions.

---

* See Note 10, Page 228.

† Since disability is usually caused by illnesses or injuries, the term "episode of illness" is often used as if it were synonomous with the term "episode of disability."

In our own work, five grades of "severity" of episodes of disability have been recognized. The most severe episodes are those which prevent an individual from carrying out his usual and primary social role. These episodes are severe enough to prevent a workman from going to work, to prevent a school child from going to school, and to prevent a house-wife from carrying out her housework. These are called "disabling episodes," or "disabling episodes of illness." People with "disabling illnesses" are sick enough so that, in terms of the sociologist, they must temporarily abandon their primary social role and assume the "sick role." Information relating to the number of days of disability, or "sick days" in a population can be obtained from data on absence from work, absence from school, number of men on the sick list of a military unit, and so forth. These data apply to special populations in industrial, educational, or military settings. Data on more general populations must be obtained from cross-sectional surveys or longitudinal surveys of selected population samples.

Episodes of disability severe enough to prevent people from carrying on their usual social roles, and requiring them to adopt the "sick role" may be recognized as having two grades of severity. In one grade are those illnesses such as the common cold, an episode of acute gastroenteritis, or a severely sprained ankle, which make it necessary for a person to give up his usual activities, but do not so disable him that he cannot carry on some activities, such as reading or feeding himself. These are by far the most common disabling episodes.

The most severely disabling episodes are those which are so prostrating that the individual is unable to do anything except be sick. All of his bodily activities are directed, in effect, to preserving his life. Under these circumstances, the active help of other skilled persons is often required and the person himself may become a "patient" who will be placed in a hospital or other facility if this is available. Lobar pneumonia or an acute myocardial infarction are examples of illnesses that often attain this severity. An acute alcoholic delirium, or a psychotic excitement also have this degree of severity. In the case of illnesses such as these, patients are placed in special institutions not only to facilitate their own care, but also to protect them and others from the consequences of their disordered actions. The prevalence of the most severe illnesses are roughly indicated by data on "hospital days" in a population, but again, survey methods must be used if a more precise determination is to be made.

In addition to "disabling episodes," "partly disabling episodes" of illness have been recognized. Episodes of illness that are associated with the serious impairment of the function of one or more organ systems can have relatively little effect on the function of the person as a whole, are regarded as "partly disabling" because the individual may be able to carry out his usual activities, but he must do so in a somewhat restricted manner.*

In general, for purposes of population surveys, the determination of the frequency and duration of "disabling episodes of illness" is most practical.

One of the problems in all measurements of disability has to do with the ambiguity of social attitudes toward disturbances of mood, thought, and behavior. In general, there is agreement in this and other societies that episodes of disability caused by environmental agents, such as bacteria, viruses, physical force, and most chemical agents, are indeed, "illnesses." There is also general agreement that disabilities caused by degenerative disorders, by the gradual failure of organ systems, and by genetic disorders are, in effect, "illnesses." But there is not complete agreement about when the disorders of the highest integrative function of the organism—those that are manifested by disturbances of mood, thought, and behavior—constitute "illnesses." When these disorders are profound, as in psychotic states, there is general agreement that they constitute "illnesses." On the other hand, when disturbed behavior is associated with sexual aggression, assault, or murder, this behavior may be regarded as a "crime." When disturbed behavior is evidenced by the stealing of property, or by the forging of checks, this also is usually defined as a "crime." Similarly, when a period of disability is caused by the ingestion of alcohol or marijuana, this is regarded not as an illness, but as the result of voluntary behavior, which may or may not be condoned, depending on the circumstances under which it occurred.

In general, for the purposes of surveys, it would appear desirable to count and measure the frequency and duration and severity of all forms of disturbed or disabling behavior regardless of how the society classifies these. In order to estimate the total amount of disability one should define "disturbed or disabling behavior" according to some arbitrary scheme which accords with the goals of the survey. One can also classify each episode according to whether the society regards it as "an illness," a "crime," "sociopathic behavior," "voluntary behavior," or "personal idiosyncrasy." In the counting of partly disabling and disabling episodes of illness, conflict often arises about how one should count absence from work which is caused by drunkeness, or disability from a "cold" which is created not so much by the viral agent which produces the cold, as by the poor morale, resentment and self-interest of the person who has the cold. It has, in general, been our policy to count as "episodes of disability" all episodes of disability, of whatever cause, whether they are the result of microbial infections, injuries, drunkeness, minor grades of depression and anxiety, poor morale, or outright malingering. In each of these instances the individual is counted as

---

* See Note 11, Page 229.

214

"disabled" because he is unable to fulfill his usual social role, and is, in this sense, disabled. However, the cause of the disability and the nature of the disability is different in each case. Having counted the disability as disability, whatever its cause, we may then attempt to describe episodes of disability, according to their nature and the causes from which they arise.

The procedure of counting all disability as disability, regardless of its cause, is useful because there is an ambiguous definition of diseases, in general, quite over and above these ambiguous definitions that pertain to disorders of mood, thought and behavior. The medical division of illnesses into nosological categories of "diseases" is a useful procedure for diagnosis, but not necessarily a helpful one from the point of understanding and counting phenomena of human health. The usual medical definitions of most diseases do not define them as discrete and independent entities. Many diseases are defined by their manifestations, and the manifestations of one disease can also be manifestations of other diseases. Nor are individual episodes of diseases independent entities in the logical sense. The occurrence of one episode of disease may seriously influence the likelihood that another will occur —in fact, it sometimes almost inevitably implies that the other disease will occur.

Thus, if a man becomes ill and has a discrete episode of "disability" which is attributed to "an acute myocardial infarction," one may, in fact, discover that this man has, in addition to coronary heart disease, generalized atherosclerosis, hypertension, obesity, diabetes mellitus, and a number of other conditions more or less closely interrelated. One may also discover that this diabetes may be regarded as a manifestation of his obesity, that obesity commonly occurs among diabetic people, that hyperlipidemia and atheroscelrosis are manifestations of diabetes, that coronary heart disease is a manifestation of atherosclerosis, that diabetic persons often have hypertension and atheroscelrosis, that hypertension predisposes to myocardial infarction, and so on. It is possible to sort out physiologically and pathologically what is going on in a given case, but the episode of "disability" is better counted and measured independently in terms of its duration and severity, regardless of its assumed cause or causes.

This is not to say that the description of the kinds of impairments and illnesses that are prevalent in populations and their probable causes is not a useful exercise. It is, in fact, a highly valuable maneuver, especially when there is reason to believe that certain aspects of an environment may be associated with the occurrence of certain special kinds of illnesses or injuries. The assessment of the incidence or prevalence of various kinds of illness in human populations is dependent upon standard epidemiological procedures.*

---

* See Note 12, Page 230.

### 3. The Measurement of the Effect of the Environment upon Human Growth and Development

The estimation of variations in human growth and development has a long standing basis in anthropology, medicine, psychology, and education. Measures are available from these various fields which yield valuable information on this point. Many of the measures that are in common use have been applied to a number of populations, and a good deal of normative data are available.

Among the indicators that can be used are the number of abortions and stillbirths in a population, the duration of pregnancies, the birth weight of infants, measures of weight, height, bone maturity, age of walking, talking, rate of growth and height and weight, age of onset of menses, final height, final weight, and various measures for their interrelationship. There are many available measures of intellectual ability, such as those represented by the various standard intelligence tests. There are many other and more complex measures of the development and maturity of the nervous system early in life, of the development of the infant's awareness of its surroundings, and of its ability to relate to people. Indications of many measureable aspects of personality characteristics are available from psychological sources.

Not to be overlooked among these measures is the information that can be obtained from the actual attainment of the individual himself, and of his performance in the social roles potentially available to him. Information relating to how far a child does actually go in school, how rapidly he progresses, how much he assimilates the knowledge that is available to him, the extent to which he moves into the various social roles that are potentially available to him, the degree to which he exhibits types of behavior which are regarded by the society as deviant or undesirable, all can be used as indicators of how a person has matured, fundamentally, and into what social roles he has entered within the environment in which he has grown.

The overall measurements of mortality, morbidity, or disability within human populations has a basis of past experience to recommend it, and some theoretical reason for assuming that more or less "complete" measurements may be made. As an overall proposition, this is probably less true in the area of human development. As compared to the psychological and social indicators of development, the physical measures are easier to use, more standardized, and have a more general applicability; but even these cannot pretend to be complete or global measures. "Global" or "overall" measurements of maturity in terms of behavior or social roles probably is not to be hoped for at this time. However, there is good reason to believe that highly reliable and comparable indicators of discrete types of performance, whether these be intellectual, behavioral, or social, can be applied to population

216

samples, and that these can be made to yield information about the possible effects of environments.

## 4. The Estimation of Environmental Constraints upon Human Activities

If the measurement of human development falls short of having any global indicators, the measurements of the effect of the environment in constraining the activities of people can be said to have no hope of a global indicator at all at this time. We have put forward the suggestion that this is a useful area of information to have about environmental interactions, without any attempt to pretend that the total number or types of human activities which might be influenced by the environment could be estimated, much less measured or described. However, this does not prevent one from studying a population in a manner which allows one to determine what the activities of its members are, and how these activities appear to be influenced by certain discrete or general aspects of the environment.

The procedure is based upon the selection of random samples of the population, the systematic recording of their activities during sample days, and the assessment of the extent to which these activities are interferred with or limited by certain aspects of the environment. The technique that we have used for this purpose is that of the "daily round of life"* which is rather like the time budget which is being used by others. (9)

## 5. The Estimates of the Effects of the Environment on Pleasure and Satisfaction

This area of environmental effects also seems to defy global measurement of an exact nature, but it too appears to be quite amenable to the discrete determination of some effects. The procedure depends upon obtaining a representative sample of the attitudes and opinions of people about various aspects of their environment or about their environment as a whole. The method to be used will undoubtedly be based upon the nature of the population sample that is obtained. Experience suggests that the selection of the sample and the methods that are used for obtaining the opinions and attitudes of the people in it will be critical determinants of the validity of the data. Sometimes the opinions and the attitudes that are *not* sought may be as important in evaluating the results as the ones that are sought.

The report of the individual respondent in the sample will be the final source of data. One can seek individual attitudes and opinions either by interviews or by questionnaire, or one can use more complex procedures that involve projective techniques, or involve the observations of behavior. In general, one must be guided by the experience

---

* See Note 13, Page 230.

and knowledge of those who are skilled at carrying out such surveys. Regardless of the pitfalls involved, the probability that the results would have great validity is attested to by the experience of those who have been engaged in marketing research and in various forms of public opinion sampling over the past few decades. (10)

## D. Some Illustrations of the Use of These Methods

We have proposed that the effect of an environment upon the people in it can be measured by its effects upon:
1. Their rates of mortality
2. Their rates of disability
3. Their growth and development
4. The constraints upon their behavior
5. The pleasure and satisfaction that they receive from the environment.

We have also indicated that when these effects are listed in the order in which they appear above, they are ranked according to their general importance to the society and to the people who live in the environment. Although these methods as a whole have not been systematically applied to the study of environments, parts of them have been applied in various contexts, and their overall application does not appear to be difficult.

### 1. Measurements of Mortality and Morbidity

When there is reason to believe that two populations are similar in the genetic, ethnic, and social backgrounds of their members, and when they have been exposed to dissimilar environments for a sufficient period of years, information which indicates the effects of these environments upon the two population groups, may already be in existence.

Tables V, VI and VII give some information relevant to the mortality and morbidity of members of the black population living in the rural south, and living in New York State during the period between 1960 and 1970. The mortality data, derived from the U.S. Vital and Health Statistics indicate that blacks living in New York State (nearly all of whom live in urban areas) have death rates and infant mortality rates that are slightly lower than those of blacks living in South Carolina, the majority of whom live in rural areas (Table V). A direct comparison between the infant mortality rates among blacks living in northeastern metropolitan areas as compared to southern rural areas indicates a similar advantage with those in the northeast. The morbidity data obtained from the National Health Survey indicates that the blacks who live in the northeast have a distinctly lower rate of disability, whether this be measured by days of bed disability, days of restricted activity, or days of work loss, and that a smaller proportion of them have three or more chronic conditions (Table VI). However, the relative fre-

218

quency of some of the causes of mortality and morbidity in the two populations are somewhat different (Table VII).

These data on morbidity and mortality suggest that regardless of the occurrence of juvenile delinquency, drug addiction, crime, and unemployment among the urban blacks in the north, this environment is healthier for them than the rural environment of the south. These figures might be buttressed by additional information relating to their growth and development, which indicate that in the northern urban environment, the birth weight of Negro children is higher, the number of impairments are fewer, and the level of schooling attained by the population is higher. The per capita income of the black population is also higher —a figure which may be of some importance, since the overall level of income of the members of the American population shows close and positive association with many indicators of their health.

When populations are relatively small and when data on their health have not been collected on an on-going basis, some of the cross-sectional methods that we have propesed can be used. Table VIII is an illustration of data obtained by this method, which we used several years ago to compare the health of a sample of men and a sample of women who work for a large industrial concern in New York City. (11) These two samples were drawn from populations of several thousand men and women who were of comparable age, who lived in New York City, and who worked for the same company in an area on the upper East Side of New York City. The data were obtained from reviewing the health of the members of these two samples over a 25 year period from age 20 to age 45, approximately, using questionnaire-guided histories, examinations, and records according to the procedure that we have described in notes 10, 11 and 12. At issue was the question of why the amount of disability experienced by the women was greater than the amount of disability experienced by the men, when the death rate among men was known to be higher than that among women at all ages.

The calculation of the mean number of days of disability (days of sickness absence) indicated that the women in the sample had indeed had more disability than the men during the observation period. The rate was 10.5 days per woman per year during the first 20 years of observation and 20.5 days per woman per year during the next 5 years when the women were in their early 40's. Comparable rates for the men were 4.30 days of disability per man per year during the first 20 years, and 7.6 days per man per year during the next five years. Table VIII indicates how the illnesses were distributed into categories according to the organ systems affected, and shows that, in general, the women had experienced more episodes of disability and recorded illness involving most of their organ systems. However, Table IX shows that the majority of these episodes of illness were relatively minor, and probably not life threatening. In Table X we have applied the concept of "seriousness" to the illnesses, multiplying the incidence of illnesses by their seriousness. The result indicates that although the men had relatively fewer episodes of disability, the overall seriousness of their illnesses was much greater. This is another way of saying that their likelihood of death from illness was greater. The existence of the greater likelihood of death was supported by the finding of a higher death rate among the men in this population. Further indication of the probable validity of this procedure was the fact that the incidence of very serious illnesses such as pneumonia, tuberculosis, hypertensive cardiovascular disease, and arteriosclerotic heart disease was $2\frac{1}{2}$ times as high among men as among women during the 20 year observation period.

Thus, the intensive study of a rather small sample of men and women drawn from a larger population appears to have yielded a reliable guide to both their morbidity and mortality, while at the same time, illustrating the extent to which these two indicators of health measure different aspects of health and well being.

These are not intended to be ideal illustrations of the use of measures of morbidity and mortality, as indicators of the effects of environment. The intent is more to show how they can be used. In actual practice one would select and define the environments to be compared in some precise manner, and would take measures to insure that the study samples of the populations which have been exposed to this environment are comparable not only in their genetic characteristics, but also in their age, and in the length and nature of their exposure, and one would take care to insure that the data relating to morbidity and mortality were obtained in an identical manner for the two populations. The same can be said for the measures of growth and development.

## 2. Measurements of the Constraints upon Human Behavior

In many instances features of the environment which are thought to have an adverse effect upon human health and well-being do not create demonstrable or measurable mortality or morbidity during a period available for observation, and any effects that they may create over the long run are obscured by the effects of other and more powerful causes of ill health. Nevertheless, such features of the environment may create powerful constraints upon human behavior. Such a situation was found during the study of the relation of Kennedy International Airport to the people of the surrounding areas of New York City. (2) The noise and the aircraft and automobile emissions that are associated with the operation of the airport did not create any excess of human death or disability which could be clearly demonstrated from the available records or from on-going observations, and the occasional death attributable to aircraft accidents in the vicinity of the airport created a relatively small risk of death compared to the vast number of deaths that were created by other causes. However, a calculation of the noise level around the airport and its effect upon the members of the surrounding population, indicated that more than 700,000 people live within an area in which the noise of the aircraft interfered with their sleep. In this same area there were 266 public and private schools, attended by approximately 275,000 pupils whose schooling was interrupted regularly by aircraft noise. It was also ascertained that within this same area church services, community meetings, outdoor conversations, and outdoor gatherings of all sorts, were inhibited or interfered with by the noise. In addition, numbers of the residents had felt that they were forced to install air-conditioning in their living quarters because the pervading noise became unbearable if the windows were open. The presence of the airport, therefore, prevented large numbers of people from carrying out activities that they wished to carry out, and it was found that the the number of people thus affected, and the types of activities that were interrupted could be counted and tabulated. Many of these people were also constrained to carry out other activities which they would not ordinarily have carried out, in the sense that some installed air-conditioning in houses, and some took other measures to soundproof them, and in many instances people gave up their present houses or apartments and moved to other areas.

A study of the community attitude towards noise, based on individual interviews with a sample of over a thousand randomly selected residents in 169 different locations within the "NEF 30"* noise level area around the airport, indicated a high level of dissatisfaction with the airport as an aspect of the environment. A method of indirect questioning was used to ascertain the level of expressed annoyance of the members of the population sample. Only 7% reported no anoyance, while 93% said they were annoyed. The sample attitudes indicated that a majority of those tested found that aircraft noise interfered with their rest and relaxation inside their homes, and prevented them from engaging in outside activities. The majority reported that the noise interfered with conversation, with telephone listening, and with sleep, and some of those questioned described symptoms such as fatigue, which might be regarded as relevant to their health.

By careful sampling procedures, the technique of the daily round-of-life and the use of questionnaire-guided interviews or psychological tests can also be used to indicate how an environment places constraints upon the behavior of the people in it, or influences their attitudes. Tables XI and XII were derived from the use of the daily round-of-life technique to study some of the daily patterns of activities of a

---

* A "Noise-Exposure Forecast Area" within which the expected community reaction against aircraft noise would not be compatible with the use of the land for residences, schools, hospitals, churches, etc.

group of men in their mid 50's, all of whom worked in the same occupation, in the same area, and for the same company. (*11*) The question at issue was the extent to which the patterns of activity of the men were influenced by their employment, and by their educational and social class background. It was evident that both of these variables influenced many aspects of the men's daily activities, and that men of different educational background might be very different in their habits and activities, even when they were of identical ages and working in the same job with the same company. Table XIII indicates some of the attitudes and feelings of these men, which were assessed by questionnaires and by directed interviews. The same variables were considered, and similar results were obtained.

## Part II Notes, Tables and Bibliography

### A. Notes

1. "Free energy," broadly speaking, is energy that is available for doing work.

2. "Information," broadly speaking, is the property of matter and energy that has to do with its degree of order, or lack of randomness. (*6*) It is the property which provides the basis for organized systems and structures, for "non-random" and apparently "purposeful" behavior, and for communication.

3. For example, most foods are highly organized organic materials with a considerable information content. Since they are only partly broken down before being absorbed, the intake of food, in itself, represents a considerable acquisition of information (order) as well as energy from the environment. (*4*) The process of "recognizing" the useful organic substances in ingested foodstuffs, and of rejecting those which are not useful, goes on within the epithelial cells of the gastrointestinal tract as a part of the process of digestion. It involves intracellular information processing of some complexity. Complex intracellular mechanisms for information processing are also involved in the immune reactions and cellular defense mechanisms that exist in some cells of the gastrointestinal tract, as well as in some cells of the skin and the respiratory tract.

4. To give examples: 1) If a man has been adapting to an air temperature considerably colder than his body tempearture by wearing heavy clothing and keeping active (as he might on a ski slope), then, if the air becomes colder, the adaptive demands upon the man may become greater; but, if the air warms up significantly, the adaptive demands upon the man that arise from a cold ambient environment may become less. 2) If a man has been working late at night at a second job

in order to support his family, the birth of another child may increase the demands upon him; but if no new child is born an increase in his income from his first job may allow him to give up the second job and reduce the demands upon him for excess hours of purposeful effort.

"Atherosclerosis" is a generic term used to describe a number of disease processes characterized by the gradual accumulation of lipid materials in the linings of the arteries. One of these processes appears to be the result of the consumption of an abundant diet, high in animal fat and protein, over a long period of time, beginning early in life. Atherosclerosis usually causes no obvious disability, whatever, until a person has lived well into the middle years of his life, at which time the gradual narrowing or occlusion of the blood vessels supplying his heart has advanced to a point at which lack of blood causes an interference with the metabolism of the heart muscle. At this time the electrical activity of his heart muscles can be easily disrupted, and he may die abruptly and unexpectedly. In this instance, the interaction between the man and his environment that leads to his untimely death is mediated largely by nature of his dietary intake, although the level of his caloric expenditure in physical activity probably affects the development of the pathological conditions to some extent.

"Arterial hypertension" is a second chronic disease of apparent environmental origin which may cause no evident disability for many years, and which may be discovered quite incidentally during the course of a routine examination of an apparently healthy person. This condition, after many years, creates a great susceptibility to the development of strokes, of "heart attacks" and of other medical disasters which may greatly shorten life. The dietary intake of salts and other minerals, over the course of many years, is thought to play a role in the development of this disorder, but it appears that another significant role in its development may be environmental influences mediated by the central nervous system. In short, there is reason to believe that people who perceive other people and other members of their social group as hostile or threatening, and who see their social role as humiliating and degrading may react with sustained, but suppressed feelings of rage which are accompanied by cardiovascular reactions that lead to or enhance the occurrence of hypertension. For this reason, the position of the Negro in American society during the past 200 years is thought, by some, to have been an important factor in the high prevalence of hypertension among members of this group.

5. A typical example of this is the common vascular headache, or migraine. Migraine headaches may recur at frequent intervals throughout the active life of a person, prostrate him for a day or two on each occasion, but not shorten his life at all. (George Bernard Shaw had severe migraine until he was beyond the age of 70, but he lived to the age of 96.) The common cold is also an example of an illness

which is associated with some disability but without any great threat to life. It has been estimated that fewer than one in 10,000 common colds is followed by the development of a fatal illness.

6. For example, in the case of the common cold, the mechanism most impotrant in the genesis of the syndrome appears to be infection with a virus, of which more than 100 are now known to be capable of causing this reaction. However, a syndrome very similar to the common cold may be caused by allergenic agents, or by toxic or irritating dust, because the nasal adaptive reactions which are initiated by these environmental agents are very similar to those initiated by viral infection. On the other hand, an illness such as migraine, appears to be based on an underlying predisposition, which is genetically determined, and to be initiated by environmental influences that arise out of the reaction of the person to the people around him and to his role in society. The reaction of the individual may involve sustained purposeful activity, arousal, sleeplessness, and intermittent periods of depression as well as the vascular phenomena that are involved in the headaches.

7. For example, if a man lives at the end of the runway of an airport, the noise of airplanes may interfere with his sleep. Sleep is a fundamental biological need. It is generally desirable that sleep be uninterrupted. Although it is evident that occasional interruptions of sleep are tolerated by people for long periods without apparent harm to them, people in general prefer not to have their sleep interrupted. The occasional noise of airplanes passing over the head of a man and interrupting his sleep does not necessarily shorten his life span, make him ill, or impair his development, but it does prevent him from sleeping when he wishes to do so. In order to have uninterrupted sleep he may have to find his sleep at times when the runway is not in use, or find it at some other place.

Similarly, if a man lives in a suburb and works in the city, he may have to travel for some time each morning and each afternoon on a train, bus or automobile, in order to get to and from his place of work. The trip does not, in itself, do him any harm; but it does represent an activity that he must undertake which he would not necessarily undertake if his home were nearer to his place of work. Examples such as this can be multiplied readily. If a house containing a family of five has only one bathroom, some members of the family may have to wait while others use the facilities in the morning. If a house does not have an installed source of hot water, those who wish to use hot water will have to warm it up on the stove, or by some other means. If there is only one bedroom for a family of four, if there are panes missing from the windows, or if there is no central heating, the people who live in this house may be, in various ways, constrained from carrying out their desired activities, or forced to carry out activities that they would not engage in otherwise.

8. One of the major problems for those who attempted to maximize the health, welfare, and freedom of action of individuals arises from the conflict between the needs of the social group, and the needs of the individual. These are not the same. Social groups behave as if the needs of the group, for cohesion and for survival, take precedence over the needs of the individual members for the satisfaction of their biological drives and their personal preferences. In the last analysis, social groups behave as if the needs of the group take precedence even over the maintenance of the health of the individual members. Under special circumstances, the needs of the social group take precedence even over the maintenance of the lives of the members.

In the biological sense, a social group is an adaptive arrangement which makes it possible for the group as a whole to cope with its environment and to provide for the protection, development, reproduction, and survival of its members to an extent that would not be possible if these were dependent upon individual action alone. The social group provides for the sharing of tasks and the assignment of roles to those members of the group who are, to a certain extent, biologically "best fitted" to carry out these roles. Although the members as a whole, and the group as a whole, benefit by this arrangement, this benefit is attained at the expense of limitations upon the freedom of action of the individuals, and upon their opportunities to satisfy their biological needs.

This is, perhaps, more obviously apparent among the rather simple social groups of the higher animals than it is among the more complex and sophisticated social groups of humans. In a primate social group, for example, the mothers, the newborn, and the immature may be given special preference with regard to protection and food, even at the expense of the group. But, in return for this, they allow themselves to be guided and dominated by other members of the group. The mature dominant males maintain almost exclusive possession of the sexually available females, but they may have to compete among themselves for this privilege, and this competition can be damaging or even fatal to the loser. These males pay for their dominant role in the group, in part, by defending the group against predators, and this role as protector of the group may be fatal to them.

Biological constraints on behavior are usually not so crude and obvious in human societies; nevertheless, all human societies are bound together by innumerable and often quite subtle constraints upon the behavior of their members. The free expression of hostility and aggressive behavior between members of human societies must be suppressed or constrained under almost all circumstances, or social groups would fall apart. Constraints upon sexual behavior, and wide-spread rules about individual possessions, precedence, and status seem to be essential features of all human societies. In nearly all societies there are a very large number of social roles, for each of which there are many learned, and largely implicit, rules governing behavior. These pervade almost every aspect of human life. All societies also have hierarchical characteristics, with rights, privileges, responsibilities, and duties unevenly distributed among their members. These are accorded to some and denied to others for various reasons. One result of this is that the exposure to, and the opportunity to make use of, various parts of the man-made environment are not equally distributed among the members of society. Indeed, the sum total of goods and services available to people is not equally distributed.

The implication of this is that the adverse or beneficial effects of the man-made environment, or portions of it, cannot be separated from the societal determinants which so largely decide who will be exposed to what portion of the environment, and in what way. Even beyond this, since restrictions upon the expression of aggression, and upon the satisfaction of sexual drives, and upon opportunities for sleep, rest, recreation, food, and the like, may have important implications for health, and since these are an inherent feature of life in any human social group, changes in the human environment which are beneficial to the health of the individual, may not be beneficial to the social group as a whole. An aspect of the environment which is "good" for the social group may be "bad" for many of the people in it, and vice versa. Efforts to "improve" the environment often encounter this dilemma.

9. This is approximately the order in which our society values environmental effects, if one can judge by the effort and attention that is given to alleviating those affects that are regarded as undesirable. In general, more concern is given to the prevention of death than to the prevention of illness. Among illnesses, more concern is given to the prevention and treatment of those that are potentially lethal than is given to the prevention and treatment of those that are merely disabling, and more concern is given to those that may be followed by permanent impairment than is given to those from which a complete recovery is the rule. In general, more concern is given to the prevention and treatment of illness, as such, than is given to providing circumstances under which the growth and development of people will proceed optimally. When there are concerns about growth and development, these are chiefly focused upon the prevention of clear-cut defects. If the general behavior of the society can be taken as a guide, the prevention and treatment, even of those illnesses from which recovery is the general rule, seems to take precedence over the provision of circumstances under which optimal human development may occur. That is to say, the society seems to act as if it is more important to eradicate measles among all children than it is to provide optimal or even ade-

226

quate public schools for all children. Yet, regardless of how much the provision for schooling may have been neglected, the provision for an adequate school system, historically, preceded public (societal) efforts for removing the constraints and disabilities placed upon people by inadequate housing, inadequate transportation, and the poor design and construction of cities. Furthermore, when public concern for housing, urban renewal, or transportation was first expressed by the construction of new facilities, these facilities were designed to eliminate the disabilities and constraints inherent in the previously inadequate artifacts, without major concern for the pleasure or satisfaction of those who might use them. Pleasure and satisfaction were placed at the very tail-end of the hierarchy of values. Possibly as a result of this, people who live in the housing developments that have been provided in the last few decades, and who ride to work on the subways, do not usually complain so much that the roofs leak, the buildings are unheated, or the subways do not travel rapidly enough, as they complain about the discomfort and the many causes of dissatisfaction that they find in their housing and means of transportation.

It is possible to rank environments, or various features of environments, according to the seriousness of their effects upon the people who are exposed to them, as we have done in the paragraphs above, but it would be wrong to suppose that people themselves always behave as if they valued all aspects of the environments in the order that we have just ranked them. In fact, people often behave quite otherwise. People continue to smoke cigarettes, drink whiskey, and drive over-powered cars at a rapid rate because of the satisfaction that these activities provide them, in spite of the abundant, and quite apparent evidence of the potentially lethal effects of these activities. A man will intoxicate himself with whiskey even though he knows quite well that on the next day he will have a transient disabling illness as a result of the alcohol that he has consumed. Unless one prevents people from doing so, they will eat raw oysters, drink unpasturized milk, and swim in sewage-filled waters, with the full knowledge that these might be followed by life endangering infectious diseases. People spend more money on their health than on their education, and more money on their houses and on their automobiles than upon their health. If people regard certain types of clothing or certain types of dwellings as beautiful or satisfying, they may use these in spite of any impracticality or discomfort that may be associated with them. Indeed, people often seek satisfaction and pleasure from activities such as sky diving, skiing, or sports car racing, not in spite of, but because of, the element of danger to life which is inherent in these activities.

The implications of this, from the point of view of measurement of the quality of the environment, is that it is probably not wise to regard one category of environmental effects upon people as being over-riding in relation to all others at all times. It seems wiser to have methods of measuring or tabulating environmental effects independently, so that the various "qualities of the environment" can be estimated without, at the same time, making an absolute value judgment among them. Yet it is also important to have a scheme for rank ordering the effect of the environment upon people and with the *caveat* we have just mentioned, we propose to use the rank order that we have just described.

10. In attempting to deal with this problem, several years ago we adopted the device of defining the "seriousness" of an episode of illness as "the likelihood that this episode of illness or its sequelae, if untreated, will lead to the death of the subject." The likelihood of death from a given episode of illness, we regarded as being indicated by that proportion of similar episodes of illness that would lead to death if an infinite sample of such illness episodes were taken. This, in turn, is regarded as being closely proportionate to the reported "case fatality rate" for untreated cases of this disease and its sequelae. The case fatality rates of episodes of illness may be expressed as probabilities from 1.0 (100% fatal) to 0.0 (never fatal). There are data available in the medical literature providing estimates of the case fatality rates of many illnesses. These are not exact, but the variations in the case fatality rates among different diseases is so great that the likelihood of death from a serious illness is orders of magnitude greater than the likelihood of death from a trivial illness. The likelihood of death from a given episode of illness is, therefore, most conveniently expressed, as a negative whole power of 10. That is to say, a disease which has an expected case fatality rate of somewhere between 10% and 100% (between 0.1 and 0.999) can be described as having a case fatality rate of $10^{-1}$. A disease which carries with it a case fatality rate between 1% and 10% can have this expressed as $10^{-2}$, and so on. (See Table I)

By this scale, for example, lobar pneumonia, or malignant melanoma (a form of cancer) which have case fatality rates greater than 10% if they are untreated, can be assigned a seriousness of $10^{-1}$, while the common cold or the common vascular headache, which are fatal in less 1 in 10,000 cases, may be assigned a seriousness of $10^{-5}$. Published case fatality rates are not available for many diseases, and for these, one must estimate rates. Fortunately, most diseases for which published rates are not available are diseases of little seriousness, and usuable estimates of case fatality rates are available for most of the serious illnesses. Because "seriousness ratings" represent powers of 10, and because the "serious ratings" of all of the episodes of illness experienced by a given period of time are to be added together, accuracy in estimating the rates for more serious illnesses far outweighs the effect of any inaccuracy in estimating the rates for those which are less serious.

Using this method of rating, and a method of examining and history taking which provides an estimate of all of the episodes of illness that have occurred in the members of a population over a given period of time, one can rate each episode of illness during this period according to its "seriousness." This "seriousness rating" may then be totaled for each person, for each year, or each period of years. This will yield a value for each person in the sample which is generally proportional to his risk of death from illness during the years of the observation period: These values, when compared from person to person, probably indicate the rank order in which they risk death. Averaged over a population and compared with another population, over a similar period of time, but in a different environmental situation, they will probably yield an indicator of the relative lethality of the effects of living in the two environments. (12)

There have been no adequate prospective studies of the use of this method under these circumstances in order to determine whether predictions will actually be born out by the observation of subsequent mortality. However, the use of methods such as this for predicting mortality for insurance purposes, and for predicting the likelihood of death from diseases, such as coronary heart disease, indicate that methods such as this do work with some accuracy. (13) There is reason to believe that the method here proposed might be a useful one for studying the relative lethal effects of various environments on various populations.

11. The scheme that we have used for measuring disability is based on five grades of "severity" as follows:

"Disabling illnesses" are of two grades of severity:

Severity 5—illnesses that are totally prostrating;

Severity 4—illnesses that prevent a person from fulfillnig his primary social role, and require him to assume the "sick role," but are not totally prostrating.

"Partly Disabling illnesses" fall into three grades of severity, of which only one, "severity 3" is usually utilized:

Severity 3—illnesses which do not prevent a person from carrying out his usual social role, but make it necessary for him to do this in a restricted manner.

Examples of such partly disabling illnesses are many episodes of peptic ulcer and diabetes mellitus, some forms of hypertensive cardiovascular disease, the common cold, and a mild vascular headache. People with diabetes can do almost anything that other people do, but some of them have to be careful of what they eat, and have to limit their activities because of the insulin they take. People with the pain of a peptic ulcer or the discomfort of a common cold, or minor headache, may continue to carry on the usual activities, but with less effectiveness.

Severity 2 and Severity 1—illnesses below the third grade of severity. Two grades of "disability" below grade three can be recognized. One of these is associated with a definite impairment of one or more organ systems, but with little or no effect upon the capacity of the individual to carry out his usual activities. Examples of this are moderate grades of obesity or the early stages of hypertension. Here, one can recognize that there are some abnormalities of the functions of the organs of the individual, but these do not impair his activities to any significant extent. A still lower grade of severity is associated with some bodily disorders that can be recognized as being present at a cellular level, but which do not impair organ function as such, to any significant degree. These are of theoretical interest only at this time. (Table II)

12. For the estimation of the overall prevalence of illnesses of all sorts in a population at a given time, and for estimating the frequency and probable causes of all episodes of illness over the past, one can utilize a cross-sectional survey with special medical historical questionnaires designed to provide appropriate estimates. We have developed such a questionnaire which we have used in a number of populations during the past ten years. It is based upon the nosological scheme used in the *Standard Nomenclature of Diseases and Operations* (*13*) which has been prepared by the American Medical Association for use in the classification of hospital statistics. This scheme is somewhat similar to one used in the *International Statistical Classification of Diseases.* (*12*) It divides illness into diseases or "syndromes," each of which is further divided into "episodes." Each episode or syndrome is classified according to which of 19 arbitrary "organ systems" is the major site of its manifestation, and according to which of 11 "etiological" categories best describes its "cause." (see Tables III and IV)

Using a scheme such as this, one can estimate, for a given individual over a period of time, the number of syndromes he has exhibited, the number of episodes of each syndrome, the number of his organ systems involved in illness, and the number of etiological categories in which his illness fell. According to a classification such as this, the "common cold" represents a "syndrome." A given "cold" lasting for, let us say three days, represents one "episode" of this syndrome. This episode would be located primarily in the "respiratory system" and the etiological category in which it would be placed is that of "infectious "disease."

13. The technique of the "daily round-of-life" is based upon the selection of probability samples of populations, and the determination of the 24 hour activities of members of these populations during selected samples of days. The days are selected so as to take into account the variations of activities with days of the week and with the seasons of the year. The gathering of this information is achieved by

230

the use of a standard questionnaire-diary review of the day's activity, beginning at the time that a person awakens and carrying him through the full 24 hour cycle until he awakens the next morning. In serial form, he is asked to describe what he does, how he does it, where he is when he does it, with whom he does it, and how he feels about it. He accounts for the entire day on an hour by hour, or even minute by minute basis.

One thus obtains from each individual in a population sample such data, for example, as how he dresses, where he sleeps, what he does before breakfast, what he has for breakfast, with whom and where he has it, where he goes at the end of his first meal, how he gets to work, what work he does, with whom he does it, what his attitude is toward it, and so on. The information samples can include representative data from work days, week ends, holidays, and at various seasons.

A great deal of information can be obtained from data of this type. One can obtain information about the nature of a person's dwelling, his relation to the people around him, the means of transportation that he uses, the nature of his occupation, his daily caloric expenditure, what he eats, how much he smokes or drinks, what his recreation is, who his companions are, and so on. Discrete areas of information from one population group can be compared with similar data from other population groups. Then, if there are questions about the nature and characteristics of a person's dwelling or of the number of people who live in it, the means of transportation he uses and the characteristics of his job, the nature of his associates, his opportunity for recreations and so on, one can obtain systematic information about these features of the world in which he lives and their apparent effect upon his daily life.

This method of surveying can be used in population samples and can be used to provide evidence bearing upon discrete questions. In surveys, during the past 10 years, we have used this mechanism in order to determine the amount and types of recreation that people engage in, the time it takes them to travel to their work, the means of transportation they use, their reaction to delays in traffic, their relations to people they work with, the amount of time they spend at lunch, and (with the help of suitable tables of caloric expenditure) their daily activity in terms of calories expended.

Such a body of information can be used to ask further discrete or general information about some of the constraints that an environment places upon those who use it. For example, if there are questions about the duration of sleep, the interruption of sleep, the privacy of sleep, these data can be obtained. If there are questions about what methods of transportation are used, how frequently they are used, how much time during the day is spent in travel and whether or not this creates fatigue, these data, too, can be obtained. A subjects attitudinal statements can reveal how he perceives his environment and what aspects of it appear to him to be most unsatisfactory and for what reason, or one can use data from this sort of survey to compare the social roles of the members to populations, the number of recreations they engage in, what they eat, and the like.

## B. Tables

### TABLE I—The Scale of "Seriousness"

| "Seriousness" rating of illness | Probability that an episode will be fatal if untreated |
|:---:|:---:|
| 1 | $P < 1{:}10{,}000 \ (< 10^{-4})$ |
| 2 | $1{:}1{,}000 > P > 1{:}10{,}000 \ (< 10^{-3} > 10^{-4})$ |
| 3 | $1{:}100 \ \ > P > 1{:}1{,}000 \ (< 10^{-2} > 10^{-3})$ |
| 4 | $1{:}10 \ \ > P > 1{:}100 \ (< 10^{-1} > 10^{-2})$ |
| 5 | $P > 1{:}10 \ (< 10^{1} > 10^{-1})$ |

The "Seriousness Rating" is obtained by adding five to the negative number indicating the power of ten that represents the probability. Thus, the "seriousness rating" of the least serious illness $(P < 10^{-4})$ becomes 5–4, or 1. In this manner "seriousness" is rated from 1 to 5, with the "most serious" illnesses having the highest mark.

232

## TABLE II—Rating the "Severity" of Illness

| "Severity" rating of illness | Characteristics |
|---|---|

1. Illnesses associated with a definite abnormality of cells or metabolic systems, but not seriously impairing the function of any organ system.

Examples: Orthostatic albuminuria; latent syphilis manifested only by sero-positivity; small benign naevus.

2. Illnesses associated with a definite impairment of one or more organ systems, but having little or no effect opon the capacity of the individual to carry out his usual activiies.

Examples: Functional constipation; moderate grades of obesity; early stages of hypertensive vascular disease.

3. Illnesses which seriously impair the function of one or more organ sysems, but which have little effect on the highest integrative functions, so that the individual may carry out his usual activities.

Examples: Many episodes of active peptic ulcer; diabetes mellitus; hypertensive cardiovascular disease; the common cold; vascular headache.

4. Illnesses which prevent an individual from carrying out his usual activities, but do not prevent all other activities.

Examples: Measles; fracture of ankle; moderately severe anxiety state; many episodes of the common cold or dysmenorrhea; any disease which causes absence from work or "bed disability."

5. Illnesses which severely impair the highest integrative functions and make it impossible for the individual to carry out any activities other than those directly associated with survival.

Examples: Meningococcus meningitis; hepatic coma; typhoid; catatonic schizophrenia.

## TABLE III—Categories of Illness
### (Organ systems)

| | | Topographic category in "standard nomenclature" |
|---|---|---|
| 1. | Congenital conditions and sequelae | 0 |
| 2. | Generalized illnesses | 0 |
| 3. | Respiratory | 3 |
| 4. | Gastrointestinal | 6 |
| 5. | Hepatic | 6 |
| 6. | Biliary and pancreatic | 6 |
| 7. | Genito-urinary | 7 |
| 8. | Cardiovascular | 4 |
| 9. | Hemic and lymphatic | 5 |
| 10. | Metabolic and endocrine | 8 |
| 11. | Articular and skeletal | 2 |
| 12. | Muscular | 2 |
| 13. | Dermal | 1 |
| 14. | Cranial | Various |
| 15. | Aural | x |
| 16. | Ophthalmic | x |
| 17. | Dental | 6 |
| 18. | Neural | 9 |
| 19. | Mood, thought, behavior | 9 |

Also tabulated:
Injuries
Surgical operations

## TABLE IV—The "Etiologic Categories"

0.  Diseases* due to prenatal influence
1.  Diseases or infections due to a lower plant or animal parasite
2.  Diseases or infections due to a higher plant or animal parasite
3.  Diseases due to intoxication
4.  Diseases due to trauma or physical agent
5a. Diseases secondary to circulatory disturbance
5b. Diseases secondary to disturbance of innervation or of psychic control
6.  Diseases due to or consisting of static mechanical abnormality (obstruction, calculus, displacement or gross change in form) due to unknown cause
7.  Diseases due to disorder of metabolism, growth, or nutrition
8.  New growths
9.  Diseases due to unknown or uncertain cause with the structural reaction (degenerative, infiltrative, inflammatory, proliferative, sclerotic, or reparative) manifest; hereditary and familial diseases of this nature
x.  Diseases due to unknown or uncertain cause with the functional reaction alone manifest; hereditary and familial diseases of this nature
y.  Diseases of undetermined cause

* In the sense of any considerable departure from the normal structure or function.

Taken from **The Standard Nonmenclature of Diseases and Operations.** 4th Ed., 1952, copyrighted by A.M.A., pub. Blakeston Div., McGraw-Hill Book Co., Inc., N.Y.

### TABLE V—Mortality Among Negroes in Northeastern and Southern Regions

|  | New York | South Carolina |
|---|---|---|
| Death rate/1,000 residents ................. | 8.3 | 10.0 |
| Infant mortality/1,000 live births ........... | 36.8 | 37.8 |
|  | Metropolitan areas Northeast | Rural areas South |
| Infant mortality/1,000 live births ........... | 37.1 | 44.5 |

Source: U.S. Vital and Health Statistics, 1967

### TABLE VI—Disability Among Negroes in Northeastern and Southern Regions

|  | Northeast | South |
|---|---|---|
| Days of bed disability * .......................... | 6.4 | 7.4 |
| Days of work loss * ............................... | 4.7 | 7.8 |
| Days of restricted activity * .................... | 14.0 | 17.3 |
| Percent of people with +3 chronic conditions ......... | 7.7 | 12.3 |

* Rate per person per year
Source: National Health Survey, 1965-67

234

## TABLE VII—Mortality Among "Non-White" Males in New York and South Carolina, 1963-67

|  | New York | South Carolina |
|---|---|---|
| Death rate/1,000 | 8.3 | 10.0 |
| Infant mortality/1,000 live births | 36.8 | 37.8 |
| Accidental deaths/100,000 |  |  |
|     Motor vehicle | 13.2 | 30.1 |
|     Other | 37.9 | 63.8 |
| Diseases of the heart/100,000 | 452.5 | 314.4 |
| Vascular lesions affecting CNS/100,000 | 76.7 | 202.5 |
| Influenza and pneumonia/100,000 | 64.9 | 87.1 |

Sources: U.S. Vital and Health Statistics and National Health Survey

## TABLE VIII—Men and Women in a Similar Environment from Ages 20 to 40
Illness Recorded Over 20 years

| Categories of illness ("organ systems") | Episodes per 100 persons per year | |
|---|---|---|
|  | Men | Women |
| 1. Generalized illnesses | 0.60 | 0.47 |
| 2. Respiratory | 68.70 | 98.96 |
| 3. Gastrointestinal | 27.58 | 47.84 |
| 4. Hepatic | 0.09 | 0.00 |
| 5. Biliary and pancreatic | 0.22 | 1.09 |
| 6. Genito-urinary | 0.69 | 16.64 |
| 7. Cardiovascular | 0.99 | 0.47 |
| 8. Hemic and lymphatic | 0.00 | 0.42 |
| 9. Metabolic and endocrine | 1.03 | 3.28 |
| 10. Articular and skeletal | 2.70 | 2.03 |
| 11. Muscular | 7.82 | 16.43 |
| 12. Dermal | 9.26 | 16.49 |
| 13. Cranial | 1.51 | 8.89 |
| 14. Aural | 2.10 | 2.81 |
| 15. Ophthalmic | 5.90 | 4.99 |
| 16. Dental | 8.53 | 9.83 |
| 17. Neural | 0.04 | 0.20 |
| 18. Mood, thought, behavior | 1.59 | 7.38 |
| 19. Congenital conditions and sequelae | 1.55 | 0.15 |
| Totals | 140.90 | 238.37 |

## TABLE IX—Men and Women in a Similar Environment from Ages 20 to 40
### Major sources of the difference in rates of disability

| Syndromes | Episodes per 100 persons per year | | |
|---|---|---|---|
| | Men | Women | Difference |
| Rate for all syndromes | 140.90 | 238.37 | 97.47 |
| Common cold, "grippe", and "sore throat" | 64.22 | 88.45 | 24.23 |
| Acute gastroenteritis | 21.64 | 48.31 | 26.67 |
| Dysmenorrhea | 0.00 | 15.24 | 15.24 |
| "Mylalgia" and myositis" | 7.83 | 16.34 | 8.51 |
| Minor abrasions, contusions, and lacerations | 0.22 | 8.10 | 7.88 |
| Headaches | 1.51 | 8.89 | 7.38 |
| Minor episodes of anxiety, tension, or other mood disturbance | 1.42 | 5.98 | 4.56 |
| Differences in rates for these syndromes | | | 94.47 |

## TABLE X—Men and Women in a Similar Environment from Ages 20 to 40
### Annual Risk of Death

Incidence of Illnesses Experienced Multiplied by Their Seriousness

| Categories of illness | Men | Women |
|---|---|---|
| 1. Generalized illnesses | 152.272 | 73.994 |
| 2. Respiratory | 653.849 | 452.903 |
| 3. Gastrointestinal | 128.686 | 104.186 |
| 4. Hepatic | 21.550 | 76.440 |
| 5. Biliary and pancreatic | 8.620 | 0.000 |
| 6. Genito-urinary | 133.623 | 165.468 |
| 7. Cardiovascular | 392.460 | 52.135 |
| 8. Hemic and lymphatic | 0.000 | 3.224 |
| 9. Metabolic and endocrine | 90.557 | 34.953 |
| 10. Articular and skeletal | 9.030 | 50.700 |
| 11. Muscular | 0.782 | 3.702 |
| 12. Dermal | 19.319 | 19.592 |
| 13. Cranial | 0.151 | 0.889 |
| 14. Aural | 1.684 | 1.029 |
| 15. Ophthalmic | 2.335 | 2.043 |
| 16. Dental | 1.823 | 2.107 |
| 17. Neural | 0.043 | 0.000 |
| 18. Mood, thought, behavior | 3.745 | 147.082 |
| 19. Congenital conditions and sequelae | 1.076 | 0.015 |
| Total | 1621.605 | 1190.462 |

## TABLE XI—Men Aged 55-60

Working for One Company in One State
Daily Round of Life Week-Days
(in percent)

| | No college | | | | College | |
|---|---|---|---|---|---|---|
| | Work-men | Fore-men | Super-visors | Mana-gers | Super-visors | Mana-gers |
| Men in category who: | | | | | | |
| Arise later than 0700 | 17 | 22 | 53 | 58 | 48 | 45 |
| Travel to work >½ hr. | 24 | 27 | 49 | 54 | 70 | 72 |
| In own car, self-driven | 67 | 71 | 56 | 38 | 30 | 20 |
| By train | 1 | 11 | 25 | 37 | 43 | 55 |
| Walk—all or part | 10 | 7 | 0 | 12 | 22 | 23 |
| During work day spend: | | | | | | |
| More than ½ of day sitting | 14 | 29 | 43 | 41 | 75 | 72 |
| More than ½ of day standing | 27 | 2 | 0 | 0 | 0 | 0 |
| More than ½ of day walking about | 27 | 24 | 9 | 10 | 4 | 3 |
| ¼ day or more driving | 18 | 21 | 21 | 20 | 4 | 3 |
| ¼ day or more in "light physical work" | 47 | 0 | 0 | 0 | 0 | 0 |
| ¼ day or more in "heavy physical work" | 8 | 0 | 0 | 0 | 0 | 0 |
| Take less than 1 hr. for lunch | 23 | 50 | 26 | 25 | 25 | 23 |
| Take more than 1 hr. for lunch | 0 | 2 | 2 | 12 | 11 | 18 |
| Work ½ hr. or more after quitting time | 8 | 42 | 36 | 48 | 30 | 39 |
| During one or more evenings/wk. | | | | | | |
| Do unpaid work from office | 3 | 20 | 33 | 39 | 28 | 52 |
| Do paid overtime work | 25 | 2 | 0 | 2 | 0 | 0 |
| Make repairs or improvement on home | 40 | 33 | 40 | 7 | 30 | 18 |
| Hold a second paid job | 8 | 5 | 5 | 2 | 6 | 2 |
| Study or take courses | 5 | 5 | 0 | 12 | 12 | 12 |
| Do educational or professional reading | 47 | 48 | 72 | 74 | 58 | 70 |
| Attend lodges, fraternal or professional organization | 27 | 16 | 22 | 22 | 22 | 24 |
| Engage in civic or charitable activities | 25 | 36 | 45 | 46 | 47 | 52 |
| Spend 3 or more evenings/wk. in all of above activities | 47 | 42 | 55 | 59 | 47 | 53 |
| Go to bed before 11 P.M. | 33 | 41 | 26 | 25 | 32 | 43 |
| Sleep more than seven hours | 30 | 24 | 29 | 44 | 34 | 45 |

## TABLE XII—Men Aged 55-60
### Daily Round of Life Week-Ends
#### (in percent)

|  | No college | | | | College | |
|---|---|---|---|---|---|---|
|  | Work-men | Fore-men | Super-visors | Mana-gers | Super-visors | Mana-gers |
| Men in category who: | | | | | | |
| Do unpaid work from office, 2 hours or more | 0 | 14 | 10 | 29 | 11 | 33 |
| Do paid overtime work, 2 hours or more | 17 | 7 | 0 | 2 | 2 | 0 |
| Make home repairs or improvements 8 hours or more | 25 | 27 | 38 | 25 | 30 | 12 |
| Study or take courses, 2 hours or more | 1 | 2 | 2 | 5 | 6 | 4 |
| Do educational or professional reading, 2 hours or more | 21 | 25 | 45 | 56 | 43 | 47 |
| Attend lodges, fraternal or professional organizations 2 hours or more | 10 | 2 | 7 | 10 | 11 | 10 |
| Engage in civic or charitable activities, 2 hours or more | 15 | 22 | 16 | 15 | 30 | 33 |
| Average 8 or more hours/ weekend in all of above activities | 43 | 47 | 50 | 38 | 50 | 35 |

## TABLE XIII—Men Aged 55–60
### Attitudes Toward Certain Aspects of the Environment
#### (in percent)

|  | No college | | | | College | |
|---|---|---|---|---|---|---|
|  | Work-men | Fore-men | Super-visors | Mana-gers | Super visors | Mana-gers |
| Men in category who: | | | | | | |
| Feel pressed for time on way to work | 22 | 29 | 36 | 22 | 37 | 27 |
| Are annoyed by traffic tie-ups | 23 | 32 | 41 | 19 | 23 | 20 |
| Feel pressed for time during work | 16 | 37 | 34 | 17 | 41 | 26 |
| Feel some tension on job | 24 | 45 | 36 | 36 | 30 | 29 |
| Work with unpleasant people more than ¼ of the time | 7 | 17 | 15 | 7 | 9 | 7 |
| Feel tired when they arrive home | 39 | 61 | 47 | 49 | 61 | 53 |
| Have to work steadily to keep up with outside activities | 31 | 47 | 28 | 30 | 31 | 28 |
| Spend more than ¼ of time off the job with unpleasant people | 34 | 27 | 14 | 14 | 12 | 7 |
| Feel some tension and worry in their daily lives | 8 | 9 | 10 | 14 | 27 | 12 |

# References

1. Train, Russell E.: *The Quest for Environmental Indices*. Science 178 (4057) :121.
2. Jamaica Bay and Kennedy Airport: A multidiciplinary environmental study Vol. II, Chapter 2 *Jamaica Bay as a Resource for the People of New York City and the Surrounding Region*. National Academy of Sciences, National Academy of Engineering. Washington, D.C. 1971.
3. WHO Expert Committee on Malaria 15th Report (Geneva 1970). Technical Report Series No. 467, 1971.
4. Schrödinger, E.: *What is Life? and Mind and Matter*. Cambridge University Press. London, 1967.
5. Shoenheimer, R.: *Dynamic Steady State of Body Constituents*. Harvard University Press. Cambridge, 1942.
6. Yockey, H. P.; Platzman, R. L. and Quastler, H. (eds) : *Symposium on Information Theory in Biology*. Pergamon, London, 1958. See especially Quastler: "A Primer on Information Theory," p. 3.
7. Dubos, R. J. et al: *Lasting Biological Effects of Early Environmental Influences*. Journal of Experimental Medicine.
   I.   Conditioning of Adult Size by Prenatal and Postnatal Nutrition. 127:783, 1968
   II.  Lasting Depression of Weight Caused by Neonatal Contamination. 127:801, 1968
   III. Metabolic Responses of Mice to Neonatal Infection with a Filterable Weight-Depressing Agent. 128:753, 1968
   VI.  Notes on the Physicochemical and Immunlogical Characteristics of an Enterovirus that Depresses the Growth of Mice. 130:955, 1969
   V.   Viability, Growth, and Longevity. 130:963, 1969
8. U.S. Department of Health, Education, and Welfare: *Interviewing Methods in the Health Interview Survey*. Vital and Health Statistics. Series 2 Number 48, 1972.
9. American Behavioral Scientist: *Multinational Comparative Social Research*. Vol. 10, Number 4, December, 1966.
   Appendix to *Multinational Comparative Social Research*. Vol. 10, Number 4, December, 1966.
10. Hinkle, L. E.; Redmont, R.; Plummer, N. and Wolff, H. G.: *An Examination of the Relation Between Symptoms, Disability, and Serious Illness, in Two Homogaseous Groups of Men and Women*. American Journal of Public Health: 50: 1327, 1960.
11. Hinkle, L. E.: *An Estimate of the Effects of "Stress" on the Incidence and Prevalence of Coronary Heart Disease in a Large Industrial Population in the United States*. Symposium on Thrombosis: Risk Factors and Diagnostic Approaches, Oslo, Norway, July 1971.
12. U.S. Department of Health, Education, and Welfare, *Eighth Revision International Classification of Diseases*, Public Health Service Publication No. 1693, U.S. Government Printing Office, Vol. 1 & 2 December 1968.
13. American Medical Association, *Standard Nomenclature of Diseases and Operations*, Richard J. Plunkett, M.D. & Adaline C. Hayden, R.R.L., eds., McGraw-Hill, New York, 1952.

## Chapter VIII

## The Residential Environment, Health, and Behavior: Simple Research Opportunities, Strategies, and Some Findings in the Solomon Islands and Boston, Massachusetts

ALBERT DAMON

While much remains to be done, both theoretically and procedurally, in formulating research design into the relationship between residential characteristics and health and behavior, there are more opportunities for research than is generally recognized. Useful results can be obtained by simple methods, without waiting for multimillion dollar grants and perfectly designed studies. I shall illustrate this statement with examples of research completed, in progress, and in prospect, pointing out some general principles, procedures, and pitfalls. Since my interests are primarily biological, I shall concentrate on the physical aspects of the environment—crowding, noise, excessive stimulation—and the biobehavioral aspects of the response, leaving to behavioral-science colleagues the details of research into the all-important psychosocial processes which mediate the associations. If relationships can be demonstrated between the residential environment on the one hand, and health and behavior on the other, people's attitudes and perceptions are likely to account for more than the purely physical aspects of the environment. If no relationships can be demonstrated, there is nothing to explain. The concern of this paper is with the existence and nature—rather than the mechanisms—of such relationships as can be explored with slight resources. It is a poor man's guide to research.

### Definitions and Methods of Study

The "residential environment" denotes the environment built or adapted by man for his habitation. While caves would qualify under this definition, I mean particularly houses and their larger groupings, from the minute hamlets of some "primitive" people to modern conurbations. "Health" signifies physical and mental well-being, and "behavior" the objective activities of a person or group. We are interested here in environmental effects on man, not the reverse, although the effect of man on his environment is an important study in its own right.

*Epidemiology.* The biomedical science dealing broadly with the health and behavior of human groups is epidemiology. A definition which restricts epidemiology to pathologic phenomena or behavior is

241

"the study of the distribution and determinants of disease frequency in man." (*1*) But the modern epidemiologist is more than a student of disease—he is a human biologist. Topics apart from disease which interest epidemiologists, and which their techniques have helped to illuminate, include multiple births, the human sex ratio, and secular trends in maturation, growth, and aging. Since the Second World War, epidemiology has expanded its scope from infectious diseases ("epidemics") to the chronic, non-infectious diseases or processes which have supplanted infections as the leading causes of illness ("morbidity") and death ("mortality") in industrialized societies like Western Europe, the United States, and Japan. Such conditions include coronary heart disease, hypertension, strokes, cancer, suicide, congenital anomalies, diabetes, peptic ulcer, and arthritis. (*2*) Interestingly, accidents are a prominent cause of death in both primitive and advanced societies.

Epidemiologic method can delineate and assess the multiple causes of the foregoing "diseases of civilization." Infections are relatively simple to study: there is a host (the patient), an agent (the micro-organism), and an environment (physical, biological, and socioeconomic) in which host and agent interact. This schema has been successfully applied to accidents as well as to infections. (*3–5*) But the distinctive diseases of civilization—which they really are, judging from their absence in increasingly sophisticated biomedical surveys of tribal peoples (*6–9*)—have many causes. Coronary heart disease, for example, the principal cause of death in European and American men, is "due" to heredity, body build, smoking, diet, physical exercise, and psychosocial factors. Peptic ulcer is "due" to heredity, temperament, gastric secretion, dietary habits, and "stress." Such risk factors can be identified and assigned relative weights, singly or combined, for a given population. We may expect that the extent of risk attributable to stimuli in the physical, built environment will differ for various times, places, and people, and that the outcome variables chosen as indicators of their effect will have many causes besides those that concern us here.

Epidemiologic method (*1, 10–12*) has four stages: description, hypothesis, analysis and experiment. The first three stages are observational. As astronomy shows, a great deal can be learned from planned observation. Epidemiologic description consists of charting disease distribution in terms of time, place ("environment"), and person ("host"). This distribution will suggest hypothesis for analytic—that is, quantitative—test. Of course if there are no associations, speculation on how the associations might be mediated, or on the reason for their absence, becomes pointless. If analytic test does sustain an hypothesis, final proof of the suspected causative factor(s) is obtained by experimental manipulation. The whole process is illustrated by the fluoridation of drinking water to prevent dental caries, or the reduction in lung cancer rates among men who stop smoking.

242

The basic epidemiologic tool is a rate—that is, a fraction with the number of cases as the numerator, and the population "at risk" as the denominator. The denominator population could be a total group, residentially defined (as by a household census), or more commonly an age-sex subset of such a population. Populations can be defined other than residentially, of course, for other purposes, such as by race, religion, occupation, or socio-economic status. In any case, there must be a denominator, which is a defined population. The epidemiologist's function has indeed been epitomized as "placing a denominator under a clinician."

Rates can be of "prevalence," describing the disease situation at a given point in time ("point prevalence") or over a period of time ("period prevalence"). Rates can also refer to "incidence," measuring the occurrence of new cases in a period of time. Point-prevalence rates are derived from one-time surveys, period-prevalence and incidence rates from repeated or continuous surveillance. The fundamental equation of epidemiology is

$$P = Id,$$

where

$P$ = prevalence
$I$ = incidence
and $d$ = duration of illness.

Like mortality, morbidity, hospitalization, or days lost from work, all of the epidemiologic indices of health rest on rates and therefore on populations defined in some specified way. Further technical procedures in epidemiology and biostatistics, such as sampling, matching, statistical analysis, inference of cause from association, and so on can be found in standard texts. (*1, 10–12*)

## Practical Implications

The foregoing outline indicates the basic requirements for a research design relating the residential environment to health and behavior. A population must be established, to serve as a base for computing rates. Coverage must be as complete as possible, since the effects we are seeking may be subtle. If they were obvious, elaborate research would be unnecessary. This means that numbers must be large enough to show the statistical significance of associations or of differences between study and control groups that may be real enough, but modest in degree. For the same reason very little "slippage," in the form of non-response, lack of information, or incomplete follow-up can be allowed. Just a few missing observations, representing a few percentage points, could obscure real but slight associations.

The need for adequate numbers imposes constraints on the choice of outcome variables. Rare events require large populations for meaningful analysis. Even leading causes of death or disability affect small frac-tions of a population. Accidents, for example, the third leading cause of death in the United States, in 1968 killed 57.7 persons per 100,000, making accidental death a poor variable for evaluating small-scale environments which affect small populations. Injury, however, defined as requiring medical attention or causing at least a day's restriction of activity, in 1968 affected 25 persons per 100 over all ages, (13) making injury a useful gauge of environmental quality even in small populations.

Relevance imposes another constraint on the choice of outcome variables. One should look for disturbances in health and behavior that might be expected to result from specific environmental (and host) features. Residential layout is more likely to induce household falls than automobile accidents, for example; and the latter affect young adults, whereas household falls affect mainly women and elderly persons. If sleep is disturbed, or if long hours of commuting by public transportation produces fatigue, one would look for such manifestations of irritability as frequent clinic visits or arrests for disturbing the peace, or for such evidence of impaired functioning as retardation of children in school grade levels.

Disability or frank disease affect relatively few people. The most appealing measures of incipient malfunction or subclinical disease, as well as the easiest to obtain, are those which occur in everyone, like blood pressure or serum cholesterol. The trouble with such measures is that they are but weakly associated with "stress" and even predict frank disease poorly. Measures of child growth and development like height, weight, dental or bone age, or stages of puberty, though good indices of health status for populations, are unlikely to differ enough among or within urban micro-environments in the United States to help in the present context. Even purported measures of stress, like the questionnaires used by A. H. Leighton (14) among adults in different cultures and by D. C. Leighton (15) among school children, may depict feelings rather than the objective behavior in which we are interested. We must avoid looking where the light is good, if what we seek lies elsewhere.

So far, three kinds of constraints have been seen to influence the investigator's choice of outcome variables: numbers, relevance, and ease of measurement. A fourth problem involves scale. Census tracts or neighborhoods are defined areas in which certain *social* indicators may be available for enumerated populations. Income, education, unemployment, overcrowded housing units, welfare recipients, broken homes, illegitimacy, divorce, arrests, crime, homicides, and suicides are examples. Occasionally, as in the New York City Health Areas, *medical* data may have been gathered on an areal basis by various agencies. Examples would be rates of mental hospitalization, of birth, stillbirth, prematurity, infant mortality, and venereal disease. Areas can be characterized socially, and health and behavior can be compared among areas. Struening and Lehmann (16) review such research, called social area analysis, and apply the concepts to new data from Health Areas in New York City, which consist of two or three census tracts. Galle et al. (17) do the same for 75 Chicago "community areas." But census tracts and even neighborhoods are residentially heterogeneous. In "Jamesville," a pseudonymous district of Boston, for example, my colleagues and I could not establish distinct neighborhoods with fairly homogeneous housing type or quality. Within any one block we found great variation in both. Even within a large housing project of 1,149 families, with uniform construction and a fairly uniform demographic mix of tenants, there were marked environmental differences, such as ambient noise levels, from one part to another.

The relationship between the residential environment and health and behavior can be sought at different levels, ranging from rural or urban areas down through the census tract; the multi-block unit mentioned by Hinkle in comparing the health status of persons living along Park Avenue, New York City, in the 70-79th street and the 100-119th street blocks; the neighborhood, the block, the individual building, and even—as in the peculiar susceptibility of poor single lodgers to tuberculosis (18, 19)—the dwelling unit or apartment. As regards crowding, micro-crowding within dwellings seems to be more important than macro-crowding among buildings or areas. Chombart de Lauwe is said (20) to have shown little relationship between the number of residents per housing unit and social and physical pathologies, but a doubled rate when the space available per person per unit fell below a threshold value, 8 to 10 square meters. Two studies in Chicago (17, 21) showed no relation between density per acre and social pathology among community areas, but floor space per person did disclose significant associations.

In our own studies on Malaita, Solomon Islands, the neighboring Lau and Baegu tribes span the human range as regards macro-crowding, from 200–250 persons per acre on artificial islets (Lau) to 10–20 persons per minute bush hamlet, miles from the nearest neighbors (Baegu). Yet their rates for tuberculosis, often associated with crowding in cosmopolitan populations, were identical—2–3% of acute tuberculosis and 18–19% of chronic or healed cases, diagnosed radiographically. (22) Within households, the average number of persons was between 4 and 6 in both tribes, with roughly 4 square meters per person among the Lau and 2.4 square meters per person among the Baegu.

Six studies, (17–22) then, including our own, underline the importance of the individual dwelling place, rather than the total residential area, in evaluating certain effects of the residential environment. The same studies also suggest that levels of tolerable crowding vary from one culture to another, and that it is the social rather than the physical aspects of crowding that matter. Further evidence to this effect comes from comparison of micro-densities in various cultures. (*17*) In Europe, lower limits of desirable floor space per person are held to be 15.3 square meters; in the United States, 30.6 square meters are considered desirable; actual figures, compatible with good health, are 2.4 to 4 square meters on Malaita, 6 to 9 in Hong Kong, and 7.6 to 9.1 in the Boston housing project to be described shortly.

## Desiderata for Research

It is now clear that in order to explore the relationship that concerns us, we need access to sizeable, defined, fully-ascertained populations whose residential environment, health, and behavior are known or obtainable in detail. Such groups are hard to find, particularly in a country like the United States, with a multiple-choice system of medical care and no record linkage from one component to another. It is easy to define groups residentially or in terms of health and behavior— for example, enrollees in a prepaid medical-care plan, clinic registrants, school dropouts, or sidewalk samples from midtown Manhattan—but the problem is then to obtain the other, biobehavioral set of data. On the whole, it is cheaper and easier to investigate environments than health. If a choice must be made, define a population already under medical or behavioral surveillance and then evaluate its environment, rather than the reverse. This may require observation in many neighborhoods, but it is still easier than trying to interview or examine many individuals.

The ideal study group is one of large size and known demographic makeup, living in a defined locality and attending one or a small number of health facilities. Such groups can occasionally be found in a university community in a small town, a retirement colony, or a housing development with a comprehensive, primary medical-care facility treating most of the group. The Leisure World Retirement Community, Seal Beach, California (*23*) or the Columbia Point Clinic in Boston (*24*) are examples. Within such communities uniformity of environment, population, or both can be turned to advantage, since some confounding variables are controlled. One can generally find a characteristic which does vary, such as density within a residential area, or noise levels, or ethnic differences, which permit these factors to be evaluated by themselves. Further details will be given later.

If limited aspects of the environment or of health and behavior are to be related, records may be available without the need for individual interview or examination. An excellent example is the demonstration, from hospital and census data, that persons living near Heathrow Airport, London, were more liable to mental hospitalization than those living farther away. (*25*) Obtaining cooperation is so difficult and subject to bias, and examining individuals is so expensive that researchers

246

on a modest budget should use records wherever possible. Records are of course more suitable for some types of data (clinic visit, hospital admission, school dropout and truancy) than for others (diagnosis of behavioral disorder or type of illness, police warnings vs. arrest). Records should be searched within each agency or facility, such as police departments, school systems, or clinics, since central linkages, whether by social workers or health, welfare, or housing agencies are notoriously incomplete. Confidentiality can be preserved by using address as the identifying index rather than name.

A general shortcoming of records is that they are rarely collected for the purpose an investigator has in mind. School or police districts, for example, usually comprise diverse neighborhoods, and facilities for curative medicine seldom collect the detailed socio-economic data crucial to the behavioral scientist. In the ideal study, populations and procedures are tailored to a specific problem. But an investigator with limited time and resources will do well to take advantage of existing data, even if it means modifying his objectives.

## Research Opportunities

Two broad kinds of community can be studied residentially and behaviorally: primitive and developed. The intermediate category, which would include a village or even a city in the underdeveloped countries of Latin America, Asia, or Africa is less suitable on both theoretical and practical grounds. Such settlements are more complex and specialized than the simpler forms of societies which can illuminate basic man-environment interactions closer to the biological level. Rapid cultural change may introduce a new factor of stress. The village of India, the African bidonville, the Latin American barrio or favela, or the Arab and Mediterranean communities, with inward-looking houses and markedly different activity patterns for the two sexes—all of these have limited relevance to American or Northwest European conditions. At the same time such towns and cities are ethnically and in other ways more homogeneous than the large industrial cities that are our chief concern. They pose different problems. This too is in part a matter of scale.

## Primitive Societies

The various geographic, cultural, and genetic isolates of the world, though fast disappearing, provide a priceless resource for evaluating the effects of residential organization on health and behavior. They permit direct observation of human response to diverse combinations of density and spatial arrangement. However stimulating or provocative of hypotheses animal observation and experiments may be, one cannot extrapolate from rodents or primates to man, nor from laboratory experiments on man to his behavior in free-living communities.

It might be argued that the very existence of a viable, functioning society proves its adaptation to its environment. Some groups function surprisingly well, in terms of work output and reproductive performance, at levels of health and nutrition that would send Western Europeans and North Americans to mass graves. New Guineans, the Chinese of Southeast Asia, Nepalese, and many African and Latin American groups come to mind. True enough, these groups have adapted, but the quality of adaptation can vary greatly. Biomedical evidence to this effect includes the increased height, earlier maturation, and higher hemoglobin levels (not to mention improved maternal and child health, lower death rates, and increased longevity) among primitive groups following public health measures such as sanitation, nutrition, and disease control. (For New Guinea and the Solomon Islands, see 9 and 26.) The height increase means that the population, though functioning, had not reached its full genetic potential in its previous environment. Small size and slow maturation may in fact be adaptive to a poor environment. Genetic potential is finite, differing from one group to another, and even the capacity to respond to a better environment ("plasticity") may be genetically determined. Beyond a point, already reached among well-to-do Americans, environmental amelioration has not increased height. (27, 28)

By analogy with risk factors in disease, we might say that the quality of behavioral adaptation will vary from one group to another, and within one group may change over time as the environment changes. Behavioral adaptation is harder to measure than biomedical adaptation. In the present context, we are interested in relating the quality of both kinds of adaptation to the residential environment.

Primitive populations, though lacking written records, can be easily specified residentially, enumerated, and known on a close personal basis. This is in fact the ethnographer's first job. The next step, seldom attempted, seems to be much more difficult—that is, to record objectively and quantitatively people's health and health-related behavior. The paucity of observations on physical health is understandable, since few ethnographers have medical training. But one would expect more systematic observation than appears in the anthropoligical literature of such broad categories of health-relevant behavior as neurosis, frank mental illness, social deviance, and signs of "stress," however defined. (Disturbance in mood, thought, or feeling would be a partial definition.) A "happiness quotient" for individuals or for a society as a whole may be too much to expect, but this is what we really need. Margaret Mead (29) has come close, for several Oceanic groups. The kinds of behavior generally recorded by social anthropologists are, however, much more abstract: cognitive, economic, religious, legal, linguistic, or family-oriented (kinship, child-rearing, courtship, and the like). There are standardized ways of assessing behavior, (14, 15, 30–33) and a beginning

248

has been made in transcultural psychiatry, (*34, 35*) but most health and health-related behavioral data on primitive people are purely anecdotal or impressionistic. This rather harsh judgment is supported by the Symposium just cited (*34*) and by my search through the Human Relations Area File with two colleagues.(*36*)

The Human Relations Area File, a cross-indexed compendium of world ethnographies, was examined for ten Oceanic societies, and two more, not yet included in the File, were analyzed from monographs. We found that ethnographers had paid detailed attention to the physical and man-made environments but had made few or no objective, quantitative assessments of health and behavior. From the ethnographic literature it is possible to compare population composition and density, residential design and layout, and patterns of daily living across cultures. Indeed, one challenging problem is why human groups in similar habitats, with similar ways of life, vary widely in village size. For example, among shifting agriculturists in Melanesia, village size varies from 10 to 20 persons among the Baegu and Kwaio of Malaita, in the Solomon Islands, to 1,500 to 2,000 in parts of New Guinea. We know next to nothing of the causes or the biobehavioral correlates of such extreme differences.

Analysis of living patterns in Middle Eastern cities from the Human Relations Area File, as well as from monographs, suggests that time is an important variable in urban life styles. Reports from other research bears this out. Time patterns of activity can enhance or reduce the effect of the environment, making a given spatial layout tolerable or intolerable. This may help explain the situation among the far-from-urban Lau of Malaita (Solomon Islands), who live on crowded artificial islets in a salt-water lagoon. With 200 to 250 persons living on one acre or less, densities on these islets exceed the 80,000 per square mile reached in parts of Calcutta, Hong Kong, or Johannesburg. Nevertheless, the Lau enjoyed robust physical health, despite trachoma and intestinal parasites, as shown by detailed biomedical examination in 1968. (*9*) Equally to the point, their mental health was excellent, according to ethnographers P. and E. K. Maranda (personal communication).

To complete the picture, as well as to complicate it, I should point out that young adult Lau had even higher blood pressure than young adults in the United States, but their blood pressure did not rise with age, unlike ours. The Lau had virtually no hypertensive or coronary heart *disease,* however. In addition to their crowding, they also consumed much salt, and salt intake has been postulated, though not demonstrated, to be a determinant of blood pressure levels in human populations. (*37*) Males at all ages and females aged 13 to 24 years, living on a more crowded islet, had higher blood pressure than those on an islet with "only" half its density, but the more crowded islet had a much stricter chief and a tense, stressful atmosphere. Blood pressure was unrelated to family size, an index of micro-crowding. In short, nothing is simple, even in a relatively simple society.

Among the Lau, several factors may offset the harmful effects usually attributed to overcrowding among animals and urbanized man. *(38)* Their absolute number of daily encounters is fairly small, and all are with kin or close acquaintances. Spatially, each islet is divided into three areas: one reserved for men, one for women, and a common portion for both sexes, containing family houses. There is easy access to unlimited, unpeopled space on the surrounding sea or on the "mainland," a few hundred yards away. New islets are continually being constructed to relieve overcrowding. Adults typically leave the crowded islets during the day, the men to fish and the women to garden and fetch water. Even on the islets, time is traded for space, with most of the men's time and much of the women's time (all of it, during menses and childbirth) spent in the uncrowded areas reserved for either sex.

Since time patterns seem to be an important mechanism of adjustment to crowding, and since disruption of biologic time patterns— altered diurnal wake-rest-sleep cycles, constant arousal and alertness, constant need for decisions—are thought to contribute to urban stress, daily rounds of life should be compared for representative persons within and across cultures. This would be a simple way to quantitate one aspect of the individual's interaction with his environment, which includes other persons and the cultural products of personal interaction, as well as the natural environment. Not only how the person spends his time, but where, with whom, and with what expenditure of energy should be recorded. Field ethnographers could make a great contribution by routinely obtaining this kind of information.

A promising study design would be to compare the time budgets—an easily obtainable facet of the life style—of pairs of siblings, one of whom has migrated to a new environment. Pairs of sisters in San Juan, Puerto Rico and New York City (as reported by Lewis, *39*), or pairs of brothers in Boston and Ireland, *(40)* or in New York City and Israel, *(41)* or rural Mississippi and Chicago, or Appalachia and Detroit are suggested. Particularly valuable would be the biomedical data, as collected by Trulson et al. *(40)* and by Segall *(41)*, on such pairs.

So far, I have proposed that ethnographers define their populations residentially, enumerate and specify them demographically, characterize their residential environment in detail (e.g., the arrangement and dimensions of dwellings, grouping of houses into larger aggregates, density within households and hamlets), record their behavior in standardized ways with regard to signs and symptoms of stress and to disorders of mood, thought, and feeling, and obtain "daily rounds of life" for representative persons. All this, of course, is in addition to the anthropological observations on larger scale "social" behavior that form the core of ethnography.

What else can this ethnographer do to explore the effect of the residential environment on health and behavior? The ideal solution would be for a biomedical team to survey each society, collaborating with the social anthropologist. Although this is being done here and there around the world—by Neel et al., (6) Salzano et al., (42) and Neel and Chagnon (43) in the Amazon Basin, Buck et al. (44) in Peru, Lee and DeVore (45) and their biomedical collaborators Truswell and Hansen (46) among the South African Bushmen, and Damon (9) in the Solomon Islands—this complex, expensive kind of research cannot begin to meet the need for some time to come. The next stage would be the intensive study of a single group by a physician acting as his own social anthropologist, as by Dunn (47) in Malaya and Sinnett (48) in New Guinea.

A third possibility, the most feasible for anthropologists in general, is for the ethnographer to make a few key biomedical observations himself. Ethnographers cannot be expected to conduct extensive biomedical surveys unaided, but they could be taught to take blood pressure—a possible index of chronic stress. (Most primitive groups have low blood pressure, but a few have high ones, even by United States standards.) There is a good training film for blood pressure measurement, produced by the United States Public Health Service, which could form part of a training package for departments of anthropology. Simple questionnaires for mental as well as physical health could be devised. Ethnographers could certainly be shown how to collect, process, and send blood and stool samples for laboratory analysis. Careful dietary observations should be made, including the food intake of three families for three days each, with weighing of portions and with later biochemical analysis of food samples. Salt intake is particularly important in relation to blood pressure. (49)

Although some anthropologists do collect dietary data, biomedical orientation and technical training are all too rare, even among ecological anthropologists. Yet few activities of anthropologists hold greater promise for helping mankind. The Public Health Service might develop its own training package for departments of anthropology and field ethnographers, furthering its own goals and strengthening the behavioral sciences at the same time.

## Research Opportunities in Advanced Societies

As in primitive societies, research here at home on the effects of the residential environment on health and behavior requires a defined, enumerated population of at least several hundred persons, a residential environment described in standardized detail, and objective, quantitative observation of health and behavior. Some such data exist in records, while some may have to be gathered directly. I have already mentioned that colleges and retirement communities are promising places for research: both contain special populations, simplifying research though limiting its ultimate application. Colleges are particularly useful since they contain buildings both old and new, a single source of health records, and standardized, quantitative data on one kind of behavior in the form of course grades and class standing.. There may also be appraisals by advisors, tutors, instructors, dormitory proctors, and the like. Students are usually easy to interview and examine. Various research strategies can be devised. The number of subjects can be increased by including a few years' experience. The health and performance of the same students can be compared before and after residence in a new dormitory of known design. Over a longer period, records could be compared of students living in various types of buildings—single-sex or coeducational, noisy or quiet, high or low density, those favoring privacy or communality, and so on. To be sure, self-selection is present, and the restricted ranges of age and of the health and behavioral criteria may obscure any associations, but the possibility should be explored.

Rarely can a representative population be found, living in a single locality, whose health and behavioral records are available. As we have seen, either the environmental or the outcome variables will be known, but seldom both. One can define populations residentially and try to measure their health and behavior, or one can define populations undergoing health and behavioral surveillance and try to describe their environments. As examples of the latter, consider participants in health insurance and maintenance programs, such as the Health Insurance Plan of New York City or the Kaiser Permanente Clinics on the West Coast. Only health records will be available for such groups and, then, mainly in connection with illness; after an initial examination, current status is not routinely followed. Few other behavioral data will be available. Confidentiality of records may pose problems.

Employees of large firms with medical departments offer some advantages, in that job performance is known, in addition to health. Current health and behavioral status could be ascertained readily for research purposes, and cooperation would be easier.

An unexploited opportunity to make this kind of observation is provided by research populations already selected to represent defined populations and already under detailed health and behavioral surveillance. Such groups might include subjects in the three age spans (adults, children, adolescents) of the National Health Examination Survey, (50) the two groups of the New York City children being followed by Langner and associates (51) at the Columbia School of Public Health, or the Harlem pregnancy series of Rush, (52) of the same institution. There are other such research populations, such as natural communities in Framingham, Massachusetts, (53) Tecumseh, Michigan, (54) and Alameda County, California, (55) or subjects in the Normative Aging Study of the Veterans Administration. (56) It would be feasible, though expensive, to evaluate the residential environments of such persons, for correlation with their health and behavior. Even with these large numbers of subjects, however, environments may be so diverse as to yield categories too small for statistical analysis.There might be an unacceptably high rate of refusal to cooperate.

If the investigator defines a group by residence and then tries to obtain his own data on health and behavior, all the difficulties are magnified—the time, cost, and effort of locating individuals, inducing their cooperation, and examining them; the refusal rate; and the possible fragmentation of end results into a welter of small categories of illness or deviant behavior.

The solution is to locate a residentially or spatially defined group for whom current health and behavioral data are available. Such groups may be found in countries with socialized medicine, like Britain and the Scandinavian countries or, in the United States, in lower-income or public housing developments served by one or very few medical facilities. Boston has two such housing developments, Columbia Point, (24) served by a clinic based at Tufts Medical School, and an area I shall call "Jamesville," served by the Breed's Hill Clinic of the Massachusetts General Hospital. (57) The rest of this chapter will present my research experience so far on the residential environment, health, and behavior in "Jamesville."*

### Research at the Jamesville Housing Project

Jamesville is a geographically distinct, low-income section of Boston where 15,000 persons live in one square mile. There is some industry, a few small shops, and—the chief economic enterprise—a large repair and shop facility of the United States Navy. Commercial docks also provide employment. Ethnically, Jamesville is 95% white and predominantly Irish Catholic as has been true for at least 50 years. In 1964 the median family income was $5,350, one of the lowest for any district of Boston.

Our first step was to evaluate the kinds of data available for correlational studies. The types of housing included the Jamesville Housing Project, with 1,149 units in 45 three-story brick and cement buildings; brick row houses varying in quality from tenements to Federal-style single-family houses restored for moderate to upper-income occupancy; modern frame, single and two-family houses; and newly constructed houses of suburban type. The quality and condition of buildings ranged from abysmal to excellent. Except for the Housing Project, it proved impossible to define neighborhoods with relatively homogeneous hous-

* This research, to be reported more fully elsewhere, was supported by the Bureau of Community Environmental Management. Participants included Lucia Cies, Sanford and Mary Jane Low, Charles M. Poster, Anne St. Goar, and Barbara de Zalduondo.

ing. Within any one block there was marked variation in the external conditions as well as the type of housing. One might have attached indicators of health and behavior to specific houses and created statistical rather than geographic "neighborhoods" for analysis, as in the proposed research designs discussed above, which might involve populations already under health surveillance. But this was beyond our limited resources and, more important, would lose sight of real neighborhoods, where people actually live.

We therefore focused on the Housing Project, a residential environment and a real neighborhood which could be described in detail. Using the survey forms of the Neighborhood Environmental Evaluation and Decision System (NEEDS) of the Bureau of Community Environmental Management, we made preliminary evaluations in the Project and in the adjoining U.S. census tract. As indicators of health and behavior, we chose school truancies and dropouts, police arrests, and visits to the Breed's Hill Clinic. It soon became clear that the Housing Project itself could provide the best denominator population for such comparisons, and that problems of interpretation would be simpler if comparisons could be made within the Project rather than between the Project and the census tract. A "natural experiment" was present within the Project, in that the noise varied from normal urban levels, around interior buildings, to well-nigh intolerable along one border exposed to heavy traffic from a main-artery, two-level bridge and from a large marginal road. Our measurements with a portable decibel meter (Octave Band Noise Analyzer, Model 1558A, General Radio Co., Concord, Mass.)* showed that noise during the day, between 6:30 A.M. and 6:30 P.M., averaged in the noisy area around 80 decibels, a condition under which over time some permanent hearing loss has been detected in industry. (58) Occasionally, in brief bursts, the noise level rose into the 90's or even exceeded 100 decibels. After 6:30 P.M., readings fell gradually to 74 decibels at midnight. A quieter, interior sector, which we used for comparison, gave readings between 5 and 10 decibels lower.

To our three initial outcome variables—rates of arrests, school delinquency, and clinic visits—we added, after some field experience, the condition of entryways within buildings, a responsibility of the tenants using each entry. Having found the NEEDS technique better suited to whole neighborhoods, its primary focus, than to individual buildings or entries, we devised our own checklist, based on cleanliness, condition of mailboxes and staircases, broken windows, and the like.

Our strategy was to compare all four outcome variables between the residents of eight buildings in the noisy area and the residents of nine buildings in the quieter, interior sector. If no differences should appear,

---

* Kindly loaned by Dr. John D. Dougherty, Harvard School of Public Health.

this could indicate that noise is unrelated to health and behavior, that the outcome variables were inappropriate, or that the sample size was too small to show any effect. With negative findings, a prudent investigator on a modest budget would do well to try another approach. If differences did appear, they would have to be interpreted. Noise might be merely associated with the outcomes, rather than a determinant of them.

Arrests in 1969 and 1970 were significantly more frequent in the noisy sector than in the quiet sector. The noisy sector averaged 44 persons arrested out of 598 residents, or 7.4% per year; the quiet sector, 24.5 out of 563 residents, or 4.4% per year; $p < 0.03$. (Persons arrested more than once, including 19 persons over the two-year period, and 57 total arrests, were counted only once per year.) The great bulk of arrests were for minor offenses, notably drunkenness, followed by minor assault. The most serious offenses were one instance of rape and a few of aggravated assault (with injury), among 119 persons arrested over a two-year period.

The age distribution in the two areas (Table 1) differed somewhat, particularly in the percentage of persons aged 10 to 19 years, who formed the largest percentage (35%) of all persons arrested. In the noisy area, 200/598, or 33%, were between 10 and 19 years of age; in the control area, 123/563, or 22%. But the higher arrest rate in the noisy area held for all age groups, not only for subadults (Table 2); in fact, the ratio of arrest rate in noisy sector to arrest rate in quiet sector was actually highest in the 5th to 7th decades of life. In epidemiologic parlance, the increased risk of arrest in the noisy area as a whole was "attributable" to the 10–19 year age group, who contributed the largest numbers to the total, but the "relative" risk of arrest was higher for older persons. The increased arrest rate in the noisy sector was therefore not an artifact of differing age distributions in the two sectors.

There was an interesting sex difference, in that in the noisy area, 22% of persons arrested were women, but in the control area, only 4% ($p < 0.01$).

In respect to condition of entryways, rated as excellent, good, fair, or poor, the 20 entries in the noisy sector were significantly worse than the 31 in the control sector ($p < 0.01$).

Annual rates of school truancy in noisy and quieter sectors were 10% and 3% ($p < 0.01$), of absenteeism 35% and 12% ($p < 0.001$), and of junior high and high school dropouts 6.3% and 4.7% ($p > 0.50$), respectively. (These rates were based on the school-age populations "at risk," namely children between ages 5 and 15 for truancy and absenteeism, and youths between 16 and 24 for high school dropouts.) All of the differences pointed in the same direction, although that for dropouts did not reach statistical significance.

As for clinic visits, 521 (87%) persons in the noisy area but only 358 (64%) of those in the quieter area were enrolled. Multiplied by duration of enrollment, these numbers served as the denominators for person-years "at risk;" the numbers of visits during the period "at risk" were the numerators. For persons living in the noisy and quieter areas, annual clinic visits for physical complaints averaged 3.6 and 4.1; for mental or behavioral complaints, 1.07 and 0.95; and for all complaints, 4.6 and 5.0, respectively. These data are inconclusive. In view of the age distribution of clinic registrants—in the noisy area, 62% of registrants were under 20, 26% between 20 and 49, and 12% over 50; in the quieter area, 53%, 26%, and 21%, respectively—one might expect more physical complaints among the elderly folk in the quieter area, as was the case.

In brief, three of our four outcome variables—condition of entries, arrests, and school attendance—showed significantly impaired functioning among persons in the noisy area. Clinic visits were unrevealing. But these associations of course tell us nothing about cause. They may reflect some aspects of the environment other than noise, or the residents of the noisy area might be more liable to arrest and might take worse care of their dwellings whatever their environment. The direct test would be to compare arrest rates for the same families before, during, and after residence in the noisy sector. Lacking such data, we compared densities and looked into the mechanics of family assignment within the project.

Density within buildings was fairly comparable in the two areas, with 82.6 square feet (7.6 square meters) available per person in the noisy area and 98.5 square feet (9.1 square meters) per person in the quieter area. As for residential assignment, tenants as well as housing officials agreed, despite anecdotes that "problem" families were sent to the noisy "jungle" area, that large families were assigned to large apartments, of which there happened to be more in the noisy area. The statistics on density and on age distribution (Table 1) within the two areas reflect this practice. While large families may be problem families, the two are not synonymous. It seems unlikely (and comparison of outcome variables among individual buildings within the noisy area confirms the belief) that family size alone can account for the associations.

### Future Research at Jamesville

One obvious direction for future research is to continue to collect records from the medical clinic. Eventually almost all of the housing project tenants will be enrolled in the clinic, making comparison more meaningful. Blood pressures should be compared between residents of the two areas, as an index of stress.

The best tool for evaluating environments is to observe health and behavior before and after environmental modification. The Jamesville Housing Project provides three such opportunities. In response to tenants' wishes, their kitchens and bathrooms were completely renovated, during 1969 and 1970, at no cost to them. Secondly, a new housing project of advanced "suburban" design is being built across the street from the present Project, into which some of the Project families will move. Despite contradictory findings from several large studies on change in health following "improved" housing (summarized by Carstairs (59) and Cassel (60)), these two leads should be pursued.

The third, ideal possibility concerns the imminent redesign of the bridge, the major source of noise. When redesign has been completed, in a few years, noise levels should be much reduced. It should be most instructive to compare the health and behavior of the same families in two environments, physically the same except for noise.

A possible pitfall in before-and-after comparison is that time trends may occur independently of the factor under study. In Jamesville the percentage of persons arrested increased from 1969 to 1970, from 5.9% to 8.8% in the noisy area, and from 3.2% to 4.8% in the quiet area. A decrease in the percentage arrested, following interior renovation of apartments, a move to better housing, or decreased noise levels would run counter to the time trends, strengthening the interpretation of the change as reflecting the changed environment. All such studies require a control group of persons who do not experience the environmental change, to rule out the post hoc fallacy.

The preliminary research at Jamesville just outlined encouraged us to look into the tenants' perceptions, attitudes, and ordinary behavior as they are affected by the Project's physical layout. This is the link between the environmental stimulus and a person's health and behavioral response. To this end a predoctoral student and his wife moved into the Project, as ethnographers would do in another society. They investigated formal and informal networks of social interaction, interviewed tenants, attended tenants' meetings, and made quantitative observations of building conditions. This research is preparatory to a study of spatial and social structure in a Peruvian barrio. Comparison of the two cultures could lead to standardized methods for evaluating environments trans-culturally and to generalizable findings of practical and scientific value. Even in the United States there are major cultural and environmental differences that planners and designers must take into account, ranging from Arctic Eskimos to Southwestern Indians and Chicanos, midwesterners in small towns, ethnic enclaves in crowded cities, and scattered suburbs everywhere. Biobehavioral guidelines are sorely needed for both established communities and new ones like those in Operation Breakthrough of the Department of Housing and Urban Development. Anthropoligists and biomedical scientists have been slow to accept the challenge.

## Conclusions

"Conclusions" may be too pretentious a term for the distillate of the thoughts, suggestions, and preliminary research presented here. "Impressions" would be more appropriate.

Research into the relationship of the residential environment to health and behavior is needed and feasible. Epidemiologic methods are appropriate. They require sizeable, defined populations, as completely enumerated and with as large a percentage as possible included in the study. Such populations can be found in both primitive and highly urbanized, industrialized societies. The ideal study group would be a natural population living in a neighborhood, with complete residential description and health and behavioral records available, hence, not requiring individuals to be examined. In the United States, college communities in small towns, or even non-college towns, come close. But this is not really where the housing action is. Large housing projects served by one or a very few medical facilities offer the best opportunity.

Literature review and personal research in the Solomon Islands and in Boston, Massachusetts, lead to the general conclusion that any effects of the built environment on health and behavior (and such effects are still to be demonstrated) result from people's perceptions and attitudes rather than from their direct response to physical stimuli. People can adapt, psychologically and socially, to almost any environment. The major component of their environment, and of their adaptation, is other people. This was dramatically shown by the difference in attitude toward architecturally similar housing projects expressed by two groups of Boston tenants we interviewed in Roxbury and in Jamesville. Neither group complained of the buildings physically. The Roxbury tenants, concerned for their safety, disliked the project because of the "new" people who had moved in; the Jamesville tenants felt more secure and were generally pleased with their environment because they liked their fellow-tenants and fellow-townsmen.

Research on the direct effects of the physical environment is nevertheless worth pursuing, since even negative findings could allay fears as to the harmful effects of residential design. Various research techniques and strategies, particularly those suited to modest budgets, have been suggested and illustrated, along with the problems that may arise. For primitive groups, it is suggested that ethnographers add to their usual descriptions of villages and houses, and to their usual demographic enumeration, the objective, quantitative observation of health and behavior. Time budgets, or "daily rounds of life," are easily obtained. Standardized recording of behavior, particularly the kinds of

258

behavior indicative of stress or maladaption, is possible, using well-tested instruments. Ethnographers could also make simple but useful biomedical observations, such as measuring blood pressure and obtaining food, blood, and stool samples.

Research experience so far in a public housing project in Boston, Massachusetts, has been presented. Data were obtained on the environment (density, building conditions, noise levels), the tenants (demography, attitudes, perceptions), and their health and behavior through medical clinic, school, and police records. Confidentiality was preserved by searching records for addresses, not named persons. Initial findings show a significantly increased rate of arrests and school absence and truancy, and significantly worse maintenance by tenants of their own entryways, in a noisy part of the project as compared to a quieter part. The rates of medical and psychiatric clinic visits did not differ, however.

Further kinds of research that could be pursued in such a setting center on person, place, or time. One could compare the health and behavior of groups of persons (new and long-term residents, young and old, employed and unemployed); or of persons living in different parts of a housing project (quiet and noisy, crowded and uncrowded); or of residents before and after a specified environmental change. Guidelines for such research have been suggested.

## Acknowledgment

I am grateful for the kind assistance of the Boston Police and School Departments and the Boston Housing Authority.

TABLE 1—Age and Sex Distribution in Noisy and Control Areas, "Jamesville" Housing Project

| | Noisy area | | | | Control area | | | |
| | Males | | Females | | Males | | Females | |
| Age | N | % | N | % | N | % | N | % |
| --- | --- | --- | --- | --- | --- | --- | --- | --- |
| 0– 9 | 80 | 31 | 58 | 17 | 71 | 32 | 52 | 15 |
| 10–19 | 94 | 36 | 106 | 31 | 63 | 28 | 60 | 18 |
| 20–29 | 20 | 8 | 34 | 10 | 23 | 10 | 38 | 11 |
| 30–39 | 12 | 5 | 31 | 9 | 16 | 7 | 32 | 9 |
| 40–49 | 20 | 8 | 45 | 13 | 14 | 6 | 27 | 8 |
| 50–59 | 9 | 3 | 26 | 8 | 14 | 6 | 29 | 9 |
| 60–69 | 9 | 3 | 21 | 6 | 11 | 5 | 43 | 13 |
| 70–79 | 11 | 4 | 12 | 4 | 6 | 3 | 39 | 11 |
| 80–89 | 5 | 2 | 5 | 1 | 5 | 2 | 19 | 6 |
| 90–99 | 0 | 0 | 0 | 0 | 0 | 0 | 1 | (0.3) |
| Total | 260 | 100 | 338 | 99 | 223 | 99 | 340 | 100 |

TABLE 2—Arrest Rates by Age, 1969 and 1970, "Jamesville" Housing Project

| Age | Noisy Area | | | Control Area | | | Arrest Rate Ratio, Noisy/ Control |
| | Population | Persons arrested, 2 yrs. | Arrest Rate/ Year (%) | Population | Persons arrested, 2 yrs. | Arrest Rate/ Year (%) | |
| --- | --- | --- | --- | --- | --- | --- | --- |
| 0–9 | 138 | 1 | 0.4 | 123 | 0 | .... | .... |
| 10–19 | 200 | 32 | 8.0 | 123 | 16 | 6.5 | 1.2 |
| 20–29 | 54 | 13 | 12.0 | 61 | 12 | 9.8 | 1.2 |
| 30–39 | 43 | 10 | 11.6 | 48 | 9 | 9.4 | 1.2 |
| 40–49 | 65 | 17 | 13.1 | 41 | 5 | 6.1 | 2.1 |
| 50–59 | 35 | 11 | 15.7 | 43 | 4 | 4.7 | 3.3 |
| 60–69 | 30 | 4 | 6.7 | 54 | 3 | 2.8 | 2.4 |
| 70–79 | 23 | 0 | 0.0 | 45 | 0 | 0.0 | .... |
| 80–89 | 10 | 0 | 0.0 | 24 | 0 | 0.0 | .... |
| 90–99 | 0 | 0 | 0.0 | 1 | 0 | 0.0 | .... |
| Total | 598 | 88 | 7.4 | 563 | 49 | 4.4 | 1.7 |

# References

1. MacMahon, B. and Pugh, T. F. Epidemiology: Principles and Methods. Boston, Little, Brown, 1970.
2. British Medical Bulletin. Epidemiology of non-communicable disease. Brit. Med. Bull. 27: 1–94, 1971.
3. Gordon, J. E. The epidemiology of accidents. Am. J. Public Health, 39: 504–515, 1949.
4. McFarland, R. A. and Moore, R. C. Human factors in highway safety: review and evaluation. N.E.J. Med. 256: 792–798, 837–845, 890–897, 1957.
5. Haddon, W. The prevention of accidents. In Preventive medicine (Clark, D. W. and MacMahon, B. eds.). Boston, Little, Brown, 1967.
6. Neel, J. V., Salzano, F. M., Junqueira, P. C., Keiter, F., and Maybury-Lewis, D. Studies on the Xavante Indians of the Brazilian Mato Grosso. Am. J. Human Genetics 16: 52–140, 1964.
7. Polunin, I. V. Health and disease in contemporary primitive societies. In Diseases in antiquity (Brothwell, D. E. and Sandison, A. T. eds.). Springfield, Illinois, Thomas, 1967.
8. Henry, J. P. and Cassel, J. C. Psychosocial factors in essential hypertension. Am. J. Epidemiol. 90: 171–200, 1969.
9. Damon, A. Human ecology in the Solomon Islands—Biomedical observations among four tribal societies. Human Ecology, 2:3, 191–215, 1974.
10. Morris, J. N. Uses of epidemiology. (2nd ed.) Edinburgh, Livingstone, 1964.
11. Taylor, I. and Knowelden, J. Principles of epidemiology. (2nd ed.) Boston, Little, Brown, 1964
12. Witts, L. J. Medical surveys and clinical trials. (2nd ed.) New York, Oxford, 1964.
13. Statistical abstract of the United States. Bureau of Census, U.S. Dept. of Commerce. Washington, D.C., Gov't Printing Office, 1970.
14. Leighton, A. H. Some observations on the prevalence of mental illness in contrasting communities. In Social and genetic influences on life and death. (Platt, R. and Parkes, A. S., eds.) Edinburgh, Oliver and Boyd, 1967.
15. Leighton, D. C. Measuring stress levels in school children as a program-monitoring device. Am. J. Public Health 62: 799–806, 1972.
16. Struening, E. L. and Lehmann, S. A social areas study of the Bronx: environmental determinants of behavioral deviance and physical pathology. Research Publication, Assoc. Res. Nerv. Mental Diseases 47: 130–138, 1969.

17. Gallé, O. R., Gove, W. R., and McPherson, J. M. Population density and pathology: what are the relations for man? Science 176: 23–30, 1972.
18. Holmes, T. H. Multidiscipline studies of tuberculosis. *In* Personality stress and tuberculosis. (Sparer, P. J., ed.) New York, International Universities Press, 1956.
19. Brett, G. Z. and Benjamin, B. Housing and tuberculosis in a mass radiography survey. Brit. J. Prev. Soc. Med. 11: 7–9, 1957.
20. Hall, E. T. The hidden dimension. Garden City, New York, Doubleday, 1966.
21. Winsborough, H. The social consequences of high population density. *In* Social demography. (Ford, T. and De Jong, G., eds.) Englewood Cliffs, New Jersey, Prentice-Hall, 1970.
22. Clouse, M. E. and Damon, A. Radiologic survey in the Solomon Islands, 1968: lungs, heart, spleen, scoliosis, bone age, and dental development. Human Biol. 43: 22–35, 1971.
23. Friedman, G. D., Wilson, W. S. Mosier, J. M., Colandrea, M. A., and Nichaman, M. Z. Transient ischemic attacks in a community. J.A.M.A. 210: 1428–1434, 1969.
24. Bellin, S. S. and Geiger, H. J. Actual public acceptance of the Neighborhood Health Center by the urban poor. J.A.M.A. 214: 2147–2153, 1970.
25. Abey-Wickrama, I., and others. Mental-hospital admissions and aircraft noise. Lancet 2: 1275–1277, 1969.
26. Vines, A. P. An epidemiological sample survey of the Highlands, Mainland, and Islands Regions of the Territory of Papua and New Guinea. Dep't. Pub. Health, Port Moresby, 1970.
27. Bakwin, H. and McLaughlin, S. D. Secular increase in height. Is the end in sight? Lancet 2: 1195–1196, 1964.
28. Damon, A. Secular trend in height and weight within Old American families at Harvard, 1870–1965. I. Within twelve four-generation families. Am. J. Phys. Anthrop. n.s. 29: 45–50, 1968.
29. Mead, M. Adult roles. *In* Transcultural Psychiatry. (DeReuck, A. V. S. and Porter, R., eds.) Ciba Foundation Symposium. Boston, Little, Brown, 1965.
30. Lin, T. Y. A study of the incidence of mental disorder in Chinese and other cultures. Psychiatry 16: 313–336, 1953.
31. Langner, T. S. A twenty-two item score of psychiatric symptoms indicating impairment. J. Health and Human Behavior 3: 269–276, 1962.
32. Srole, L., and others. Mental health in the metropolis. The Midtown Manhattan Study. New York, McGraw-Hill, 1962.
33. Dupuy, H. J. and others. Selected symptoms of psychological distress. Public Health Service Publication No. 1000-Series 11-No. 37. Washington, D.C., Gov't. Printing Office, 1970.
34. Ciba Foundation Symposium. Transcultural psychiatry. (DeReuck, A. V. S. and Porter, R., eds.) Boston, Little, Brown, 1965.
35. Hare, E. H. and Wing, J. K. Psychiatric epidemiology. London, Oxford, 1970.
36. Damon, A., Poster, C. M., and Gerald, A. B. Residential design, health, and behavior. Final report, Contract C.P.E. 70–103, Bureau of Community Environmental Management (Mimeographed.) 1969.
37. Evans, J. G. and Rose, G. Hypertension. Brit. Med. Bull. 27: 37–42, 1971.
38. Stott, D. H. Cultural and natural checks on population-growth. *In* Culture and the evolution of man. (Montagu, M. F. A., ed.) New York, Oxford, 1962.
39. Lewis, O. La vida: a Puerto Rican family in the culture of poverty—San Juan and New York. New York, Random House, 1966.
40. Trulson, M. F., and others. Comparisons of siblings in Boston and Ireland. J. Am. Dietetic Assoc. 45: 225–229, 1964.
41. Segall, A. J., Harvard School of Public Health (Epidemiology). Personal communication.

42. Salzano, F. M., Neel, J. V. and Maybury-Lewis, D. Further studies on the Xavante Indians. Am. J. Human Genetics, 19: 463–488, passim, 1967.

43. Neel, J. V. and Chagnon, N. A. The demography of two tribes of relatively unacculturated American Indians. Proc. Nat. Acad. Sci. 59: 680–689, 1968.

44. Buck, A. A., Sasaki, T. T., and Anderson, R. I. Health and disease in four Peruvian villages. Baltimore, Johns Hopkins, 1968.

45. Lee, R. B. What hunters do for a living, or how to make out on scarce resources. *In* Man the hunter (Lee, R. B. and DeVore, I., eds.) . Chicago, Aldine, 1968.

46. Truswell, A. S. and J. D. L. Hansen. Medical and- nutritional studies of Kung Bushmen in Northern Botswana. S. Afr. Med. J. 42: 1338–1339, 1968.

47. Dunn, F. L. Epidemiological factors: health and disease in hunter-gatherers. *In* Man the hunter (Lee, R. B., and DeVore, I., eds.) . Chicago, Aldine, 1968.

48. Grace, C. S., Sinnett, P. F., Whyte, H. M. Blood fibrinolysis and coagulation in New Guineans and Australians. Australias. Ann. Med. 19: 328–333, 1970.

49. Prior, I. A. M. and others. Sodium intake and blood pressure in two Polynesian populations. N.E.J. Med. 279: 515–520, 1968.

50. U.S. National Center for Health Statistics. Origin, program, and operation of the U.S. National Health Survey. Public Health Service Public. no. 1000-Series 1-No. 1 (reprinted) . Washington, D.C., Gov't Printing Off., 1965.

51. Langner, T. S. Columbia School of Public Health (Epidemiology) . Personal communication.

52. Rush, D. Columbia School of Public Health (Epidemiology) . Personal communication.

53. Gordon, T. and Kannel, W. B. The Framingham study, 20 years later. *In* The community as an epidemiologic laboratory. (Kessler, I. I. and Levin, M. L., eds.) Baltimore, Johns Hopkins, 1970.

54. Napier, J. A., Johnson, B. C. and Epstein, F. H. The Tecumseh, Michigan community health study. *In* The community as an epidemiologic laboratory (Kessler, I. I. and Levin, M. L., eds.) Baltimore, Johns Hopkins, 1970.

55. Hochstim, J. R. Health and ways of living. *In* The community as an epidemiologic laboratory (Kessler, I. I. and Levin, M. L., eds.) Baltimore, Johns Hopkins, 1970.

56. Bell, B., Rose, C. L., and Damon, A. The Normative Aging Study—an interdisciplinary, longitudinal study of aging. Aging and Human Devel. 3: 5–17, 1972.

57. Connelly, J. P. Harvard Medical School (Pediatrics) . Personal communication.

58. Dougherty, J. D. and Welsh, O. L. Community noise and hearing loss. N.E.J. Med. 275: 759–765, 1966.

59. Carstairs, G. M. pp. 134–135, *In* Transcultural psychiatry. (DeReuck, A. V. S. and Porter, R., eds.) Ciba Foundation Symposium. Boston, Little, Brown, 1965.

60. Cassel, J. Present volume.

# Chapter IX

# Residential Environment and Health of the Elderly: Use of Research Results for Policy and Planning

Kermit K. Schooler, and
Neal S. Bellos

It has been noted that those who have the responsibility for making and executing plans affecting the lives of many human beings frequently do not profit from the knowledge of those same topics obtained by those engaged in social and behavioral research. It might be added that it is also very likely that the researcher does not profit from the experience of the practitioner and planner, either. Some of the reasons for this lack of communication and understanding will be discussed later in this document. In this paper, a large body of data collected in a well-executed research project dealing with effects of the environment on the aged will be examined to show how data on environmental effects can be usefully analyzed and to determine how the implications of that data analysis might be applied. The first section of the paper will be a brief description of the research project, the analysis methodology used, and some *selected* relevant findings. The second section, will examine the implications of such research results for the planning of programs and services resulting in the main from local efforts, and will conclude with an examination of the implications of such research for the establishment and execution of national policy.

## Part I. Description of the Research

The research to be described here has its roots in two independent areas of concern for social scientists. The first is the concern for understanding the ways in which man-made environment effects the health and well-being of people, while the second is a concern for the detection of causal factors affecting adjustment of the elderly. While each of these areas of concern is reflected in a body of literature consisting of relatively small, highly localized studies, the literature is relatively empty of systematic large-scale studies concerned with the impact of man-made environment on the process of aging. Not only is the evidence inconclusive regarding the existence of the main effect itself, but where the bits of evidence do seem to support the contention that environment has an impact on the adjustment of the elderly, generalizability of those data appears to be questionable. This study, therefore, represents an attempt to establish the relative importance of environmental characteristics with respect to the process of aging, to delineate the nature of such relationships, and to do so on a sample of such size and character as to permit generalizations heretofore unwarranted. Relationships among four sets of variables are examined: 1) characteristics of the residential environment; 2) the maintenance of social relationships; 3) health and 4) morale. The methodology has been described elsewhere (1) in considerable detail and is presented here only in summary form. An area probability sample of nearly 4,000 persons, 65 years of age and over, not living in institutions, was drawn. The sampling procedure gives some assurance that the data will be reasonably representative of that universe of elderly persons. An interview of approximately two hours duration was conducted with each member of the sample. Questions were asked pertaining not only to the four principal domains just mentioned, but also pertaining to demographic characteristics, residential mobility, and knowledge and use of social services.

Formulation of hypotheses pertaining to the concepts of environment, social relations, health, and morale is easily accomplished. However, the step from conceptualization to measurement is a long one which can only be accomplished by the translation of the names of concepts into specific operations. Consider, for example, the concept of morale.

"At one extreme, the investigator, recognizing that morale is a multi-faceted concept, feels compelled to use a large number of measures of his dependent variables, one for each facet, so as to be sure that each meaningful aspect may be investigated and analyzed and that all relevant relationships may be discovered. The risk to the investigator is manifold. The detail of the measurement process may be tedious, the manipulation of data and subsequent analysis may be burdensome and the extraction of meaning may be nearly impossible. Moreover, when the investigator hopes that his findings will have implications for policy formation and implementation, there is a risk that some relationships will run contrary to each other in such a way that while to implement policy which would have favorable consequences in the light of one set of relationships, unfavorable consequences will ensue with respect to other sets of relationships. At the other extreme, the avoidance of such risks by over-simplifying the measurement of morale carries with it its own risk that only one or a few facets of the concept will be tapped and that they will be the 'wrong' facets in terms of policy recommendation.

"A resolution to the dilemma may be achieved through the use of factor analytic procedures which, by their nature, will identify underlying concepts shared in common by a multitude of measures of what seems on the face of it to be separate facets of the main concept. Such a procedure has been undertaken in this study of an elderly sample." *(2)*

The logic of this argument regarding the operationalization of the concept of morale may be applied to the other principal domains (environment, social relations, health) as well. That is to say, in the case of each of the four principal domains relatively large numbers of single questionnaire items have been condensed into or represented by a smaller number of factors. Much of the analysis of the data was then accomplished by converting the factors into factor scores for each individual. The factor scores could then be treated as variables.

At this point, then, it is appropriate to describe the outcome of the factor analytic approach, since so much of the subsequent analysis of data was based on the results of those factor analyses.

## A. Environment Factors

The *first* environmental factor extracted was loaded high on such items as distance to the bank, a barber, stores, public transportation, etc. This is the "distance to facility" factor. The *second* environmental factor was loaded high on questionnaire items and interviewer observations dealing with the condition and state of repair of the dwelling unit, surrounding grounds, style, size and condition of furniture, and the impressionistic comparison of the respondent's structure with others in the neighborhood. This is the "condition of dwelling unit" factor. The *third* environmental factor required respondent judgment about the convenience of his location to facilities such as those in Factor 1, as well as to friends and relatives. It has been called the "convenience" factor. The *fourth* factor in this domain was a mixture of items, some characterizing the dwelling (particularly apartment houses) with regard to safety and convenience features (adequate hallway illumination, maintenance, etc.) and some feature dealing with opportunities for socializing (outdoor recreation and visiting areas, social room, and laundromat). In addition, the number of dwelling units and floors in dwellings were loaded high on this factor. To simplify, call it the "features" factor. The *fifth* factor concerns items related to the respondent's awareness of the availability of various social and supportive services—personal counseling, overnight companionship, employment guidance, visiting nurse, etc.—11 services in all. The final, *sixth,* factor deals with measures of the size of the dwelling unit and the structure, and some other structural characteristics.

## B. Social Relations Factors

Seven factors were also extracted from the social relations domain. The *first* represents the number of friends, frequency of visiting or being visited, etc. This factor is termed "neighboring." The *second* social relations factor contains group and organization membership and attendance items (number of organizations, meetings attended, number where majority of members are 65 or over, or whether the organization maintains programs for the elderly). This is the "organization" factor. Factors *three* and *five* are similar, pertaining to frequency and recency of contact with children, the difference between the factors being accounted for mainly by family size; that is, the *third* factor refers to contact with the respondent's first and second mentioned child, while the *fifth* refers to contact with the respondent's third, fourth, fifth, and sixth mentioned child. The clustering in the *fifth* factor of items seems to be an artifact of the coding system where those who had, say, no fifth child were coded with those that had no contact with the fifth child. The *third* factor, referring to contact with the first and second mentioned children is no doubt less influenced by family size and consequently may be more useful as a separate factor. Factor *five* is, therefore, not used in the analysis described here. The *fourth* factor is a function of original family size, depending on the number of siblings and the frequency they are seen. The *sixth* social relations factor concerns indirect (telephone and letter) contact with children. The *seventh* factor is a measure of contact—recency of visiting friends and church, visits to the bank or post office, and a crude estimate of total number of people that the respondent had at least minimal contact with during the typical week.

## C. Morale Factors

The *first* morale factor is comprised of seven items contained in a scale developed and refined by M. Powell Lawton. *(3)* These particular items are seeemingly based on day-to-day fears and worries and upsets. For convenience, this is referred to as the "fears and worries" factor. The *second* factor includes four items from what is commonly known as the Srole Anomie Scale. *(4)* Morale factor *III* includes three more Lawton items, as well as the respondent's self-image (whether he views himself as young, middle-aged, old) and his self-appraisal of how he differs from others of the same age. It also contains two items based on the interviewer's observation of respondent alertness, understanding of interview procedures and over-all reaction to the procedure, on the scale from enjoyment and involvement through boredom, lack of concern, to being visibly upset. Factor *IV* is loaded on some items referring to respondent's feelings about life-long accomplishments. The *fifth* factor again is a subset of Powell Lawton's items, specifically in contrast with the first factor, concerned with more sustained unhappiness and dissatisfaction. Finally, the *sixth* factor, which for a variety of technical reasons was not used in the analysis, is loaded on items comparing one's financial situation with others.

## D. Health Factors

The items in the *first* health factor tend to be related to the amount of difficulty performing certain day-to-day activities. Questions asked were in the form of "Do you have any trouble. . . .;" the specific areas involved in this factor: ". . . getting around the house, washing and bathing, going outdoors, dressing, working in the house, cutting toenails, climbing stairs, and cooking meals." A final item asks whether or not the respondent needs help because of his health. For convenience, this factor is referred to as "Disability I." The *second* health factor deals with health as it is commonly considered: items related to inactivity due to health, self-rated current health, chronic health problems, hospitalization, restriction of activities, number of visits to a doctor, visits to a medical clinic, and comparison of present health to last year's and to age 60. This factor is referred to as "General Health." The *third* health factor is called "Disability II." The majority of items in this factor relate to the respondent's ability to perform certain tasks: painting furniture, driving a car, fixing appliances, planting and gardening, and taking a plane or train. Also included is the distance the respondent can walk, how often health restricts his activities, and whether or not he has a lasting health problem. There was another health factor entitled "Use of Other Health Services." This factor is of a somewhat different order than the three discussed above and it consists of only two items.

## E. Analysis of Relations Among the Factors

It is obvious that such a large number of variables can produce an inordinately large number of relationships among them, especially when one allows for relationships beyond the zero-order. A more complete reporting of the analysis of these data can be found elsewhere, but the purpose of this paper can best be served by a judicious selection, chosen to illustrate the following principles:

1. The dependent variable, a measure of which we would, in some sense, want to optimize as a consequence of social intervention, can have a unitary name (for example, "health"), but can be defined in more than one way. Relations of other variables to the dependent may vary according to the choice of definition of the dependent variable.

2. A similar argument can be made in the case of the principal independent variable, in the present instance "environment." There are many facets of environment that can be studied, but it may be asserted here that not all facets are related in the same way to any particular measure of health. This point in conjunction with the previous one suggests readily that, if one would attempt to effect changes in health by intervening with respect to some environmental characteristics, the consequence of such intervention will depend on how one chooses to define environment and how one chooses to define health.

3. If it is indeed true that in some ways environment influences health, consideration must be given to the likelihood that that process of influence from environment to health varies with or is contingent upon characteristics of the population. That is, hypothetically, the relation for the wealthy may be different from the relation among the poor. Males may respond differently from females, etc.

Irrespective of the way in which data are collected, there is a question of the most effective way of analyzing large quantities of data in order to understand complex relations among many variables. Multiple regression can be useful in demonstrating how the combination of all variables, intervening and independent, predict the ultimate dependent variable. However, that approach in itself does not permit the investigator to make inferences about causal links among the several predictors. In contrast, in order not only to make inferences regarding the effect of several predictors on one criterion, but to be able to draw inferences about the relative importance of links between predictor variables, one may resort to the technique known as path analysis. *(5)*

To apply path analysis one begins with a causal model in which the links between pairs of variables are specified and the causal direction pertaining to each link is also specified. A model employed in the study just described implies, for example, that health may be predicted from morale, social relationships, environment, and a set of demographic characteristics. It suggests, further, that the environment factors themselves directly "cause" social relations, morale, and the dependent variable, health. The model tested also suggests that social relations and morale, in that order, intervene between environmental characteristics and measures of health. Finally, the model states that all of these sets of variables are to some extent determined by a set of demographic characteristics. The technique of path analysis allows us to apply numerical values, called path coefficients, which are indicative of the relative importance of each of the links in the causal model. The remainder of this section will be devoted to a discussion of some selected findings based on the path analysis.

Earlier it had been noted that a variable, or concept, such as health can be defined in several ways; and that the relation between combinations of variables and the criterion-measure, health, will itself vary according to the definition of health used. In the present instance, the multiple correlation between each of the health factor scores and the set of predictors (including morale, social relations, environment, and demographic attributes) varies from about .4 to about .6, or, as shown in Table 1, $R^2$, which may be interpreted as a percentage of variance of the dependent variable accounted for by the combination of predictors, varies from .159 to .323. In other words, these predictors account for almost one-third of the variance of the Disability II factor but only half as much of the Disability I factor. To elaborate this point somewhat further, note in Table 2 the zero-order relations between each of the predictor variables and two of the four health criteria. Age, marital status, sex, and race do not significantly predict the general health factor but do predict Disability II. Population, on the other hand, does significantly correlate with the general health factor but not with the disability factor. As one scans the Table, ones sees that correlations with the third health factor are higher than those with the second health factor, but this is to be expected considering that the multiple correlation with the third health factor is substantially higher as shown in Table 1.

Of especial concern to this particular paper are the correlations between the environmental factors and the health factors. The first environmental factor is the only one which correlates higher with the second health factor than with the third health factor. It should be noted further that the second, third, fifth, and sixth environmental factors all seem to correlate significantly with the third health factor (disability), yet only the second and first environmental factors correlate significantly with the second health factor (general health). Thus it would appear that if at this simple level one wanted to recommend intervention at the environmental level in order to effect changes in levels of health, justification for that intervention would depend on how, indeed, health was measured and which combinations of characteristics of the environment one were to consider as predictors. It will be shown shortly that the situation is even more complex.

Let us turn our attention now to the consideration of the process by which environmental factors might be mediated as they effect level of health. In this part of the analysis we will compare the path analysis for the third health factor with the path analysis for the second health factor in order to demonstrate that the process varies as the definition of "health" changes. It has already been shown that the second, third, fifth, and sixth environmental factors have significant correlations with the third health factor. Table 2 corresponds with the bottom row of Table 3 and Table 4. The next-to-bottom row of each of those tables represents the direct path between each of the predictor variables and the criterion. Since, in most instances, those numbers are substantially lower than the total effects, the inference is drawn that much of the effect of the predictors is indirect, that is, mediated through other variables.

Thus we see that the second environmental factor is mediated through the second and sixth social relations factors and the second and fourth morale factors. In contrast, the third environmental factor is mediated through the first and seventh social relations factors and the third and fourth morale factors. A similar set of observations can be made for the prediction of the second health factor. In this instance we are primarily interested in the effect of the second environmental factor and note that its effect is mediated by the second, the third and the sixth social relations factors, as well as the second and fourth morale factors. One notes further that the second social relations factor is mediated by the third morale factor and it is indeed this factor which significantly predicts self-reported general health.

The mediating process just described is contained, in effect, by the right-hand side of Tables 3 and 4. However, since we have started with the attempt to explain the influence of environment on health, is it not appropriate to try to understand other more immediate determinants of these environmental characteristics? To do this we turn to the left-hand side of Tables 3 and 4, where the relations of several demographic characteristics to the other predictors are shown. In the case of Table 3, environmental factor II is predicted significantly by race, income and education, whereas environmental factor III is significantly predicted by age and, to some extent, sex. The fifth environmental factor does not appear to be predicted well by any of the demographic characteristics while the sixth is very significantly predicted by the population size of the sampling point. In the case of the prediction of the second health factor (Table 4) it is noted that the second environmental factor is best predicted by income and education and race.

Noting the causal effects of demographic characteristics, the importance of considering classes or categories within these demographic variables becomes apparent. We will consider in this context further path analyses of the effects on the third health factor (Disability II) within categories of three of the demographic characteristics: sex, race, and the urban-rural dichotomy. Comparing Tables 5 and 6, representing males and females respectively, it is seen that the total effect of environment on health is noticeably greater among males than among females, especially with respect to environment factors II, III, V and VI. Moreover, the mediating effects of social relations and morale are also shown to be somewhat different. But of somewhat greater interest to the investigator examining possibilities for intervention are the data from the left-hand side of the table, where it can be shown, for example, that in the case of males, income is twice as important a predictor of the second environmental factor as it is for females, whereas population-of-sampling-point is a substantially better predictor of the second environmental factor for females than it is for males. A similar mode of comparison shows that the prediction of environmental factor III does not vary significantly between males and females, age being by far the most important predictor shown.

Turning to a comparison by race, we note in Tables 7 and 8 that the first environmental factor is a better predictor of health for non-whites than for whites, while the fifth and sixth environmental factors are better predictors of health for whites than for non-whites. These observations notwithstanding, it is apparent that for both classes, the best

270

predictors are environmental factors II and III. In the case of whites, environmental factor II is significantly predicted by income and education, whereas for non-whites, size of location, in addition to those two predictors, has an effect on environmental factor II. In regard to environmental factor III, it is interesting to note that income is a rather significant predictor among non-whites but not so among whites. It is instructive also to examine the process by which the second and third environmental factors are mediated. For example, the effect of the second environmental factor on the second social relations factor is twice as strong among non-whites as among whites. A similar difference obtains with respect to the sixth social relations factor. With regard to the third environmental factor it will be noted that the effects on the morale factors are substantially higher in the non-white sample.

Turning now to an analysis shown in Tables 9 and 10 pertaining to the rural and non-rural samples, it is seen that the demographic determinants of the second and third environmental factors are not appreciably different between the two samples, with the exception of the stronger effect of race on environmental factor III in the rural sample than in the non-rural. Further examination does not reveal that the mediating process in non-rural areas is substantially different from that in rural areas.

*Summary:* To this point, using Schooler's data for illustration. we have argued as follows: (a) A criterion such as health can be defined in several ways. The manner and extent to which this criterion can be predicted or explained by other variables, such as environmental characteristics will vary, depending on the terms of the definition. (b) Different environmental characteristics predict health differentially. (c) The mediating process by which environment effects health varies. (d) The mediating process varies in relation to the characteristics of the sample being attended to.

## Part II. The Policy and Planning Process: Implications for Utilization of Research

This section of the paper examines the policy and planning process in order to develop a frame of reference within which to discuss the implications for utilization of research on environment and health such as that just described. This discussion only scratches the surface of the subject, opening up areas that indicate applicability of this research, as well as identifying issues beyond the scope of particular research findings, extending to larger questions of social science research.

The literature on policy introduces an apparent hodgepodge of differing definitions and various elements. Implicit in these discussions is the nature of the relationship between the processes of planning and policy, an explication of which, however, is not within the scope of this paper. For the purposes of drawing out some implications for the utilization of social research, the authors have settled on a particular usage of the terms planning and policy. The Lindblom thesis (6) posits that the major elements of the policy and planning process can be grouped around either issues related to a *rational, analytic* process or issues related to a *power-influence-political* process. We will refer to the issue set of the former being encompassed by *planning*, and those of the latter as *policy*.

In addition we look at social planning as a process whose purpose is the design and implementation of specific activities to improve the social well-being of vulnerable population groups, within a locality relevant context. The social policy process is interpreted in the context of influencing major decisions on social affairs extending to the national arena.

## A. The Planning Process and its Limitations

In its infancy, social planning struggled for legitimacy in a society resistant to the very concept. (7) Beset by a lack of money, knowledge, and/or consensus, social planning efforts in recent years have had, at best, a modest record of success, as in the cases of juvenile delinquency programs or anti-poverty activities. In actuality, social planning could be described as a searching, problem-solving process; social programming is a more appropriate term for developing projects. Many projects have been established to deal with social problems—bad health, unemployment, poverty, etc. Too often they have a prefabricated quality, with little evidence of thoughtful construction.

Underdeveloped as the social planning enterprise may be, a matching of its rational model with the constraints of practice can uncover several areas where social planning could be enhanced by the social research enterprise.

In theory the social planning process follows a generic problem-solving model consisting of the following steps:

a. *Data Collection*—this phase consists of collecting the important information pertaining to the problem.

b. *Problem Definition and Goal Formulation*—here the data collected are assessed and interpreted, the problem stated, and objectives defined to cope with the problem.

c. *Selection of Actions*—this phase develops a variety of means of achieving objectives. These alternatives are weighed, and that one chosen which has the most promise of achievement of the objectives.

d. *Implementation*—the chosen alternative is enacted.

e. *Evaluation*—the results are measured. If objectives are not achieved, the cycle repeats itself.

The social planner, in the real world, seldom, if ever, has the opportunity of putting a rational planning model into operation. He is beset with a variety of limitations. These limitations in turn define specific areas where social research is important—data availability, goals, means, and new techniques.

## 1. Data Availability

The planning model indicates that the first step to be undertaken is the collection of pertinent data. The social planner, here, finds himself faced with considerable constraints. First are the time limits placed on his activities. Having to face deadlines, he must necessarily limit the time required to collect his data. If his activities are related to federal programs, then his time may be further shortened by the all-too-often urgent nature of planning for federal funding.

Second, the planner may not have the resources to generate his own data. The gathering of information is a costly process, and only sophisticated planning organizations have such a capacity. Therefore, the planner is often in the position of borrowing data.

Third, the social planner not only plans, but most of the time he is engaged in community organization or organizational maintenance activities. The goals of his employing organization, the nature of the task, community influence patterns, and the planner's own style call for a variety of role behaviors above and beyond rational planning. Jack Rothman defines enabler, or technician, or social actionist roles. (8) Francine Rabinowitz, in *City Politics and Planning*, describes a technician, broker, and mobilizer role. (9) The activities implied by these differing roles all add up to the need to take time away from data handling.

Fourth, the social planner must have a variety of skills to fill a variety of roles. The setting in which he operates may place a premium on his community organization responsibilities (and many, if not most, do). These organization responsibilities call for administrative, public relations, coordinating, and political skills. Therefore, it is understandable that many persons filling social planning slots do not have the necessary social science background for the collection and analysis of data.

For reasons of lack of time, resource, other responsibilities, and skill, the social planner may not be able to have access to pertinent data. He must then rely on available and borrowed data. Some social issues such as education, race, and poverty have a currency that has produced a plethora of data. Less visible and/or popular issues, such as aging, do not have such attention. So, for example, the aging planners are required to borrow data in an area where there is not much available information.

The planner also requires that, in addition to being available, his data are applicable. The product of the planner is a commitment to action. The information he uses must lay the base for projecting future actions. Therefore, the planner looks for data that give firm direction.

He finds, however, that most research findings are couched in qualification. For example, levels of significance are a meaningful interpretation standard for the researchers, but the planner requires a way of translating the research qualifications into estimates of outcomes.

## 2. Goals

Goal setting (i.e., choice of ends) is a perplexing yet crucial task for planners. Without goals of sufficient specificity implementers have little to guide their service activities. Without goals of a measurable nature, what of substance can be evaluated? Yet that very area which seems to call for objectivity is surrounded by conflicts of value and of self-interest. Facts are interpreted differently by different people. As such, the same facts lead to different problem definitions; and it is axiomatic in the planning field that he who defines the problem is also defining the solution.

Social planners do not alone set the goals for their planning outcomes. The planning process involves citizens, public officials, and a variety of interest groups. From this variety of interests stems potential goal conflict. While conflict can be functional, it can also be dysfunctional. The record of O.E.O. and its local C.A.A. affiliates attests to the negative side of conflict. The controversies generated by trying to achieve the goal of "maximum feasible participation" influenced or determined the demise of the war on poverty.

## 3. Choice of Means

The major criteria for program selection today are: what the potential consumer may wish (if citizens are involved in the planning process), what the various power centers won't veto, and the availability of money to fund the program, rather than a measure of which program can do the best job. According to H. A. Simon, the planner "satisfices." Today, however, satisficing is no longer satisfactory for the planner and his public. The planner wishes that the goals of his planning are achieved. He is holding himself accountable. Moreover, his publics are holding him more and more accountable, be they citizens or the Federal government. Downs (10) states that the bureau leader is a utility maximizer. Rather than satisficing, if the costs are right, he will move to a maximum position. According to Dror, (11) even maximizing as a concept is inadequate: the standard should be optimizing. If Downs is describing reality, and if Dror is stating a desirable position, both still are based on an assumption that the individual decider has some measure of what is maximum or what is optimal.

The planner, then, by reasons of responsibility and of self-interest is in need of better ways for choosing among means.

### 4. New Techniques

It has been mentioned previously that citizens have been participating in the planning process. More recently the spirit of this participation has been to include representatives of the consumer group for whom a particular social service is being planned. This concept of participation, which is gaining currency, has evidenced many operational problems and questions. One of the major questions to arise is "how representative are the representatives?" Obviously, the relatively small number of consumers who participate in planning activities are not representative of the universe of consumers. If their participation is sought to truly represent consumer needs and desires, the present small numbers of participants will not give an accurate view.

The consumer of social services could be viewed differently in a market context. Market enterprises design their goods with the notion of consumer utility. If the consumer finds that a particular product has no utility for him, he won't buy it. Hence, no profit for the company. It would be interesting to transfer this concept to social services. The design of social programs and services would then be based on a notion of whether the consumers would find utility in the program. If the consumer found no utility in the program, then the program will have little effectiveness.

To operationalize this concept, consumer preference could not be measured from the small numbers of present planning participants. Market research seems to be a tool more applicable in this situation. For social planning this would represent a new approach for not only design implications, but also for citizen participation in planning.

Planning in the field of aging also proposes a question for techniques. The aging population is one about which it is most difficult to generalize. Individuals are never more different than when they grow older. The obvious implication of this fact is that services to the aging must cover a range of alternatives if it is expected that a reasonable number of persons are to be reached by such services.

Yet the experience in designing social programs has been one that has produced a single set of services, inherently based on the assumption that most of the consumers have basically similar characteristics. The continuation of this pattern for the aging guarantees unserved numbers.

To cope with this situation, the planner needs a technology that will help him handle and design for a range of alternative programs.

## B. Utilization of Research to Improve the Planning Process

The above discussion of the planning process in light of the realities of social planning has identified four areas where social research and social researchers can make valuable contributons:

a. The social planner has definite limits in collecting and interpreting planning data.
b. The social planner needs better criteria by which to select goals (ends).
c. The social planner requires better ways for selecting means to achieve agreed upon goals.
d. The planner needs new techniques (1) to test for consumer utility and (2) to handle alternative designs.

Based on this summary of issues in social planning, the following discussion notes how the research project might be instructive in the planning process.

## 1. The Social Planner Has Definite Limits in Collecting and Interpreting Planning Data

Frequently the social scientist is accused of being "too ivory tower." The stereotype depicts him as being concerned primarily with "pure" research, the findings of which are of interest solely to other social scientists in the universities. Though, for many, the debate surrounding the choice between "pure" and "applied" research had been laid to rest long ago, it is worth noting that even if the debate and the issues debated were real, a single research enterprise may embody concepts and data which are relevant to both the pure social scientist and the applied practitioner. That is to say, the inclusion of planning-relevant data is not antithetical to the inclusion of social-science-relevant data within the same study and the same set of instruments. Even where one could make such distinctions, the marginal cost of inclusion of survey questions relevant to the planner in a study having principal value to the social scientist, is quite small. At the same time, we note that the marginal cost of satisfying the needs of the planner is relatively small. Further, when large sample surveys are involved valuable data can be provided from which planners in local situations can draw inferences not otherwise obtainable independently. Thus, for example, in the study reported here, the 4,000 interviews could be collected at, say, a unit cost of $50. The cost of such a study is feasible at a national level once, or twice, but hardly feasible for each of, say, 50 Model Cities, planning budgets. It ought to be possible, however, for the local planner to be made aware of the existence of this pool of data. The question might arise, for example, "In what way are the black elderly in the model neighborhood likely to be different from the white elderly in the same area?" It is noted that the research reported here is based on a sample which includes more black elderly (approximately 400) than were included in any of the samples upon which most of what we know about the black elderly are based. (12) To be more explicit, the planner who must take into consideration the characteristics of his target population, such as the black elderly, could obtain a complete analysis of a subsample, matched on the known characteristics of his own target population. And even if he were required to pay for that special analysis, it could be demonstrated that the cost would be substantially lower than the cost of obtaining those data in his own account. An issue to be confronted is the designation of the locus of authority to establish a clearinghouse for such studies and data.

## 2. The Social Planner Needs Better Criteria by Which to Select Goals (Ends)

At the outset it should be apparent that social research alone cannot establish the priority among values. Nevertheless, recognizing that social planning and the establishment of social policy is frequently characterized by the conflict of ends, social research can be useful to the participants in some ways as they engage in the debate. First, research may show that a concept which is spoken of as if it were unitary, as a goal or end to be achieved by successful planning, is really not unitary but pluralistic. Specifically, it is not unreasonable to suppose that the environmental planner hopes or expects to maximize satisfaction of the residents of the area for which he is planning. The research described here demonstrates that a concept such as Health is not unitary but has many facets. Consequently, the importance of being more specific in the delineation of goals is suggested by the further observation that not only are there several facets to the concept of Health, but, indeed, the relationships of each of the facets to a characteristic of the environment may be different from each other.

This point was illustrated earlier when it was shown that the third health factor, Disability II, correlated with (was predicted by) the third environmental factor, Convenience to Services, whereas the second health factor, General Health, was not so correlated. Should the planner incorporate such services into his design for a neighborhood or community? The answer is "yes" if he wants to maximize Health Factor III, and "it is a matter of indifference" if his criterion of success is measured by Health Factor II. The consequence of this observation is that if the planner-builder changes the environment in one way he may maximize one facet of health while in fact having no effect on one or more other facets of health.

There is a second way in which social research can assist the planner in the process of goal selection and especially in the process of mediating goal conflicts. Let us suppose that one faction believes that the objective of the urban redevelopment program is to improve health among the residents of the area, while another faction professes to be less concerned about health but more concerned about improving and sustaining morale. As the earlier analysis showed, in such a hypothetical conflict, the researcher can mediate by demonstrating that the two goals may in fact not be in conflict with each other at all, that one does not maximize health at the expense of morale.

### 3. The Social Planner Requires Better Ways for Selecting Means to Achieve Agreed Upon Goals

Suppose that the goals conflict has already been resolved and the planner must now determine the most effective or efficient means of achieving the goals. As a first step the planner may take note of the correlational analysis provided by the research. These data suggested that if one is interested in improving health, one might achieve better results by rebuilding the environment so as to make the array of services conveniently located relative to the residence itself, or by improving the quality of the dwelling unit as represented by the items of the second environmental factor, rather than the improvement in those items making up the fourth factor. (Such an observation is, of course, simplistic. However, it has been refined and elaborated through the analysis itself, the basic relationship having been observed within various relevant sub-classes of the population.) Again, noting the relationship between morale and health, the planner may determine that it is efficient for him to attempt to maximize health indirectly by doing those things which will have the direct effect of improving morale.

The planner, looking for better ways for selecting among means to agreed upon goals, can, through the use of path analysis, not only determine the tenability of a single causal model, but may also compare alternate causal models with relatively little additional effort or expenditure.

A discussion of the technique of path analysis has been included in order to illustrate a way in which social research can be useful to the planner in his attempt to make rational choices among sets of means to an agreed upon end. One might note further, however, that the systematic analysis of path models may also benefit the planner in his efforts to resolve goal conflicts. By introducing the concept of differential cost in implementing the means, in conjunction with the estimates of the path coefficients, the planner may deduce that a less preferred but, let us say, almost as good end may be more readily achieved through a different set of means. In other words, research can assist the planner in achieving efficiency (in contrast to effectiveness).

### 4. The Planner Needs New Techniques to Test for Consumer Utility and to Handle Alternative Designs

Much of social planning or talk about social planning is directed towards segments of the population which are easily described and characterized by single labels, such labels usually being categories of a demographic variable. Thus, there is social planning for the poor, social planning for the elderly, for the adolescent, the ill, the mentally ill, etc. All too frequently the planner acts as if the population-at-risk, because it can be described by a single label, is necessarily homogeneous. On the basis of the assumption that the population is homogeneous, a unitary

278

policy or plan is viewed as sufficient to meet the needs of the population. The case has been made elsewhere by Schooler (13) that such populations-at-risk, and particularly the aged population, are not homogeneous, and that what is needed is a pluralistic rather than unitary social policy and set of plans. The planner, recognizing the validity of that assertion, is in a position once again to turn to the researcher for assistance. It is not sufficient to know that the population-at-risk—say, the elderly—is defined by a multitude of characteristics. Rather, the analysis must be carried a step further to show that responses to the chosen means (e.g., changes in the environment) vary in some predictable manner in accordance with those characteristics that differentiate among sub-classes of the elderly.

Research such as that described in this paper offers only a partial solution. A complete array of demographic characteristics has been included in that study and it is a simple matter to show how relationships between, for example, environmental characteristics, health, and morale might vary within demographic categories. A review of the description of Tables 7 and 8 thus illustrates, perhaps simplistically, how the development of plans for environmental intervention might vary, depending on whether the target population was predominantly white or non white. Distance to services such as a bank, stores, clinic, park, doctor, etc. is a better predictor of health among non-whites (compared with whites); while availability of social services (counselling, visiting nurse, housekeeping, employment, etc.) and some characteristics of the dwelling (size and age of the building, number of rooms in the dwelling unit, etc.) are better predictors among whites (compared with non-whites). Furthermore, the data pertaining to the mediating effect of organizational participation suggest that environmental change which could enhance such participation might be especially effective in non-white areas. Such analysis is useful is sensitizing the planner to the pluralistic nature of his target population.

The planner, it is hoped, will be induced to develop plans (plural) rather than a plan (singular). The large sample study at one point in time can only suggest what is likely to ensue, should plans be implemented. It is rather through the evaluation of a "test market" (experiment) that one determines the most probable outcome. "If research based residential planning is undertaken seriously—just as in the de-sign and marketing of other consumer goods—a mixed rather than a unitary strategy will probably be required . . . It goes without saying that at the policy and design specification levels, guidelines to planners should be sufficiently flexible to permit such design variability." (14) But for the research to be truly effective, it is not sufficient that the planner be prepared to develop the variations for differing segments of his total market. The planning process will be improved greatly when the concept of the test market, so common in other areas of consumer goods manufacturing, is accepted in the social planning arena. At that time the full array of researchers' skills, from the concept of experimental design to the powerful new procedures of multivariate analysis, can be brought to bear.

## C. Policy and Research

As was suggested at the beginning of Part II, political-governmental decision-making is central to the policy process. The following discussion raises issues regarding the interface of the research process and the political aspects of the policy process.

### 1. A Variety of Publics

Several authors on policy (15) utilize aspects of a systems notion to describe the policy process. Their writings illustrate how the various stages of the policy process are influenced by a variety of individuals, audiences or publics.

At the input stage there are clients, real or potential; potential or active supporters; potential or actual resisters. The conversion process comprises all phases of the political and governmental web, from local to national levels, organized around political parties. The milieu of output is the governmental bureaucratic apparatus. If social research is to be applied in these stages, the question that arises is can we, and how do we, direct social research findings of differing audiences?

Some research efforts may be independently generated, but most are financed by resources other than those of the researcher. Government is a major sponsor of social service research. Under what circumstances does this situation place limits upon extending the findings of research to other audiences? Most research findings, as published, have a limited audience. Reaching out to other audiences requires the use of varied media. What are the additional problems or issues this circumstance raises for the researchers? More important, however, there are certain facets of utilizing social research in policy-making which add a dimension to the *role* of a social researcher—and that dimension is *active engagement*. If social research findings are to be utilized by political or policy leaders and, as the Lindblom analysis showed, policy leaders utilize those analytic findings which support their position, then the social researcher who wishes to market his product here must locate the particular leaders whose stance is compatible with that of the research findings. Further, the researcher has to convince that leader, through direct or indirect means, that the research will be of importance in the play of power.

Or, the research might be valuable to client groupings. Representatives of client groups are playing increased roles in policy decisions these days. More and more they are looking to the planner and researcher as advocates. In a similar vein, Wildavsky calls attention to a surrogate function. (16)

In the case of either of these examples the researcher will be placed in a more action-oriented stance. But in taking a more activist stance, can the researcher attempt to provide information impartially to all the policy publics? Or will he have to choose that public with which he identifies? Or does he have much choice? Rein comments that while social science offers a rational argument for choices, it does not make the rules of choosing. (17)

Germane to these questions is a decision the social researcher has to make: Whose agent will he be? If he is an agent of government, he becomes a technocrat. As an agent of client group, he is an advocate, a Nader-like critic. Possibly other publics would develop other roles.

## 2. Values and Conflict

The definitions of policy indicated values and conflicts underlie most policy-making. Policy, as Rein reminds us, is wrapped up with the notion of social purposes or values. This may not only re-emphasize the debate regarding value-free social science in general, but more importantly raises the question of how social science research can form a link with social purpose.

Value considerations point to the conflict nature of policy process. What then is the posture of the researcher when exposed to conflict? Can he anticipate some of the conflict-inducing aspects of his findings? If he can, what should he do about it? What should his response to conflict be?

## 3. Goals

If the social researcher believes his work would be of importance in creating policy, he is still faced with the problem of what kinds of goals he sets for himself. Daniel Moynihan (18) criticizes the social scientists for their active participation in the policy direction in the early days of O.E.O. He sees the social scientist only having a role in the measurement of the effects of social policy. At the heart of his argument is a criticism of decision based solely on one factor or of a social science prescription based on a shaky and questionable theoretical base. The question here is how far can the social researcher extend himself in prescribing to deal with social problems, when his findings have certain limitations.

Should the researcher avoid reliance on definitive remedies? Perhaps it is more in keeping with methodological limitations for the researcher to quest for the delineation of alternatives, coupled with estimates of the costs attached to these alternatives.

In either case, the determining factor may be the goals the researcher sets regarding how his research is to be used.

## 4. Toward a Better Policy Process

Most of the policy literature describes policy-making as it is. Dror develops a model for policy-making as it ought to be—"a complicated three-stage, eighteen-step approach to achieve optimal policies." *(19)*

The achievement of this model is dependent upon a large interdisciplinary undertaking. The traditional social sciences have much to offer, but a host of newly emerging fields must also be considered.

The achievement of interdisciplinary approaches to complex problems is highly desired. Unfortunately, this principle has more support verbally than in practice, so that it has a theoretical quality. How can an interdisciplinary effort be mounted by and for those social scientists who have an interest in policy? Sherif & Sherif point to some of the answers. *(20)*

*Summary.* There are larger questions for the social researcher to grapple with if he wishes to engage in the policy process. Whose agent is the researcher? How will he deal with matters of value and conflict? What goals does he set for his research? How can an interdisciplinary process be organized?

## D. Some Afterthoughts:

This discussion has identified ways in which social research can be utilized in the policy process, and has raised some larger questions for the social researcher. There remains some further related observations, which will be sketched out here by way of conclusion.

One might say that the social policy process in America has been deficient for two reasons. First, there are a variety of constraints on the governmental decision-making enterprise that inhibit use of the body of social research already available. This problem transcends a social research concern.

Second, and more pertinent to the social researcher, is that social research findings are still not sufficient to meet the needs of those who are responsible for making and implementing decisions. Research findings, such as those reported in this paper, are useful to the planner, in that they provide insights for some pathways to problem solution. But such findings still do not guarantee the outcomes the planner wishes to achieve. Moreover, the planner, assuming he is oriented to social problem solution, requires research that deals with the causality of social problems. From such a premise, it is reasonable to suggest that much of social research is still not sufficiently relevant to the planning and policy process.

On the other hand, the social researcher who inquires into the nature of causality needs opportunities for experimentation if his findings are to be applicable to the user. The large number of social programs operating in this nation may provide the experimental base the social researchers seek. The possible joining of interests, however, is deterred because the researcher may not be aware of the existence of relevant programs, he may not have a ready access to those he can identify, and his activities may be out of phase with the planning activity.

Finally, it is suggested that social purpose is inherent in the policy process. To expect that social research would have an influence on social policy is to suggest that research activities must be directly related to stated social purposes well beyond our present haphazard conditions. This nation has had and is having experience in grappling with large scale, managed, goal-oriented activities. Witness NASA's contribution toward this process. Implicit in the efforts to reach the moon is a successful research management program, conceptualized and linked to solve all the problems connected with a successful round trip. If research is to influence policy in a meaningful way, highly individualized enterprises at different levels must be organized into a complex network of related activities aimed at a common social purpose.

TABLE 1—Multiple Correlation ($R^2$) of Health Factors with a Set of Predictors Including Morale, Social Relations, and Environmental Factors, and Demographic Characteristics

| Health factor | $R^2$ |
|---|---|
| I. Disability I | .159 |
| II. General health | .186 |
| III. Disability II | .323 |
| IV. Use of other services | .200 |

TABLE 2—Correlation Coefficients Between a Set of Predictors and Two Health Factors

| | Correlation Coefficient (r) | |
|---|---|---|
| | Health 2 | Health 3 |
| Age | —.011 | —.271 |
| Marital status | —.002 | .228 |
| Sex | —.012 | —.291 |
| Race | —.006 | .122 |
| Population | —.062 | .001 |
| Income | —.093 | .290 |
| Education | —.069 | .223 |
| Env. 1 (distance to services) | —.090 | —.002 |
| Env. 2 (condition of dwelling) | —.102 | .213 |
| Env. 3 (convenience to services) | —.058 | .228 |
| Env. 4 (structural I) | —.019 | .068 |
| Env. 5 (availability of services) | —.038 | .103 |
| Env. 6 (structural II) | —.046 | —.113 |
| Soc. Rel. 1 (neighboring) | —.053 | .034 |
| Soc. Rel. 2 (groups and organizations) | .075 | —.131 |
| Soc. Rel. 3 (contact with children) | —.009 | .072 |
| Soc. Rel. 4 (contact with siblings) | .011 | .050 |
| Soc. Rel. 6 (contact with children, indirect) | —.006 | —.068 |
| Soc. Rel. 7 (contact outside home) | .069 | —.311 |
| Morale 1 (transient response to external events) | —.205 | .143 |
| Morale 2 (anomie) | —.069 | .093 |
| Morale 3 (age related) | .301 | —.379 |
| Morale 4 (sustained unhappiness) | —.095 | .090 |

**TABLE 3—Path Analysis**
**General Health (Total sample)**

| Variables effected | Effected by | | | | | | | | | | | |
|---|---|---|---|---|---|---|---|---|---|---|---|---|
| | Age | Mar | Sex | Race | Pop | Inc | Ed | E1 | E2 | E3 | E4 | E5 |
| Inc | -.168 | -.271 | -.125 | .135 | .131 | | | | | | | |
| Ed | -.093 | -.098 | .064 | .198 | .059 | | | | | | | |
| E1 | .042 | .061 | .051 | .019 | .497 | .025 | -.012 | | | | | |
| E2 | -.028 | -.048 | .026 | .241 | .066 | .153 | .237 | | | | | |
| E3 | -.188 | -.035 | -.093 | .045 | -.054 | .073 | .065 | | | | | |
| E4 | -.034 | .060 | -.048 | .016 | .180 | .073 | -.019 | | | | | |
| E5 | -.014 | .036 | -.009 | .051 | .057 | .060 | .066 | | | | | |
| E6 | .025 | -.011 | .048 | .025 | .346 | -.099 | -.050 | | | | | |
| S1 | .001 | -.015 | .045 | -.076 | -.178 | -.013 | .012 | -.062 | .001 | .118 | -.091 | .027 |
| S2 | .031 | -.122 | -.190 | -.001 | .010 | -.082 | -.204 | -.073 | -.109 | -.067 | -.050 | -.077 |
| S3 | .028 | -.046 | -.068 | -.008 | .035 | -.027 | .106 | -.004 | -.150 | -.014 | -.001 | -.028 |
| S4 | -.156 | -.065 | .041 | .042 | -.076 | .016 | -.164 | -.029 | .009 | .070 | -.055 | .004 |
| S6 | .023 | .055 | -.086 | -.104 | -.048 | .001 | -.062 | -.026 | -.128 | -.061 | -.004 | .050 |
| S7 | .114 | .109 | .069 | -.032 | -.042 | -.068 | -.066 | -.032 | -.044 | -.330 | -.007 | -.076 |
| M1 | .092 | .072 | -.162 | -.026 | .001 | -.001 | .142 | .028 | .053 | .076 | .024 | .001 |
| M2 | -.020 | .020 | .042 | .067 | -.000 | .057 | .143 | -.003 | .123 | -.060 | .030 | .032 |
| M3 | .201 | .048 | -.003 | -.034 | .007 | -.041 | -.101 | -.059 | -.049 | -.102 | -.058 | -.044 |
| M4 | -.008 | -.208 | .013 | -.086 | -.054 | .010 | -.046 | .005 | .149 | .116 | -.069 | .030 |
| H2 direct | -.103 | -.054 | -.043 | .048 | .012 | -.051 | .072 | -.048 | -.044 | .015 | .034 | -.015 |
| H2 Total | -.011 | -.002 | -.012 | -.006 | -.062 | -.093 | -.069 | -.090 | -.102 | -.058 | .019 | -.038 |

| | Effected by | | | | | | | | | | | |
| | E6 | S1 | S2 | S3 | S4 | S6 | S7 | M1 | M2 | M3 | M4 | $R^2$ |
|---|---|---|---|---|---|---|---|---|---|---|---|---|
| Inc | | | | | | | | | | | | .204 |
| Ed | | | | | | | | | | | | .067 |
| E1 | | | | | | | | | | | | .251 |
| E2 | | | | | | | | | | | | .217 |
| E3 | | | | | | | | | | | | .086 |
| E4 | | | | | | | | | | | | .044 |
| E5 | | | | | | | | | | | | .019 |
| E6 | | | | | | | | | | | | .129 |
| S1 | −.146 | | | | | | | | | | | .115 |
| S2 | −.033 | | | | | | | | | | | .161 |
| S3 | −.314 | | | | | | | | | | | .120 |
| S4 | .092 | | | | | | | | | | | .081 |
| S6 | .068 | | | | | | | | | | | .075 |
| S7 | .060 | | | | | | | | | | | .253 |
| M1 | −.012 | .030 | .050 | .056 | .025 | −.032 | −.007 | | | | | .074 |
| M2 | .017 | −.017 | −.037 | −.001 | −.049 | −.009 | −.042 | | | | | .099 |
| M3 | −.002 | −.031 | .124 | −.028 | −.017 | .016 | .130 | | | | | .220 |
| M4 | .020 | .091 | −.021 | −.089 | .021 | .003 | −.050 | | | | | .136 |
| H2 direct | −.047 | .096 | −.029 | −.025 | .014 | −.039 | −.017 | −.215 | −.090 | .365 | −.138 | |
| H2 Total | −.040 | .053 | .075 | −.009 | .011 | −.006 | .069 | −.205 | −.069 | .301 | −.095 | .186 |

## TABLE 4—Path Analysis
### Disability II (Total sample)

| Variables effected | Age | Mar | Sex | Race | Pop | Inc | Ed | E1 | E2 | E3 | E4 | E5 |
|---|---|---|---|---|---|---|---|---|---|---|---|---|
| | | | | | | Effected by | | | | | | |
| Inc | -.168 | -.271 | -.125 | .135 | .131 | | | | | | | |
| Ed | -.093 | -.098 | .064 | .198 | .059 | .025 | -.012 | | | | | |
| E1 | .042 | .061 | .051 | .019 | .487 | .153 | .237 | | | | | |
| E2 | -.028 | -.048 | .026 | .241 | .066 | .073 | .065 | | | | | |
| E3 | -.188 | -.035 | -.093 | .045 | -.054 | .073 | -.019 | | | | | |
| E4 | -.034 | .000 | -.048 | .016 | .180 | .060 | .006 | | | | | |
| E5 | -.014 | .036 | -.009 | .051 | .057 | -.099 | -.050 | | | | | |
| E6 | .025 | -.011 | .048 | .025 | .346 | -.013 | .012 | | | | | |
| S1 | .001 | -.015 | .045 | -.076 | -.178 | -.082 | -.204 | -.062 | .001 | .118 | -.091 | .027 |
| S2 | .031 | -.122 | -.190 | -.001 | .010 | -.027 | .106 | -.073 | -.109 | -.067 | -.050 | -.077 |
| S3 | .028 | -.046 | -.068 | -.008 | .035 | .016 | -.164 | -.004 | -.150 | -.014 | .001 | -.028 |
| S4 | -.156 | -.065 | .041 | .042 | -.076 | .001 | -.062 | -.029 | .009 | .070 | -.055 | .004 |
| S6 | .023 | .055 | -.086 | -.104 | -.048 | -.068 | -.066 | -.026 | -.128 | -.061 | -.004 | .050 |
| S7 | .114 | .109 | .069 | -.032 | -.042 | -.001 | .142 | -.032 | -.044 | -.330 | -.007 | -.076 |
| M1 | .092 | .072 | .162 | -.026 | .001 | .057 | .143 | .028 | .053 | .076 | .024 | .001 |
| M2 | -.020 | .020 | .042 | .067 | -.000 | -.041 | -.101 | -.003 | .123 | -.060 | .030 | .032 |
| M3 | .201 | .048 | -.008 | -.034 | .007 | .010 | -.046 | -.059 | -.049 | -.102 | -.058 | -.044 |
| M4 | -.008 | -.208 | .010 | -.086 | -.054 | .045 | .032 | .005 | .149 | .116 | -.069 | .030 |
| H3 direct | -.119 | .007 | -.259 | .016 | -.032 | | | .019 | .076 | .032 | .028 | .049 |
| H3 Total | -.271 | .228 | -.251 | .122 | .001 | .290 | .223 | -.002 | .213 | .228 | .068 | .103 |

286

|  |  | | | | | Effected by | | | | | |  |
|  | E6 | S1 | S2 | S3 | S4 | S6 | S7 | M1 | M2 | M3 | M4 | $R^2$ |
|---|---|---|---|---|---|---|---|---|---|---|---|---|
| Inc | | | | | | | | | | | | .204 |
| Ed | | | | | | | | | | | | .067 |
| E1 | | | | | | | | | | | | .251 |
| E2 | | | | | | | | | | | | .217 |
| E3 | | | | | | | | | | | | .086 |
| E4 | | | | | | | | | | | | .044 |
| E5 | | | | | | | | | | | | .019 |
| E6 | | | | | | | | | | | | .129 |
| S1 | −.146 | | | | | | | | | | | .115 |
| S2 | −.033 | | | | | | | | | | | .161 |
| S3 | −.314 | | | | | | | | | | | .120 |
| S4 | .092 | | | | | | | | | | | .081 |
| S6 | .068 | | | | | | | | | | | .075 |
| S7 | .060 | | | | | | | | | | | .253 |
| M1 | −.012 | .030 | .050 | .056 | .025 | −.032 | −.007 | | | | | .074 |
| M2 | .017 | −.017 | −.037 | −.001 | −.049 | −.009 | −.042 | | | | | .099 |
| M3 | −.002 | −.031 | .124 | −.028 | −.017 | .016 | .130 | | | | | .220 |
| M4 | .020 | .091 | −.021 | −.089 | .021 | .003 | −.050 | | | | | .136 |
| H3 direct | −.030 | .021 | −.092 | .035 | .037 | −.021 | .125 | −.073 | .046 | −.230 | .018 | |
| H3 Total | −.113 | .034 | −.131 | .072 | .050 | −.068 | −.311 | .143 | .093 | −.379 | .090 | .323 |

287

## TABLE 5—Path Analysis Disability II (Males)

|  | Effected by | | | | | | | | | | |
|---|---|---|---|---|---|---|---|---|---|---|---|
| Variables effected | Age | Mar | Race | Pop | Inc | Ed | E1 | E2 | E3 | E4 | E5 |
| Inc | -.180 | -.161 | .168 | .132 |  |  |  |  |  |  |  |
| Ed | -.121 | -.048 | .202 | .100 | .021 | -.020 |  |  |  |  |  |
| E1 | .049 | .036 | -.003 | .543 | .201 | .260 |  |  |  |  |  |
| E2 | .004 | -.038 | -.203 | -.005 | .093 | .011 |  |  |  |  |  |
| E3 | -.184 | -.060 | .054 | -.043 | .071 | -.020 |  |  |  |  |  |
| E4 | -.066 | .118 | .051 | .124 | .062 | .043 |  |  |  |  |  |
| E5 | -.031 | -.029 | .078 | .012 | -.206 | -.017 |  |  |  |  |  |
| E6 | -.013 | .013 | .005 | .350 | .020 | -.044 |  |  |  |  |  |
| S1 | -.017 | -.041 | -.047 | -.166 | -.048 | -.158 | -.115 | -.008 | .046 | -.154 | -.015 |
| S2 | .031 | -.093 | .035 | -.004 | -.027 | .125 | -.089 | -.131 | -.027 | -.004 | -.153 |
| S3 | .031 | .029 | .006 | .063 | .003 | -.131 | -.010 | -.170 | .018 | -.049 | .002 |
| S4 | -.166 | .008 | .030 | -.055 | .011 | -.067 | -.062 | .013 | .070 | -.092 | .035 |
| S6 | -.021 | .040 | -.134 | -.025 | -.094 | -.077 | -.029 | -.158 | -.076 | .000 | .039 |
| S7 | .058 | .087 | .027 | .060 | -.030 | .116 | -.074 | -.082 | -.333 | -.005 | -.036 |
| M1 | .103 | .040 | .089 | .030 | .059 | .102 | .046 | .080 | .054 | -.004 | -.020 |
| M2 | -.049 | .059 | .024 | .001 | -.040 | -.145 | .007 | .151 | -.076 | .039 | .027 |
| M3 | .183 | -.001 | -.028 | -.028 | .016 | -.036 | -.057 | -.012 | -.118 | -.041 | -.082 |
| M4 | .061 | -.290 | -.069 | -.049 | .017 | .024 | -.044 | .147 | .103 | -.000 | -.009 |
| H3 direct | -.089 | .028 | .013 | -.034 |  |  | .016 | .119 | .088 | .056 | .035 |
| H3 Total | -.233 | -.089 | .132 | -.026 | .239 | .241 | .003 | .250 | .234 | .075 | .123 |

| | Effected by | | | | | | | | | | | |
| | E6 | S1 | S2 | S3 | S4 | S6 | S7 | M1 | M2 | M3 | M4 | R² |
|---|---|---|---|---|---|---|---|---|---|---|---|---|
| Inc | | | | | | | | | | | | .120 |
| Ed | | | | | | | | | | | | .071 |
| E1 | | | | | | | | | | | | .302 |
| E2 | | | | | | | | | | | | .231 |
| E3 | | | | | | | | | | | | .070 |
| E4 | | | | | | | | | | | | .037 |
| E5 | | | | | | | | | | | | .022 |
| E6 | | | | | | | | | | | | .149 |
| S1 | −.136 | | | | | | | | | | | .127 |
| S2 | −.039 | | | | | | | | | | | .108 |
| S3 | −.369 | | | | | | | | | | | .132 |
| S4 | .061 | | | | | | | | | | | .072 |
| S6 | .061 | | | | | | | | | | | .086 |
| S7 | .045 | | | | | | | | | | | .207 |
| M1 | −.002 | .038 | −.006 | .028 | .055 | −.027 | .018 | | | | | .063 |
| M2 | .062 | .041 | −.039 | −.024 | −.034 | −.031 | −.038 | | | | | .088 |
| M3 | −.046 | −.048 | .105 | −.026 | .017 | .016 | .177 | | | | | .222 |
| M4 | −.036 | .075 | −.049 | −.060 | .067 | .018 | −.070 | | | | | .177 |
| H3 direct | −.077 | .026 | −.103 | .066 | .040 | −.043 | −.177 | .065 | .035 | −.221 | .022 | |
| H3 Total | −.159 | −.039 | −.170 | .081 | .045 | −.103 | −.305 | .089 | .089 | −.369 | .095 | .279 |

289

**TABLE 6—Path Analysis**
**Disability II (Females)**

| Variables effected | | | | | Effected by | | | | | | |
|---|---|---|---|---|---|---|---|---|---|---|---|
| | Age | Mar | Race | Pop | Inc | Ed | E1 | E2 | E3 | E4 | E5 |
| Inc | -.163 | -.340 | .116 | .135 | | | | | | | |
| Ed | -.073 | -.123 | .196 | .029 | .032 | | | | | | |
| E1 | .035 | .075 | .032 | .449 | .106 | -.010 | | | | | |
| E2 | -.050 | -.056 | .267 | .117 | .068 | .224 | | | | | |
| E3 | -.195 | -.014 | .039 | -.059 | .064 | .096 | | | | | |
| E4 | -.008 | .015 | -.006 | .222 | .061 | -.017 | | | | | |
| E5 | -.003 | .074 | .032 | .091 | .004 | .086 | | | | | |
| E6 | .058 | -.007 | .041 | .340 | -.025 | -.074 | | | | | |
| S1 | .009 | .002 | -.092 | -.188 | -.125 | .046 | -.027 | .006 | .153 | -.041 | .057 |
| S2 | .035 | -.156 | -.025 | .011 | -.040 | -.242 | -.060 | -.094 | -.083 | -.077 | -.032 |
| S3 | .027 | -.086 | -.016 | .018 | .012 | .096 | -.004 | -.142 | -.030 | .026 | -.044 |
| S4 | -.149 | -.103 | .053 | -.082 | -.001 | -.184 | -.009 | -.002 | .094 | -.040 | -.013 |
| S6 | .052 | .058 | -.088 | -.063 | -.046 | -.062 | -.027 | -.103 | -.052 | -.007 | .061 |
| S7 | .154 | .119 | -.077 | -.105 | .026 | -.064 | -.084 | -.016 | -.332 | -.018 | -.104 |
| M1 | .089 | .069 | -.093 | -.024 | .063 | .157 | .021 | .050 | .085 | .041 | .019 |
| M2 | -.001 | -.001 | .097 | .003 | -.041 | .171 | -.006 | .106 | -.044 | .032 | .042 |
| M3 | .211 | .068 | -.040 | .025 | -.003 | -.085 | -.051 | -.072 | -.096 | -.074 | -.036 |
| M4 | -.052 | -.158 | -.099 | -.056 | .051 | -.050 | .039 | .146 | .116 | -.116 | .024 |
| H3 direct | -.152 | -.004 | .021 | -.024 | | .043 | .025 | .053 | .007 | .008 | .057 |
| H3 Total | -.306 | -.180 | -.000 | .115 | .250 | .243 | .030 | .196 | .186 | .045 | .094 |

| | Effected by | | | | | | | | | | | |
| | E6 | S1 | S2 | S3 | S4 | S6 | S7 | M1 | M2 | M3 | M4 | $R^2$ |
|---|---|---|---|---|---|---|---|---|---|---|---|---|
| Inc | | | | | | | | | | | | |
| Ed | | | | | | | | | | | | .216 |
| E1 | | | | | | | | | | | | .068 |
| E2 | | | | | | | | | | | | .211 |
| E3 | | | | | | | | | | | | .215 |
| E4 | | | | | | | | | | | | .076 |
| E5 | | | | | | | | | | | | .057 |
| E6 | | | | | | | | | | | | .026 |
| S1 | −.155 | | | | | | | | | | | .123 |
| S2 | −.021 | | | | | | | | | | | .121 |
| S3 | −.284 | | | | | | | | | | | .149 |
| S4 | .107 | | | | | | | | | | | .107 |
| S6 | .072 | | | | | | | | | | | .094 |
| S7 | .074 | | | | | | | | | | | .069 |
| M1 | −.026 | −.015 | −.068 | .074 | .009 | −.032 | −.021 | | | | | .269 |
| M2 | −.022 | −.063 | −.030 | .016 | −.060 | .004 | −.037 | | | | | .075 |
| M3 | .039 | −.022 | .135 | −.024 | −.038 | .015 | .093 | | | | | .119 |
| M4 | .082 | .105 | −.013 | −.100 | −.005 | −.010 | −.046 | | | | | .232 |
| H3 direct | .001 | .026 | −.093 | .016 | .037 | −.007 | −.095 | .086 | .059 | −.254 | .010 | .138 |
| H3 Total | −.055 | .043 | −.226 | .027 | .070 | −.079 | −.264 | .120 | .125 | −.402 | .063 | .262 |

291

**TABLE 7—Path Analysis**
**Disability II (Whites)**

| Variables effected | Effected by | | | | | | | | | | |
|---|---|---|---|---|---|---|---|---|---|---|---|
| | Age | Mar | Sex | Pop | Inc | Ed | E1 | E2 | E3 | E4 | E5 |
| Inc | -.168 | -.265 | -.138 | .115 | | | | | | | |
| Ed | -.093 | -.100 | .063 | .055 | | | | | | | |
| E1 | .049 | .057 | .061 | .487 | .033 | -.020 | | | | | |
| E2 | -.037 | -.048 | .032 | .047 | .163 | .227 | | | | | |
| E3 | -.189 | -.053 | -.091 | -.056 | .058 | .067 | | | | | |
| E4 | -.042 | .064 | -.068 | .156 | .044 | -.000 | | | | | |
| E5 | -.100 | .038 | -.021 | .043 | .060 | .063 | | | | | |
| E6 | .037 | -.011 | .058 | .330 | -.095 | -.056 | | | | | |
| S1 | -.003 | -.020 | .046 | -.172 | -.011 | .015 | -.063 | -.006 | .127 | -.103 | .028 |
| S2 | .027 | -.124 | -.196 | .008 | -.073 | -.209 | -.081 | -.097 | -.079 | -.040 | -.086 |
| S3 | .025 | -.042 | -.077 | .025 | -.026 | .114 | .014 | -.133 | -.022 | -.002 | -.037 |
| S4 | -.170 | -.053 | .041 | -.079 | .025 | -.174 | -.018 | .006 | .065 | -.056 | .006 |
| S6 | .046 | .045 | -.072 | -.051 | .000 | -.040 | -.010 | -.084 | -.061 | .004 | .060 |
| S7 | .112 | .102 | .057 | -.041 | -.065 | -.068 | .032 | -.051 | -.343 | -.022 | -.082 |
| M1 | .087 | .071 | -.193 | -.019 | -.006 | .134 | .004 | .063 | .061 | .027 | -.002 |
| M2 | -.028 | .030 | .057 | .018 | .045 | .157 | -.061 | .120 | -.026 | .009 | .050 |
| M3 | .211 | .036 | -.010 | .011 | -.040 | -.107 | -.001 | -.069 | -.098 | -.053 | -.057 |
| M4 | -.017 | -.218 | .003 | -.056 | .001 | -.048 | .009 | .121 | .095 | -.055 | .029 |
| H3 direct | -.125 | .006 | -.262 | -.022 | .041 | .030 | | .080 | .042 | .022 | .058 |
| H3 Total | -.282 | -.223 | -.296 | -.001 | .275 | .203 | -.014 | .192 | .225 | .064 | .110 |

| | | | | | Effected by | | | | | | | |
|---|---|---|---|---|---|---|---|---|---|---|---|---|
| | E6 | S1 | S2 | S3 | S4 | S6 | S7 | M1 | M2 | M3 | M4 | R² |
| Inc | | | | | | | | | | | | .183 |
| Ed | | | | | | | | | | | | .027 |
| E1 | | | | | | | | | | | | .253 |
| E2 | | | | | | | | | | | | .121 |
| E3 | | | | | | | | | | | | .084 |
| E4 | | | | | | | | | | | | .034 |
| E5 | | | | | | | | | | | | .012 |
| E6 | | | | | | | | | | | | .124 |
| S1 | −.163 | | | | | | | | | | | .118 |
| S2 | −.028 | | | | | | | | | | | .156 |
| S3 | −.321 | | | | | | | | | | | .124 |
| S4 | .094 | | | | | | | | | | | .087 |
| S6 | .066 | | | | | | | | | | | .037 |
| S7 | .055 | | | | | | | | | | | .250 |
| M1 | −.002 | .046 | −.057 | .084 | .023 | −.019 | −.007 | | | | | .085 |
| M2 | .008 | −.009 | −.022 | .010 | −.052 | −.022 | −.027 | | | | | .082 |
| M3 | .003 | −.021 | .114 | −.026 | −.013 | −.009 | .111 | | | | | .199 |
| M4 | .017 | .095 | −.027 | −.100 | .017 | −.010 | −.065 | | | | | .140 |
| H3 direct | −.038 | .015 | −.047 | .024 | .037 | −.024 | −.122 | .081 | .033 | −.223 | .011 | |
| H3 Total | −.125 | .047 | −.120 | .080 | .056 | −.043 | −.299 | .156 | .066 | −.364 | .094 | .317 |

293

**Table 8—Path Analysis**
**Disability II (Non-whites)**

| Variables effected | | | | | Effected by | | | | | | |
|---|---|---|---|---|---|---|---|---|---|---|---|
| | Age | Mar | Sex | Pop | Inc | Ed | E1 | E2 | E3 | E4 | E5 |
| Inc | −.169 | −.341 | −.044 | .260 | | | | | | | |
| Ed | −.101 | −.105 | .088 | .093 | −.019 | | | | | | |
| E1 | −.008 | .082 | −.012 | .483 | .180 | .039 | | | | | |
| E2 | .022 | −.061 | .000 | .140 | .180 | .346 | | | | | |
| E3 | −.168 | .068 | −.110 | −.064 | .245 | .034 | | | | | |
| E4 | .032 | .037 | .053 | .293 | .042 | −.136 | | | | | |
| E5 | −.028 | .006 | .062 | .138 | −.105 | .083 | | | | | |
| E6 | −.049 | −.025 | −.029 | .453 | −.050 | .004 | | | | | |
| S1 | .028 | .021 | .040 | −.243 | −.185 | −.013 | −.034 | .038 | .079 | −.025 | .038 |
| S2 | .082 | −.158 | −.153 | −.014 | −.056 | −.138 | −.000 | −.187 | .005 | −.099 | −.005 |
| S3 | .031 | −.069 | −.035 | .109 | −.069 | .057 | −.107 | −.176 | .032 | .022 | .009 |
| S4 | −.094 | −.131 | .039 | −.018 | −.012 | −.059 | −.110 | −.003 | .112 | −.038 | −.016 |
| S6 | −.058 | .098 | −.141 | −.064 | −.120 | −.198 | −.086 | −.173 | −.040 | −.027 | .027 |
| S7 | .144 | .124 | .141 | −.096 | −.008 | −.033 | .092 | −.019 | −.279 | .087 | −.029 |
| M1 | .147 | .046 | .016 | .109 | .145 | .151 | −.002 | −.031 | .149 | −.016 | −.007 |
| M2 | .010 | .020 | −.040 | −.115 | −.023 | .065 | −.014 | .110 | −.209 | .133 | −.014 |
| M3 | .158 | .122 | −.001 | −.027 | .005 | −.123 | −.058 | .098 | −.148 | −.086 | .031 |
| M4 | .072 | −.161 | .061 | −.071 | .064 | −.060 | .056 | .268 | .201 | −.181 | .018 |
| H3 direct | −.097 | .021 | −.234 | −.095 | .298 | .058 | .107 | .039 | −.018 | .069 | .015 |
| H3 Total | −.237 | −.209 | −.265 | .058 | | .207 | .080 | .175 | .201 | .082 | .012 |

| | | | | | Effected by | | | | | | | |
| --- | --- | --- | --- | --- | --- | --- | --- | --- | --- | --- | --- | --- |
| | E6 | S1 | S2 | S3 | S4 | S6 | S7 | M1 | M2 | M3 | M4 | $R^2$ |
| Inc | | | | | | | | | | | | .038 |
| Ed | | | | | | | | | | | | .242 |
| E1 | | | | | | | | | | | | .247 |
| E2 | | | | | | | | | | | | .240 |
| E3 | | | | | | | | | | | | .080 |
| E4 | | | | | | | | | | | | .168 |
| E5 | | | | | | | | | | | | .043 |
| E6 | | | | | | | | | | | | .195 |
| S1 | −.044 | | | | | | | | | | | .096 |
| S2 | −.038 | | | | | | | | | | | .223 |
| S3 | −.297 | | | | | | | | | | | .110 |
| S4 | .067 | | | | | | | | | | | .061 |
| S6 | .126 | | | | | | | | | | | .166 |
| S7 | .114 | | | | | | | | | | | .259 |
| M1 | −.002 | −.062 | −.043 | −.092 | .047 | −.094 | −.025 | | | | | .104 |
| M2 | .046 | −.084 | −.078 | −.049 | −.026 | .019 | −.073 | | | | | .151 |
| M3 | −.048 | −.096 | .201 | −.048 | −.043 | .131 | .239 | | | | | .336 |
| M4 | .105 | .064 | −.050 | −.026 | .031 | .069 | .012 | | | | | .167 |
| H3 direct | .020 | .059 | −.052 | .107 | .030 | −.004 | −.155 | .051 | .106 | −.255 | .061 | |
| H3 Total | −.013 | .006 | −.155 | .061 | .037 | −.080 | −.333 | .052 | .134 | −.402 | .088 | .316 |

295

## TABLE 9—Path Analysis
### Disability II (Urban)

| Variables effected | Effected by | | | | | | | | | | |
|---|---|---|---|---|---|---|---|---|---|---|---|
| | Age | Mar | Sex | Race | Inc | Ed | E1 | E2 | E3 | E4 | E5 |
| Inc | -.179 | -.285 | -.144 | .119 | | -.113 | | | | | |
| Ed | -.084 | -.112 | .053 | .193 | | | | | | | |
| E1 | .051 | .008 | .042 | -.016 | -.024 | .230 | | | | | |
| E2 | -.039 | -.041 | .029 | .243 | .150 | .062 | | | | | |
| E3 | -.205 | -.051 | -.045 | .024 | .064 | -.025 | | | | | |
| E4 | -.030 | .071 | -.045 | .002 | .097 | .066 | | | | | |
| E5 | -.016 | .041 | -.015 | .045 | .058 | -.061 | | | | | |
| E6 | .039 | .005 | .070 | -.013 | -.042 | | | | | | |
| S1 | .014 | -.021 | .079 | -.068 | -.039 | .026 | -.052 | -.017 | .147 | -.131 | .022 |
| S2 | .019 | -.125 | -.208 | -.007 | -.083 | -.211 | -.057 | -.100 | -.094 | -.065 | -.060 |
| S3 | .021 | -.060 | -.079 | .003 | -.045 | .120 | -.009 | -.148 | .002 | .007 | -.028 |
| S4 | -.156 | -.072 | .046 | .061 | .003 | -.151 | -.021 | -.002 | .072 | -.081 | .018 |
| S6 | .014 | .058 | -.086 | -.090 | .005 | -.094 | -.036 | -.098 | -.063 | -.013 | .057 |
| S7 | .108 | .104 | -.062 | -.050 | -.074 | -.035 | -.026 | -.072 | -.352 | -.004 | -.094 |
| M1 | .077 | .069 | -.157 | -.025 | -.003 | .155 | .072 | .034 | .076 | .025 | .016 |
| M2 | -.040 | .020 | .041 | .075 | .045 | .147 | .007 | .140 | -.053 | .040 | .035 |
| M3 | .198 | .056 | -.015 | -.036 | -.039 | -.105 | -.029 | -.051 | -.115 | -.060 | -.025 |
| M4 | .008 | -.205 | .015 | -.086 | .006 | -.051 | -.016 | .156 | .137 | -.086 | .032 |
| H3 direct | -.109 | .035 | -.270 | .017 | .032 | .049 | -.001 | .078 | .036 | .030 | .036 |
| H3 Total | -.266 | -.224 | -.302 | .122 | .286 | .229 | -.066 | .208 | .247 | .066 | .092 |

| | Effected by | | | | | | | | | | | |
| | E6 | S1 | S2 | S3 | S4 | S6 | S7 | M1 | M2 | M3 | M4 | $R^2$ |
|---|---|---|---|---|---|---|---|---|---|---|---|---|
| Inc | | | | | | | | | | | | .212 |
| Ed | | | | | | | | | | | | .064 |
| E1 | | | | | | | | | | | | .024 |
| E2 | | | | | | | | | | | | .205 |
| E3 | | | | | | | | | | | | .092 |
| E4 | | | | | | | | | | | | .012 |
| E5 | | | | | | | | | | | | .014 |
| E6 | | | | | | | | | | | | .018 |
| S1 | −.237 | | | | | | | | | | | .094 |
| S2 | −.028 | | | | | | | | | | | .157 |
| S3 | −.310 | | | | | | | | | | | .130 |
| S4 | .067 | | | | | | | | | | | .073 |
| S6 | .053 | | | | | | | | | | | .065 |
| S7 | .062 | | | | | | | | | | | .272 |
| M1 | −.020 | .017 | −.061 | .076 | .007 | −.132 | .003 | | | | | .079 |
| M2 | .018 | −.007 | −.022 | −.013 | −.052 | −.008 | −.032 | | | | | .102 |
| M3 | .013 | −.032 | .116 | −.001 | −.032 | −.006 | .130 | | | | | .216 |
| M4 | −.004 | .093 | −.027 | −.064 | .036 | .019 | −.049 | | | | | .135 |
| H3 direct | −.032 | .040 | −.077 | .039 | .060 | −.015 | −.140 | .069 | .050 | −.235 | .027 | |
| H3 Total | −.124 | .055 | −.119 | .087 | .077 | −.054 | −.333 | .142 | .097 | −.381 | .103 | .333 |

297

**TABLE 10—Path Analysis**
**Disability II (Rural)**

| Variables effected | Effected by | | | | | | | | | | |
|---|---|---|---|---|---|---|---|---|---|---|---|
| | Age | Mar | Sex | Race | Inc | Ed | E1 | E2 | E3 | E4 | E5 |
| Inc | -.130 | -.230 | -.066 | .165 | | | | | | | |
| Ed | -.136 | -.050 | .103 | .201 | | | | | | | |
| E1 | .051 | .141 | .024 | -.011 | .043 | .131 | | | | | |
| E2 | .016 | -.079 | .003 | .212 | .200 | .274 | | | | | |
| E3 | -.124 | .004 | -.088 | .127 | .077 | .081 | | | | | |
| E4 | -.057 | .033 | -.090 | .025 | .055 | .037 | | | | | |
| E5 | -.016 | -.017 | -.004 | .074 | .023 | .032 | | | | | |
| E6 | .007 | .014 | -.026 | .050 | -.045 | .083 | | | | | |
| S1 | -.027 | .029 | -.062 | -.037 | .080 | -.034 | -.128 | .011 | .064 | -.129 | .016 |
| S2 | .065 | -.131 | -.128 | .024 | -.103 | -.179 | -.091 | -.161 | .014 | .048 | -.170 |
| S3 | .046 | .014 | -.040 | -.055 | .024 | .052 | -.009 | -.125 | -.071 | .031 | -.028 |
| S4 | -.163 | -.031 | .032 | .009 | .023 | -.217 | -.125 | .029 | .077 | -.024 | -.081 |
| S6 | .062 | .044 | -.085 | -.137 | -.028 | .039 | -.008 | -.236 | -.019 | -.038 | .008 |
| S7 | .110 | .129 | .097 | .049 | -.038 | -.171 | .041 | .037 | -.271 | -.093 | .014 |
| M1 | .133 | .100 | -.176 | -.029 | .028 | .112 | -.053 | .153 | .029 | .024 | .005 |
| M2 | .060 | .027 | .024 | .044 | .092 | .142 | -.092 | .060 | -.073 | -.057 | .015 |
| M3 | .195 | .023 | .004 | -.016 | -.056 | -.136 | -.161 | -.025 | -.078 | -.112 | -.136 |
| M4 | -.052 | -.211 | .008 | -.072 | .010 | -.044 | .011 | .110 | .079 | -.068 | -.020 |
| H3 direct | -.155 | -.080 | -.220 | .025 | .091 | -.018 | -.050 | .052 | .035 | -.027 | .052 |
| H3 Total | -.291 | -.256 | -.270 | .121 | .290 | .175 | -.015 | .212 | .170 | .073 | .127 |

298

| | Effected by | | | | | | | | | | | |
|---|---|---|---|---|---|---|---|---|---|---|---|---|
| | E6 | S1 | S2 | S3 | S4 | S6 | S7 | M1 | M2 | M3 | M4 | R² |
| Inc | | | | | | | | | | | | .131 |
| Ed | | | | | | | | | | | | .074 |
| E1 | | | | | | | | | | | | .042 |
| E2 | | | | | | | | | | | | .240 |
| E3 | | | | | | | | | | | | .071 |
| E4 | | | | | | | | | | | | .018 |
| E5 | | | | | | | | | | | | .011 |
| E6 | | | | | | | | | | | | .011 |
| S1 | −.128 | | | | | | | | | | | .045 |
| S2 | −.025 | | | | | | | | | | | .190 |
| S3 | −.270 | | | | | | | | | | | .109 |
| S4 | .035 | | | | | | | | | | | .105 |
| S6 | .074 | | | | | | | | | | | .120 |
| S7 | −.027 | | | | | | | | | | | .223 |
| M1 | −.042 | .045 | −.015 | −.019 | .075 | −.020 | −.027 | | | | | .098 |
| M2 | −.012 | −.057 | −.111 | .029 | −.033 | −.032 | −.077 | | | | | .095 |
| M3 | −.084 | −.027 | .122 | −.121 | .019 | .091 | .146 | | | | | .272 |
| M4 | .058 | .095 | .017 | −.166 | −.024 | −.046 | −.035 | | | | | .158 |
| H3 direct | −.076 | −.039 | −.122 | .013 | −.022 | −.025 | −.072 | .102 | .023 | −.215 | −.018 | |
| H3 Total | −.059 | −.001 | −.159 | .023 | −.004 | −.101 | −.213 | .143 | .063 | −.358 | .054 | .307 |

299

# References

1. Schooler, K. K., *Residential Physical Environment and Health for the Aged,* (Final Report of USPHS Grant No. EG00191) Mimeo, 1970
2. *Ibid.*
3. Lawton, M. P., "The Dimension of Morale," in Kent, D. P., R. Kastenbaum, and S. Sherwood, (eds) *Research Planning and Action for the Elderly,* Behavioral Publications, N.Y.C., 1972
4. Srole, L., "Social Integration and Certain Corollaries; An Exploratory Study," *American Sociological Review,* 1957, Vol. 22, 670–677
5. Duncan, O. D., "Path Analysis: Sociological Examples," *American Journal of Sociology,* Vol. 72, 1966
6. Lindblom, Charles E., *The Policy-Making Process,* Prentice-Hall, Inc., Englewood Cliffs, New Jersey, 1968.
7. Stewart, Jon G., "The Policy Process—The Limits of Knowledge in the Pursuit of Understanding: A Review Essay," *Midwest Journal of Political Science,* Vol. XIV, No. 1, February, 1970, pp. 139–157.
8. Rothman, Jack, "Three Models of Community Organization Practice," from National Conference on Social Welfare, *Social Work Practice 1968,* New York: Columbia University Press, 1968
9. Rabinowitz, Francine, *City Politics and Planning,* Atherton Press, New York, 1969, pp. 79–117
10. Downs, Anthony, *Inside Bureaucracy,* Little, Brown, and Co., Boston, 1967, p. 2
11. Dror, Yahezekel, *Public Policy-Making Re-examined,* Chandler Publishing Co., San Francisco, 1968, pp. 129–213
12. Schooler, K. K., op. cit.
13. Schooler, K. K., "Effect of Environment on Morale," *The Gerontologist,* Vol. 10, No. 3, 1970
14. *Ibid.*
15. Sharkansky, Ira (ed.), *Policy Analysis in Political Science,* Markham, Chicago, 1969
16. Wildavsky, Aaron, *The Politics of the Budgetary Process,* Little, Brown and Co., Boston, 1964, pp. 64–66 and p. 157
17. Rein, Martin, *Social Policy: Issues of Choice and Change,* Random House, New York, 1970, p. ix
18. Moynihan, Daniel P., *Maximum Feasible Misunderstanding,* The Free Press, New York, 1969
19. Dror, Y., op. cit., pp. 163–164
20. Sherif, M. and C. Sherif, *Interdisciplinary Relationships in the Social Sciences,* Aldine, Chicago, 1969

# Chapter X
## Some Implications of These Papers

LAWRENCE E. HINKLE, JR.

There are a number of theses which recur in many of these papers that are implicitly accepted by almost all of the authors, and are of very great importance if they are correct.

The first of these is the thesis that it is the social environment and not the physical environment which is the primary determinant of the health and well-being of people who live in cities. In other words, within wide limits it is not the physical condition of the house, neighborhood, or human settlement that determines a person's health so much as his own social background, his perception of his environment, his relation to the other people around him and to his social group. Cassel states this thesis most directly; Hinkle accepted it and describes the physiological mechanisms that make it possible; Kasl, reviewing the literature, finds a great deal of evidence to support it; Burden's observations and those of Schooler are not in conflict with it.

The implications of this thesis, if it is correct, are fundamental. It has been evident for some time that the well-to-do who live in Manhattan are healthier than the poor who live alongside them, even though they share the same dirty air, the same noise, the same subway, and the same density of people per acre of land, or even per dwelling unit. The correlates of social position are not limited to education, occupation, income, and type of dwelling; they include maternal health, infant mortality, child care, family size, frequency of family disruption and of major family problems, and all of the habits, attitudes, and behavior that a person learns from the social milieu in which he grows up. These, it seems, are more important determinants of his health and behavior than the physical characteristics of the buildings he lives and works in, of the surrounding neighborhood, or of the cities. It appears that the well-to-do and well-educated who live among the noise and dirt of Chicago or Detroit are healthier than the poor who live amid the quiet natural beauties and clean air of Appalachia or rural Mississippi. The importance of the social milieu is such that the dislocation and disruptions of social relations that are produced when one moves a family from a dilapidated dwelling to a modern apartment may have adverse effects upon health and behavior that are not off-set by the clean, comfortable, and convenient new dwelling. "Absolute physical values" become relative biological values because of the importance of human perceptions. Four members of a cohesive family who choose to live together in two rooms of a vacation cottage may enjoy good health and not perceive their dwelling as "overcrowded;" while two people isolated and in conflict, sharing a two-room apartment may be quite unhealthy and may regard themselves as miserably crowded. Simple efforts to improve human health and well-being by improving the physical characteristics of the environment or the neighborhood are unlikely to succeed, unless the social and psychological implications of re-housing, removal, or relocation, which, as Hinkle points out, are also the biological implications of these acts, are taken into consideration. Because of these factors, "improvements" in the man-made environment may have adverse, rather than the intended beneficial, effects upon health and behavior. In fact, as Burden has clearly stated, the intended effects may not be accomplished at all, unless the community that is affected by them becomes involved in their accomplishment.

An implication which flows from this thesis, which is clearly stated by Kasl, is that meaningful studies of the effects of the man-made environment upon people can be carried out only if the social variables and the psychological variables, as well as the physical variables, are considered. The designs of such investigations require much more careful thought and sophisticated planning than has been customary in the past. The analyses of the data that are derived must depend upon multivariate techniques of sophistication adequate to disentangle the many confounding effects creating the high degree of intercorrelation of the input variables. Precisely what variables affect what outcomes and in what way may be difficult to determine, even with the most carefully conceived design. As all of the authors have pointed out, to obtain better information in this area it is essential that investigators be given the opportunity to study longitudinally the "natural experiments" which occur so frequently in our society as new buildings are built, old neighborhoods are changed or destroyed, and new neighborhoods, or even whole new cities, are constructed.

In the past, investigations in these areas have been seriously hampered by our inability to identify and measure relevant variables of input and of output. Gutman and Geddes have made significant contribution to the identification of the input variables, insofar as these are related to the physical characteristics of the environment that men construct. The use of a schema such as theirs in a systematic way should make it possible to compare man-made buildings and neighborhoods in relation to these variables, and also to relate these variables to some of the outcome variables of human health and behavior.

All of the authors, including Gutman and Geddes, have agreed that the physical variables of the man-made environment affect human

302

health and behavior primarily as they are modified and mediated by the social and psychological characteristics of the people who use the environment. Gutman and Geddes have suggested some of the psychological input variables that it may be important to consider in such a study. Kasl and Schooler likewise have suggested some of the variables that may be important. Unfortunately, none of the authors has chosen to consider these variables at length. Our discussions in our later meetings indicated, however, that the relevant social variables will include: (a) the cultural and social backgrounds of the people who occupy and use the physical environment; (b) the precise characteristics of the social groups primarily involved in its use; (c) the social meaning of the activities and symbols that are associated with the buildings or neighborhoods under consideration; (d) the particular characteristics of the smaller social groups, such as families that are intimately associated with the environment; (e) the relationships among them; and (f) the relationships among their members. All of the authors have agreed that the social-psychological variables that affect men's reactions to their environment include their perceptions of it and their attitudes toward it, but no one has attempted to outline a general schema of the relevant psychological variables or to state the theoretical reasons why these are relevant. These are topics which merit extended consideration in the future.

There appears to be an unexpected degree of agreement about the nature of the output variables of health and behavior, and how these may be measured. Hinkle, Damon, and Cassel all draw upon the epidemiological experience, and find no difficulty in adapting to this use the well-known measures of mortality, morbidity, and growth and development which have become standard among epidemiologists and human biologists as measures of health during the past century. Hinkle makes the useful distinction that many of the effects of the environment upon people cannot be considered to be "health effects" strictly speaking. He describes "constraints upon behavior" and suggests a method of measuring them, or at least of tabulating them, by the use of the "daily round of life" or "time budget" technique. He also indicated that what he calls the "pleasures and satisfactions" that people derive from their environment can be tabulated and measured by the use of psychological testing and survey techniques like those that are already in widespread use for other purposes. Hinkle's suggestions appear to be compatible with the schemes outlined by Gutman and Geddes; and, in their general outlines, acceptable from the point of view of Damon, Schooler, and Kennedy.

It may well turn out that in the measurement of the effects of man-made environments upon human behavior, the identification of peoples' attitudes toward their environment, and their perception of it, and the measurement of the pleasures and satisfactions they do or do not obtain from it, may be the major features of future "environmental assessment" when it is carried out along the lines suggested by Gutman and Geddes. If, as most of the authors suggest, mortality and morbidity are more related to social variables or to physical variables such as infectious agents, toxic substances, diets, and hazards that directly create injuries, one can expect that these variables, except for some of the safety hazards, will not be greatly influenced by the design and construction of cities or neighborhoods. Mortality and morbidity, therefore, may be poor indicators for measuring the effects of the man-made environment except in the case of certain special structures such as highways, mines, or factories. But the effectiveness of human interactions, the facility with which these are carried out, the degree to which a portion of the man-made environment abets or deters the social functions for which it was intended, the constraints that it places upon human behavior, and the pleasure and satisfaction that it provides for those who use it, might vary widely with different environmental designs, and the measurement of these variables may become quite important.

Perhaps the most important implication of this work is derived from the relative coherence and the implied consistency of the whole body of papers. This group of collaborators, representing fields as diverse as anthropology, architecture, engineering, epidemiology, medicine, psychology, and sociology were able to establish a fruitful communication with each other. They exchanged ideas, comprehended each others' concepts, and incorporated these concepts into their own thinking. They developed a framework of agreement on some points that one might have expected to be quite elusive at the onset of their deliberations. Approaching a common field of interest which was diffuse and undefined, they were able to identify types of variables which all agreed were important. They began to develop means of identifying and measuring some of these variables, and hypotheses about how they are interrelated. They suggested a remarkably similar group of strategies for taking advantage of spontaneously occurring opportunities to learn more about the central question of how the cities, neighborhoods, and individual buildings that men construct affect their health and behavior.

The entire effort gives promise that this field of interest, which seems to be so important to the future of mankind, is not so diffuse and ethereal as it once appeared. There is reason to believe that it can be, in fact, defined; that the important features of it can be identified; that the mechanisms of interaction among its important variables can be understood; and that, ultimately, meaningful analyses can be obtained which will enable people in the future to proceed in a rational way to construct the world in which they live so that it will predictably meet their needs.

# Appendix

## EPIDEMIOLOGICAL CONTRIBUTIONS TO ENVIRONMENTAL HEALTH POLICY
### Housing and Health

Rodney R. Beard, M.D., M.P.H.
Stanford University, California

A paper presented at the 100th Annual Meeting of the American Public Health Association at Atlantic City, November 14, 1972

This work was supported, in part, by the Bureau of Community Environmental Management, United States Public Health Service, Department of Health, Education, and Welfare.

### Introduction

There are shortages of housing in almost every part of the world. The deficiency is increasing, and will become worse, even if current rates of population increase were to diminish. The variety of adaptations which people can make in response to this situation is limited. They include accelerated programs of new building, remodeling of existing structures to accommodate more inhabitants, and at worst, the crowding of additional families into dwellings designed for single family occupancy. In all of these options, well-informed, judicious planning is needed. There will be pressures for haste, or at least for speed, in development and construction of new homes; above all, since the demand will inevitably exceed the capabilities of the construction industries, and the demand for funds will exceed the easily-obtainable supply, there will be a demand for economy (cheapness) and for simplicity of construction. Established practices, and political codes which govern housing, will be challenged. There will be strong pressures for quick decisions on the acceptability of new materials, new methods, and new standards. Public health workers must be prepared to respond, to make the most of the opportunity to optimize the health-producing relationships of housing, and to prevent the degradation of housing codes where they are realistically based on health protection. This report will review the relationship of housing codes to our knowledge of the effects of housing on health, and will suggest epidemiological strategies for the development and application of new knowledge in this field.

This report was stimulated by a seminar on the epidemiological aspects of housing and health held at Stanford University in March 1972, under sponsorship of the Bureau of Community Environmental Management, United States Public Health Service, Department of Health, Education, and Welfare, in which reports were heard from several experts who had prepared position papers for the Bureau and the American Public Health Association. Much of the following discussion reflects the exchange of ideas which took place in that meeting. Several of the position papers are listed in the references, and one is printed in this volume.

## New Concepts of Housing and Health

Recent years have seen growing emphasis on the idea that an adequate characterization of a dwelling includes its surroundings, as well as its interior. Major physical factors have been given attention for a long time, stress being laid on adequate drainage, provision of open space, siting to take account of sunlight and wind, adequate water supplies, etc. (1, 2) Now it is being recognized that factors such as transportation, access to shops and recreational facilities, appropriate location of school, separation of pedestrian walks from vehicular traffic, and many similar factors have effects upon health. (2, 3) In some communities, at least, it appears that the neighborhood facilities and ambience are no less important than the quality of individual dwellings for determining the satisfaction of the inhabitants. Among working-class people in Boston's West End, Hartman (4) found that those people who enjoyed the general environment also were satisfied with their dwellings, irrespective of the objective housing quality. This observation gains significance in the light of new concepts concerning disease and social and psychic attributes. Cassel (5) has noted "One of the more widely held and cherished notions in medicine is that the spread of infectious disease is facilitated by crowdng. This assumption underlies many of the research endeavors seeking to establish a relationship between housing and health . . . Under certain circumstances, crowding may be related to an increased incidence of communicable disease, but under other circumstances no such relationship has been discovered." He provides documentation to show that increased infectious disease rates are not necessarily associated with crowding.

De Groot (6) also reviewed the available evidence, searching for materials which could be used by public officials to sustain the legality of existing housing codes. While reiterating his belief that there is an association between good housing and good health, he had to conclude that there is nothing in the literature of epidemiology to support the importance of overcrowding as a factor in the incidence of infectious disease.

Predictably, de Groot's paper has been criticized and rejected by some concerned people. It should be recognized that the review was directed to a specific purpose, and it would have been misleading and harmful to attach significance to reports which could be challenged for incomplete observations or inaccurate analyses. Also, de Groot appropriately limited his comments to studies which would be relevant today, when typhoid, yellow fever, and smallpox are no longer major threats, and when even tuberculosis has subsided to a point where many believe that overcrowding in homes is no longer an important epidemiological factor in its persistence.

Such evidence as we have for the effects of overcrowding on the spread of communicable disease indicate that risks occur when people are clumped together very closely; when one passes the level of about 50 square feet per occupant, further spacing will have little effect on communicable disease. This is not to say that other factors associated with increased dwelling space may not be valuable for health. These would be factors associated with psychosocial stress, nutrition, ventilation, recreation, education, and the like.

Wilner and Baer (7) recently reviewed the impact of crowded housing upon socio-cultural factors, and concluded that there was very little evidence that crowding, per se, had any perceptible effect. Rather, they thought, poor housing was an expression of the total life-status of the occupants.

Similar views have been expressed by several others, such as Lemkau (8) and Cassel. (5) The latter gives extensive considerations to the experimental epidemiology of animal behavior in overcrowded situations, as reported by several experimenters. In controlled colonies, where genetic stock, diet, temperature and sanitation were kept constant, as the number of animals housed together increased, there were concomitant increases in maternal and infant mortality, the incidence of arteriosclerosis, susceptibility to a wide variety of external stressers, and of neoplasms. Also, lack of territorial control was shown to lead to the development of hypertension in mice, decreased resistance to infection, and diminished longevity. Behavioral changes noted were characterized by failure of the animals to produce appropriate reciprocal responses to the actions of their companions, and blurring of characteristic obligations and responsibilities. However, some animals exhibited withdrawal from the group, remaining isolated for periods of hours. These animals were reported not to show the pathologic changes characteristic of the main group. Another pattern was the formation of deviant groups which ignored the behavioral codes of the main group; variations in pathology among these animals was not stated. Based on these lines of evidence, Cassel developed a hypothesis that "in human populations, the circumstances in which increased susceptibility to disease would occur would be those, in which . . . individuals are not receiving any evidence (feedback) that their actions are leading to desirable and anticipated consequences (i.e., in situations analogous to the first category of animal responses). In particular, this would be true when these actions are designed to modify the individual's relationships to the important social groups with whom he interacts." Tyroler and Cassel (9) tested this hypothesis in relation to heart disease in human populations which were undergoing changes in culture and found a stepwise increasing gradient of disease with each increase in the index of urbanization (cultural change). They also found excess illness of various kinds in mill workers undergoing urbanization, as compared to men from the same stock who were second-generation workers in the same place. (10)

Cassel further extends his hypotheses to say that "health changes which are dependent upon the presence of other members of the same species will not be universal and will depend on the importance of the relationships that become disordered, the position of the individuals . . . in the status hierarchy, the degree to which the population . . . is unprepared by previous experience . . . , and the nature and strength of available group supports." Note that he dropped the concept of crowding for one of social interaction in circumstances where relationships are disturbed.

The formulation offered by Cassel is more detailed than most others, but the basic concept is not unique. There is wide agreement with him and his colleagues that "any specific stimulus can have a variety of reactions . . . Conversely, any reaction may have as its antecedents a variety of stimuli." (11) This is reminiscent of Sydenham's theories of non-specific causes of epidemics, but with a difference.

It should be noted that Cassel has not drawn direct inferences of human behavior from the studies of crowding in lower animals; those studies served him as a basis for developing an hypothesis about social relationships and disease. He has taken into account the greater range of susceptibilities of mankind, and man's capacity for adaptation through manipulation of his environment.

Despite a certain disenchantment with the evidence for specific relationships between poor housing and diseases, there are several particular examples which cannot be forgotten. One is the lead poisoning of children by ingestion of paint which flakes from the interiors of old houses. Boredom leading to the habit of nibbling on anything at hand, lack of supervision, and hunger are presumptive contributory factors, but the presence of lead is the necessary factor in this tragic disease. The greater tragedy is that there are instances in which the child, convalescent after hospital treatment, is returned to the environment which caused his illness. Richter (12) points out that childhood lead poisoning has been reported characteristically from poverty homes, although the persistence of lead paint is very widespread. Many high-rental homes in Manhattan are in old buildings and have multiple layers of lead paint on their walls; they are, however, well-maintained, paint-flaking is not prevalent, close attention is given to the children, who are well fed, and lead poisoning is not observed.

It is also clear that accidental injuries are associated with dilapidated housing, children playing in roadways, and with the lack of supervision for children and of adequate help for the elderly. It is also likely that the life style of which poor housing is but an expression plays a part in the genesis of accidents, but the physical hazards to life and limb are conspicuous.

Much of the accident risk derives, not from poor design and construction, but from deterioration. This is a factor of outstanding importance at the present time, as housing is becoming dilapidated at a rate much higher than that at which new housing is being built. In New York City in 1965–1968, 107,000 dwelling units housing about 428,000 people were abandoned by their owners and occupants. During the same period, 10,115 low-rent housing units were constructed. Sixty-eight percent of 1,750 buildings demolished by the City of New York in 1968 were structurally sound. It is inferred that their rehabilitation for occupancy was economically not feasible. Richter (12) has reported striking achievements in coping with this problem in one of the nation's most difficult areas, East Harlem in New York City. The key to the success of the program has been a subsidy from the State to provide training stipends for young men of the community to enable them to serve as apartment building superintendents with the skills necessary to make routine repairs. They replace faucet washers, patch plaster, paint, repair window frames and guards, and so forth. Tenants and landlords have responded favorably, and the men are being employed at a profit, although the cost of their services is at a level which is acceptable to the landlords. This is a solution which may be appplicable in other depressed central city areas. Competition from building trades unions should be anticipated, but might be slight, since if union rates had to be paid, the jobs would not be done, and because the union members, in many places, would be reluctant to enter the districts. While there might be doubts about the wisdom of such an approach for a long-term solution, the problem is immediate, and it is certain that injuries can be avoided and lives saved by this approach.

Richter mentions the importance of involvement of the residents of the houses and of the whole neighborhood. This is an element which has only recently begun to be appreciated as widely as it should be, though it was stressed by Clair Turner and Beryl Roberts as an essential factor in health education twenty and thirty years ago. To get lasting results, when one wants to help people, he must work with them, not merely for them, and certainly not upon them. This is an element which has often been overlooked in housing improvement programs. Too frequently, housing code enforcement worsens the plight of those it is intended to help. Sometimes the cost to the tenants of improved housing is met by the sacrifice of recreation, clothing, or adequate nutrition. Redevelopment programs have usually been planned with only cursory consideration of the opinions of the residents of the affected areas, often with the assumption that they will be better off in a "project," and if they don't know what's good for them, that can't be helped. Perhaps our greatest need in a public health approach to housing is to consider the people and their desires. The dignity acquired through participation in decision making may, for some, initiate a change in the total life pattern.

## Epidemiologic Research

Despite the lack of proof of specific associations of poor housing and ill health, there is widespread agreement that there is a great deal of interaction among these factors and the others mentioned earlier. The information which exists is poorly organized. The communication of this information is quite inadequate. The obvious responses to this should be an effort to improve the exchange of ideas and information. This will require some form of professional organization which will be ready to interact with the public. Such an organization should be prepared to inform the people, but it must also have mechanisms through which the people can be heard, and through which professionals and the public can jointly reach decisions about courses of action.

Students of the health effects of housing have long been aware of the paucity of data in the field. For example, when Wilner and others (13) prepared "The Housing Environment and Family Life" in 1961, they found only forty reports which seemed worthy of review and quotation. Even these, all based on direct observation or analyses of public records, were deficient in controls, range of observations or other important ways. Very often, the consideration of socio-economic factors was incomplete. In fact, it was not until Wilner and his colleagues carried out their observations upon a group of families moved from poor to good housing in Baltimore, beginning in 1950, that there had been an adequately controlled investigation. New strategies are available for epidemiological studies of housing and health. They call for the combined efforts of several disciplines, including sociology, psychology, and economics, at least. Most of the efforts of the past have failed to test their hypotheses adequately because of inept consideration of variables from these allied fields.

In understanding a prospective epidemiologic study, it must be recognized that the study will, of itself, affect the community; this is inescapable, because the study cannot proceed without some kind of community organization. The study should be planned so that it will help to engender the organization of an effective community.

The demands for new housing, and more broadly, for better formulations of neighborhood relationships, especially in deteriorating inner city areas, cannot wait for observational research to clarify our concepts of the interactions of poverty, malnutrition, social handicaps, housing and health. Cassel responds with a call for partnership between those agencies of society charged with improving the quality of the urban environment and research scientists, a partnership which should have the responsibility for introducing changes in the physical aspects of housing and the residential neighborhood but would use this entree as a means for deliberate alteration in some of these social factors as variables. He has outlined plans for such "intervention research," listing the responsibilities of the scientists and a skeleton protocol of important observations which should be made.

Just as every rational therapeutic plan for the treatment of an illness is experimental, offering an opportunity to learn more about the disease and about the methods for treating it, every housing development is a venture into the unknown. To the greatest possible extent, every such venture should be accompanied by planned observations which will help us to understand why some projects become successful in raising levels of satisfaction, health, and social adjustment, while others fail.

The approaching years will see numerous developments of new neighborhoods, and none of these will be quite the same. Plans should be made to carry out studies in these communities, starting from the model of Wilner's Baltimore investigation and improving upon it. It should be recognized that such studies cannot be done in a short time. In most instances, a minimum of ten years should be anticipated. The design should include a highly sophisticated statistical approach, since multivariate analysis will be involved. In this area, we have much to learn from the sociologists, who have extensively adopted a technique known as *path analysis. (14)*

Path analysis was introduced by the geneticist Sewall Wright (*15*) in 1921; the referenced articles give his experienced explanations and evaluations. Blalock (*16*) has also contributed extensively to the method, and it has been discussed also by Tukey. (*17*) The method requires a logical ordering of observations of interacting events. It tests whether the proposed set of observations is consistent throughout. Wright wrote, "Path analysis is an extension of the usual verbal interpretation of statistics, not of the statistics themselves." John R. Goldsmith has called attention to it as a potentially strong epidemiological tool. The conditions under which this method is applicable are demanding and will serve as guides for the design of sound epidemiological research.

The integration of disciplines and cooperative effort which is envisioned will not come about easily, nor is it likely to be spontaneous. There must be recognition of the potential benefit and the need for this kind of effort by agencies which can provide resources for planning and carrying out the studies, and there must be professional leadership from scientists who are capable of team efforts and who are committed to sharing their ideas and their work with people from other disciplines. There are many barriers to be surmounted, not least of which is that independent research is likely to be a quicker vehicle to academic success. Even so, the idea is worthy of exploration through the development of seminars which will bring the different disciplines together for an exchange of ideas and the planning of research.

The new wave of housing construction, including subdivision and remodeling of old buildings, will produce many situations in which comparative, prospective studies on the interaction of various factors upon health can be carried out. In addition to the openings for research which will arise from new housing developments and altered community relationships, there are a number of other opportunities, somewhat less demanding of time and organization.

One of the promising areas for study is that relating to so-called mobile homes. Neutra (3) has quoted statements indicating that in 1969, half of all the single-family housing units started in the USA were of mobile homes, and that most of these were accounted for by six manufacturers. Are there significant differences in the products of the several manufacturers or among the several models produced by one of them? Presumably, the identity of the purchaser of each unit is recorded by the manufacturer. This list defines a population which can be followed with relative ease, since the larger mobile homes are not really very frequently moved, and in some states, registration as road vehicles is required, so that families can be followed and changes of ownership noted from available records. There will undoubtedly be an expansion of other kinds of mass-produced housing, in which various kinds of new technology will be introduced. New materials and specifications will challenge old building codes, and at least some of the new ways will break through. It will be important to evaluate their impact on health as rapidly as possible. On a larger scale, new technology will appear in housing tracts and new towns, and there will inevitably be significant variations for which comparisons of effects upon health and its associated factors will be important. For example, there is discussion of the relative value of the use of high-density dwelling units for families, high-rise apartments, with large areas of open space readily accessible, in contrast to the usual American practice of building single-family homes, each with its small private patch of open ground. The former is widely accepted European practice. Does it have advantages for us? Can such housing be acceptable for an even higher population density?

Richter (*12*) has said that semi-public areas, those outside the premises of individual families, but not truly public, like the streets, present very difficult maintenance problems and are often neglected. There may also be a need for intensive policing of the elevators and hallways of apartment buildings, if neighborhood relationships fail to develop. In Great Britain, Fanning (*18*) noted that housewives who lived in flats had much less social contact with their neighbors than the women who lived in individual houses. There are undoubtedly cultural variations in this respect, with a greater tendency for mingling among the Latin peoples than among those of the northern nations. Renato Pavanello has said that some of the southern people cannot bear isolation, that they require awareness of their neighbors to assure them that all's right with the world.

Another area in which investigation will be profitable is the effects of various commercial products. Poisonings from various materials used in the home—cleansers, disinfectants, cosmetics, vermin-control agents, and many others—are known to be troublesome, but the circumstances under which they can be used safely have not been defined. Insecticides constitute a category of particular interest, especially as the chlorinated hydrocarbons, relatively non-toxic for man, are phased out in response to concerns about their total ecological effects. There is reason for concern about the many materials which are dispensed in the home as aerosols from pressurized containers. The droplet nuclei from these are of a size range to reach the alveoli and be retained in the lung. While the exposure appears to be very brief, the particles which are produced are likely to remain suspended indefinitely. The risk of intoxication may be small, but the possibility of hypersensitization is real, and should be evaluated. Accidental burns and the role of clothing in limiting or aggravating them is another fruitful area.

Despite the dreary aspects of the surveys which have been quoted, there is a considerable body of evidence, incomplete or presumptive though it may be, which associates ill health with poor housing. Such associations are quite clear for accidents and for contact infections, and they are highly presumptive for air borne infections. The association of enteric diseases with unsanitary waste disposal and with inadequate or impure water supplies is well established, and it is also known that these relationships can occur readily in the context of the residential environment, i.e., on a neighborhood or a dwelling unit basis. More importantly, there is an undeniable association of ill health with the combined factors of poor housing, poverty, malnutrition, and social handicaps, such as lack of education or ethnic minority status. Each of these major factors reinforces the others. Improvements in any of them will lead to some amelioration of the others. Among these four major determinants of health, the one most readily susceptible to modification is housing.

It is evident that improvement is needed in all of the fields mentioned, and that public health workers have a part to play in all of them. Among them, modification of the residential environment stands high in its promise for quick success. Historically, environmental manipulation has been the most effective tool of public health. Long experience has established that public health benefits are most surely and most rapidly achieved through the application of design, engineering, and construction practices which eliminate specific hazards. The mechanistic approach is likely to have the more favorable benefit-cost ratio when compared to educational or sociological methods. Accordingly, improvement in housing appears to be an efficient way to attack the multifaceted problems of poverty and ill health. It should not be the exclusive method, but it should not be neglected because of the enchantment of other lines of attack. The consequences of housing improvements should be measured with care, in depth, and with broad vision.

## Conclusion

New concepts of the relationships of housing and health are based on the occurrence of nonspecific responses, in which a given cause may give rise to various health patterns, and a given syndrome of physical or emotional maladjustment may arise from various combinations of several causes. Poverty, malnutrition, social handicaps, and poor housing usually interact, and the separate identification of one or another as the causal agent for illness is impossible; nevertheless, the relative importance of each in any situation may be estimated through the use of multifactorial analysis. The method of path analysis appears very promising for this. New housing developments, innovations in technology, both of materials and construction, and a broad array of new manufactured products offer many opportunities for study. The participation of the people who are involved in the planning of epidemiological studies should make important contributions to the validity of the work. To avoid errors often made in the past, epidemiological studies of neighborhood health should be done by teams of epidemiologists, economists, social scientists, and others, working harmoniously with the studied populations. At present, the need is to establish seminars in which these disciplines and others will be represented, to exchange ideas, to learn to think together, and to plan studies which will, as quickly as possible, provide guidance for community planners and other public policy makers, so that neighborhood reconstructions and new housing ventures will provide optimal environments for human health.

# References

1. WHO Expert Committee: *Environmental Health Aspects of Metropolitan Planning and Development*. World Health Organization Technical Report Series No. 297, WHO, Geneva, 1965.

2. APHA Program Committee on Housing and Health: "Basic health principles of housing and its environment," *American Journal of Public Health 59*:841–853, 1968.

3. NEUTRA, Raymond and Ross McFarland: *Accidents and the residential environment*. Report to the Bureau of Community Environmental Management and the American Public Health Association, undated, (1970).

4. HARTMAN, Chester W.: "Social values and housing orientation," *Journal of Social Issues 19*, April 1963.

5. CASSEL, John: "The relation of the urban environment to health: towards a conceptual frame and a research strategy." Chapter V this volume.

6. DeGROOT, Ido and Robert Mason: "Epidemiological evidence for use in hearings and court testimony relating to provisions of the APHA–PHS Recommended Housing Maintenance and Occupancy Ordinance. Report to the Bureau of Community Environmental Management and the American Public Health Association, undated, (1970).

7. WILNER, Daniel M. and William G. Baer: *Sociocultural factors in residential space*. Report to the Bureau of Community Environmental Management, March 1970.

8. LEMKAU. Paul V.: *Mental health and housing*. A report to the Bureau of Community and Environmental Management, February 1970.

9. TYROLER, H. A. and John Cassel: "Health consequences of culture change: The effect of urbanization on coronary heart mortality in rural districts of North Carolina." *Journal of Chronic Disease, 17*:167–177, 1964.

10. CASSEL, John and H. A. Tyroler: "Epidemiological studies of culture change. I. Health status and recency of industrialization." *Archives of Environmental Health, 3*:25, 1961.

11. CASSEL, John, Ralph Patrick and David Jenkins: "Epidemiological analysis of the health implications of culture change: a conceptual model." *Annals of the New York Academy of Sciences, 84*:938–949, December 1960.

12. RICHTER, Elihu: "Housing and health: a new approach." Presented before the American Public Health Association at Minneapolis, 12 October 1971.

13. WILNER, Daniel M., et al: *The Housing Environment and Family Life*. The Johns Hopkins Press, Baltimore, 1962.

14. BORGATTA, E. F. and G. W. Bohrnstedt (Eds.): *Sociological Methodology 1969*. Chapters by K. D. LAND, D. R. Heise, and O. D. Duncan. Jossey-Bass, San Francisco, 1969.

15. WRIGHT, Sewall: "Path coefficients and path regressions: alternative or complementary concepts?" *Biometrics 16*:189–202, 1960; "The treatment of reciprocal interaction, with or without lag, in path analysis," *Biometrics 16*:423–445, 1960.

16. BLALOCK, H. M.: *Causal Inferences in Non-Experimental Research*. University of North Carolina Press, Chapel Hill, 1964.

17. TUKEY, John W.: "Causation, regression, and path analysis," in KEMPTHORNE, Oscar, et al: *Statistics and Mathematics in Biology*. Iowa State College Press, Ames, 1954.

18. FANNING. D. M.; "Families in flats." *British Medical Journal 4*:382–386, 1967.